The Medication Interest Model

How to Talk with Patients About Their Medications

2ND EDITION

The Medication Interest Model

How to Talk with Patients About Their Medications

2ND EDITION

Shawn Christopher Shea, MD
Director
Training Institute for Suicide Assessment and Clinical Interviewing (TISA)
Private Practice
Keene, New Hampshire

Wolters Kluwer

Philadelphia • Baltimore • New York • London
Buenos Aires • Hong Kong • Sydney • Tokyo

Acquisitions Editor: Rebecca Gaertner
Development Editor: Kristina Oberle
Editorial Coordinator: Alexis Pozonsky
Marketing Manager: Rachel Mante Leung
Production Project Manager: David Orzechowski
Production Coordinator: Sadie Buckallew
Design Coordinator: Joan Wendt
Manufacturing Coordinator: Beth Welsh
Prepress Vendor: S4Carlisle Publishing Services

Second edition

9 8 7 6 5 4 3 2 1

Printed in China

Library of Congress Cataloging-in-Publication Data

Names: Shea, Shawn C., author.
Title: The medication interest model: how to talk with patients about their medications / Shawn Christopher Shea.
Other titles: Improving medication adherence
Description: Second edition. | Philadelphia: Wolters Kluwer Health, [2019] | Preceded by Improving medication adherence: how to talk with patients about their medications / Shawn Christopher Shea. 2006 | Includes bibliographical references and index.
Identifiers: LCCN 2018016231 | ISBN 9781451185201 (paperback)
Subjects: | MESH: Medication Adherence | Interviews as Topic | Physician-Patient Relations
Classification: LCC R727.3 | NLM W 85 | DDC 610.69/6—dc23 LC record available at https://lccn.loc.gov/2018016231

LWW.com

RRS1804

Dedicated to the memory of

Former Surgeon General of the United States

C. Everett Koop, MD, ScD

whose bedside manner, innovation, and sense of mission

embodied what it means to be a physician.

Also with much gratitude to all those clinicians

who have participated in MIM workshops

for your wisdom is reflected

in the pages of this book.

Foreword to the First Edition

Let me begin with a bias – a strong one. After four decades of clinical practice and 25 years of monitoring it from the sidelines (eight of them from the best seat in the house as Surgeon General), I have become convinced that the cornerstone of all healing in medicine lies within the mysterious bond that grows between the physician and the patient. Call it what you will – *bond, alliance, relationship* – it is the heart and soul of medicine.

It is one of the reasons that I was so pleased to be the Senior Scholar of the C. Everett Koop Institute created at Dartmouth Medical School, dedicated to understanding these mysteries. It has been my goal to explore these mysteries, to honor those protocols that, by their nature, must remain mysterious and to delineate and teach those processes that can be discerned, made operational, and taught.

I have arrived at a second conclusion – as has the author of this book – a conclusion that is so obvious that it is often not recognized as critical to discuss or even to mention. No medication works inside a bottle. Period. Now let me bridge the relationship between my two conclusions.

Our patients reach for their pill bottles, unscrew their caps, and reap the benefits of our medications almost purely because of the power of their bond with us. They either trust us or they don't. They either feel they have been well informed or they don't. They either feel we care or they don't. All of these patient opinions are the reflection of the ongoing nuances of the physician-patient relationship as it defines itself.

Unfortunately, far too little time is spent in our medical school education, our residency training, and in our ongoing continuing medical education on this most practical of all interviewing skills: talking with patients about their medications. When time is spent on these topics, it is often, in my opinion, wasted with clichés and admonitions to "be empathic" and to build "collaborative relationships." Such goals are laudable, but what is needed is a probing, tenacious attempt to uncover the specific interviewing techniques, choices of words, strategies, nuances, and experiences that talented clinicians use to convey empathy and to build these relationships, not just talk about the need to do so.

I know of no book that has ever addressed this critical set of interviewing skills regarding the specific task of how we talk with our patients about their medications. By necessity, I leaned heavily on my own experience when I led the program, *Take Time to Talk*, giving tips to patient and physician alike about talking to each other; I let each group see and hear what I said to the other.

You are holding in your hands the first book, as far as I know, in the history of medicine, that admonishes physicians to take the time to talk with patients about their medications. It does so with remarkable readability, practicality, and elegance. Reading this book never feels like one is reading a textbook of medicine. Instead, one feels that one is talking informally with a trusted mentor while doing bedside rounds – a mentor who believes in the mission, understands the complexities of the work, and genuinely both enjoys and loves his patients.

Hopefully, Shea's philosophy of enhancing "medication interest," as opposed to enforcing "medication compliance," will become second nature to generations of future medical and nursing students, as well as residents from primary care to psychiatry. I believe his book will become standard reading in all medical and nursing classes on medical interviewing or the physician-patient relationship because it covers a critical topic in medical interviewing that is often overlooked – how to talk with patients about their medications.

Improving Medication Adherence is filled with a remarkable number – around 40 – specific interviewing techniques and strategies for talking to patients about their medications and their side effects, in a collaborative fashion in the primary care setting, psychiatry, and elsewhere. The principles are equally relevant for talking with our patients about antihypertensives, oral hypoglycemic agents, and antidepressants.

Curiously, the book has come not from a family practitioner or internist but from a psychiatrist, who, in my opinion, did two wise things: (1) He brought the keen observations and principles that are useful in discussing psychiatric agents – notoriously difficult to get patients interested in taking – to the discussion table, and (2) he has distilled his interaction with thousands of primary care clinicians across the country in over 150 workshops, culling from them their very best interviewing techniques concerning all classes of medications, techniques that have proven themselves in the hectic confines of contemporary primary care clinics. Thus, this book, in essence, is written by a psychiatrist but contains the input of hundreds of primary care clinicians, who know what works and what does not work in actual practice no matter what class of medication is being discussed.

I also like the no-nonsense attitude that Shea takes when he emphasizes that the techniques he describes are not offered as the right way to interview (as if there was a cookbook manner for talking to patients correctly about medications). Instead, he describes them as reasonable ways. He hopes that the reader picks and chooses those techniques that appeal to each specific clinician, for we are all different and must develop our own styles.

Shea also achieves what I view as an even more remarkable goal. He not only engenders in the reader a genuine excitement about interviewing, but also provides a foundation in the principles that are necessary for creating new and effective interviewing strategies. From these principles, the clinician can develop his or her own unique techniques throughout the ensuing years of his or her career, long after he or she has put the book down. Shea invites the reader to become an innovator, and he gives the reader the necessary tools to be one.

Long ago I learned the power of interviewing technique to enhance my relationships with my patients. For years, I had been taught to always address the parents of my patients (I was a pediatric surgeon) by their last names and to be addressed vice versa. So I did. Pediatrics, as opposed to pediatric surgery, is much more homey and first names are "in."

So as the years progressed, I began to realize that when talking with people about life and death decisions about their children or other loved ones, our relationship was not some pseudo-professional exchange of ideas, but an intimate discussion, the closest bond you can have, between people who were building a unique relationship while collaboratively battling frightening diseases and scary surgical procedures, so last names often didn't cut it.

Consequently, when I first introduced myself to a parent or patient, I always addressed them by their last names. But then, I did something special; I gave them control of how I should address them. I simply asked, "Mrs. Jones, how would you like me to address you, by your last name, your first name, or whatever you like?" With this simple question the bond between the healer and those seeking his or her help began.

By the way, if the patient's parents told me they preferred his or her first name, I was not averse to being called by my first name as well – I've been called a lot worse! Also, if the patient insists on being addressed formally by their last name, I simply reciprocate, "It's probably best to call me Dr. Koop."

Over the years I have found that patients enjoy this collaborative work on an important relationship issue – how we want to be addressed – that opens the door to the recognition that we are entering a most special alliance, one where we will be discussing the most intimate of details, sometimes talking about frightening news, such as the presence of cancer or the approach of death, and brainstorming on options, and realizing, together, that sometimes there are no further options. Such are the moments when it is powerful and reassuring to use first names and to even shed a tear or two. In the last analysis, healing is about being human, learning how to allow our science to be guided by our compassion.

In the following pages, you are in for a treat. You are about to enter the very soul of what we do, and you could not find a better guide. With sophistication, wit, astute clinical observation, and a vibrant sense of compassion, Shea throws a brilliant new light on one of the most crucial topics in medicine – improving medication adherence. Packed with practical interviewing techniques and no-nonsense strategies, this little book, in my opinion, is destined to fill a giant void in the training of all medical and nursing students, as well as becoming a classic read for experienced clinicians in search of the art of medicine. My advice is simple – read it.

C. Everett Koop, MD, ScD
Former Surgeon General of the United States (1981–1989)
Senior Scholar, C. Everett Koop Institute at Dartmouth
Elizabeth DeCamp McInerny Professor of Surgery

Preface

The purpose of life is to serve and to show compassion and the will to help others. Only then have we ourselves become true human beings.

Albert Schweitzer, MD

It has been nearly 12 years since former Surgeon General C. Everett Koop, MD, ScD, penned the words that you just read in his most gracious foreword to the first edition of this book. With his passing, we lost one of the greatest, if not the greatest, Surgeon Generals we have been blessed to have. He is not present to write the foreword to the second edition of this book on the Medication Interest Model (MIM) of which he was a great believer. As a point of gratefulness and respect, it seemed only fitting to let his first foreword herald this second edition as well. If he were alive today, I can only hope that Dr. Koop would be thrilled with this new edition and its presentation of the exciting recent developments in the MIM.

Let me begin by saying that, first, and foremost, this is a book about the therapeutic alliance. It highlights the pivotal role that skilled medical interviewing plays in shaping this alliance, indeed, gives it birth. A major component of that skill set lies with the ability to use shared decision making and collaborative exploration to help patients approach the daunting task of deciding whether it is a good idea to put a medication inside their bodies, and if they do so, should they continue to do so? The answer to this question is unique to each patient. Sometimes it is a good idea. Sometimes it is not.

Moreover, this conversation regarding the use of medications is a surprisingly complex process. It is determined by an extensive array of factors including illness beliefs, wellness beliefs, family opinions, cultural biases, personal experiences with taking medications, financial limitations, the benefits of the medications, the side effects of the medications, and the enormous variations in how patients weigh the pros and cons of taking medications. Decades of clinical experience have taught me that to expect medical, nursing, and other allied health care students to somehow magically know how to navigate these waters without intensive training is naïve at best and unfair at worst to both the students and their future patients.

The overarching goal of this book is to help medical, nursing, physician assistant, and clinical pharmacy students to learn about this process, become adept at its navigation, and be able to effectively, and compassionately, engage in this conversation in the extremely hectic environments of outpatient clinics, hospital units, and emergency rooms. Research has clearly indicated that the number one reason for treatment failure across most diseases is that patients do not take their medications as prescribed. The amount of human suffering resulting from this dilemma is truly unsettling.

Consequently, I think it is fair to say that it is of immense importance to address – in the training of medical, nursing, and other allied health care students – the complex issues that will arise for them on a daily basis as they talk with their future patients about the use of medications. In the following pages, we will give this critical topic the attention it so richly deserves.

I don't believe that it is an overstatement to say that from the very first days in courses devoted to pharmacology to the numerous days spent in introductory courses on communication skills and the creation of the clinician/patient therapeutic alliance, students from all allied health care fields should be thinking about how they intend to talk with patients about their medications in a collaborative and compassionate fashion.

Traditional approaches such as motivational interviewing and cognitive therapy have significantly advanced our abilities to enhance medication motivation, but empirical research indicates that there is much more to be learned about enhancing medication motivation and use. Moreover, as any experienced clinician knows there is more to talking with patients about their medications than addressing their motivation for use.

A plethora of hidden traps and roadblocks regarding the discussion of medications await students once they step into their clinical rotations and, ultimately, step into their first jobs and residencies following graduation. In my opinion, these traps and roadblocks warrant careful discussion and ongoing training from more experienced clinicians.

Questions that require such discussion and mentoring are numerous and include examples such as: What is my own personal philosophy about the use of medications? Do I need to share that philosophy with my patients? If so, when should I do so? What are some of the ways that experienced clinicians have found to effectively share their prescribing philosophies? What are some of the most effective ways to present patients information about side effects? How do you sensitively and effectively talk with a patient about a medication whose side effect might be death? How do you spot a patient who is hesitant to share their concerns about their medications? What questions help such patients to share their real concerns and fears? What types of questions are most effective in uncovering – in a sensitive fashion – whether doses are being missed or a medication has been unilaterally stopped? What are the cross-cultural issues that arise regarding medication use (such as the use of medications during Ramadan with Muslim patients or when is it necessary to share information about binding ingredients that may be problematic to a patient's religious beliefs such as porcine products with Jewish patients)? How does one approach a patient's interest in alternative and complementary interventions? What are the best interviewing techniques for providing education about medication dosing and scheduling? What are the typical concerns of family members? What are some of the best questions for sensitively uncovering these concerns?

The list goes on and on.

Even more disturbing is the realization *that a breakdown in the therapeutic alliance along any one of these questions* might result in a patient losing interest in using a medication or effectively following through with it.

And here is where I must share some personal excitement about the book you are about to read. Since its introduction in the first edition of this book 12 years ago, the Medication Interest Model (MIM) has expanded, become better conceptualized, and has grown to include over twice as many interviewing techniques as in the first edition. The MIM currently uses a well-defined and popular motivational model – the Choice Triad – specifically designed to reflect motivational gains regarding medication interest and use. Within the framework of the MIM, over 100 specific interviewing techniques have been described and named all of which are easily understood, demonstrated, learned, and tested for competence if so desired.

Readers of the first edition will be glad to know that I have tried to keep intact whatever elements of the first edition reader feedback has suggested were most effective, while approaching the topics of each chapter with the same informal writing style that readers seemed to enjoy so much in the first edition. As they say, don't fix what isn't broken.

Over six chapters have been added on topics not addressed thoroughly in the first edition. I am particularly excited about new chapters such as "The First Script," "Pills and People: Assessing Cultural Beliefs About Medication," and "Medication Interest: The Impact of Family, Friends, and the Digital World," which address the types of questions listed above with the thoroughness I think they deserve. Indeed, the MIM has evolved into an easily taught and distinctive model, hence the change in the title of the book itself.

Further enhancements from the first edition await the reader in the three appendices. A "bonus chapter" – *The Next Step: A Concise Guide to Enhancing Medication Follow-through* has been added as Appendix A. Such a chapter was not present in the first edition for, technically, the topic is not part of the MIM per se for it does not directly relate to *interviewing techniques regarding patient choice, motivation, and conversation related to medication management*.Complementing the interviewing tips of the MIM described in the previous fourteen chapters, this new bonus chapter provides the student with knowledge regarding a variety of answers (pillboxes, cell phone apps, digital reminders, behavioral tailoring, Medication Therapy Management provided by pharmacists, ongoing medication support via case managers, etc.) to the following question: "Once a patient has chosen to take a medication – and is motivated to do so – how does one help a patient to navigate the external factors that often lead to medication problems and discontinuance such as forgetting to take the medication, being confused about the medication's dosing schedule, not being able to cut pills in half if required to do so, lacking transportation to the pharmacy, and not having enough money for the medications?"

The second appendix – "The Tip Archives: Quick Reference" – has been moved in this second edition to the state-of-the-art, free e-book, which automatically accompanies the paperback, appearing as Appendix B. This movement to a digital version greatly improves a student's ability – as he or she first steps onto inpatient units during clinical rotations – to quickly access a concise listing of all the interviewing tips previously described in the text.

When accessing Appendix B, the exact wording of each tip immediately appears on-screen for quick reference. In addition, cross-referencing to the text pages – where the original discussion of each tip appeared – is provided if a more detailed immediate review is desired by the student. Thus, a concise summary of the over 100 interviewing tips of the MIM is only as far away as a click or two on the student's tablet, cell phone, or other mobile device.

The third appendix was added specifically for faculty interested in learning innovative ways of teaching the MIM as well as researchers interested in designing research to quantitatively and qualitatively study the impact of MIM techniques on clinical outcomes as well as the efficacy of various training approaches both didactic and experiential (one of my hopes is that the publication of this book will lead to the type of research which I believe the MIM warrants). Toward this end, a popular article from the journal *Professional Case Management* has been reprinted exactly as it appeared in the journal. This digitized reprint – *The "Medication Interest Model" An Integrative Clinical Interviewing Approach for Improving Medication*

Adherence—Part 2: Implications for Teaching and Research – appears as Appendix C in the e-book.

A few comments are in order regarding the text itself and the unique method in which large parts of the MIM were created. Although clearly designed as a textbook for medical, nursing, and other allied health provider students, it is my hope that the book will also be of value to residents and other more experienced clinicians. If I've done my job well, as an experienced clinician reads on, he or she will find interviewing techniques and strategies that validate his or her current practice, provide a handful of immediately useful ideas for his or her future practice, and, most importantly, stimulate him or her to find new answers born from their own clinical wisdom.

Moreover, the techniques in this book are not provided as the "right way" to increase our patients' interest in their medications but merely as suggestions of various ways of tackling these difficult and sometimes vexing problems. The reader is invited to check out the following techniques, adopt the ones that he or she likes, discard the ones that he or she doesn't, and create ever more powerful solutions that resonate with his or her own interviewing styles and the unique needs of his or her patients.

Before I turn the reader loose to follow up on my invitation, I should mention where many of the interviewing tips, that fill the pages of this book, have originated.

Over the past 20 years, as the Founder and Director of the Training Institute for Suicide Assessment and Clinical Interviewing (TISA) – information available at http://www.suicideassessment.com – it has been my privilege to present over 200 workshops on the MIM to primary care physicians, specialists (such as cardiologists, endocrinologists, neurologists, and psychiatrists), staff nurses and advance practice nurses, clinical pharmacists, and case managers (on teams managing diseases as diverse as CHF and diabetes to schizophrenia) from around the United States and Canada. At each workshop, I ask my workshop participants to stop me if any of the ideas that I suggest to them appear to be impractical in the setting of a hectic primary care clinic or hospital unit. In the following pages, I share only those ideas that have passed the "acid test" of their discerning judgment.

More importantly, I always invite the participants of my workshops to share the tips that they have found to be most useful in their daily practices – their private cache of practical interviewing gems. Thus, the MIM is an ever-growing model of which a large part is the direct result of these ongoing workshops and input from the participants who attend them or who visit our website.

In this sense, the MIM holds the distinction of being a motivational model for improving medication adherence that was created by directly observing and learning from the physicians, nurses, physician assistants, clinical pharmacists, and case managers who prescribe, discuss, and monitor medications on a daily basis. It is a compilation of the practical tips – suggested at my workshops – coupled with the lessons that I've learned in my own clinical practice over the years.

Finally, I should add that for over 30 years, it has been my great pleasure to study and write about the art of interviewing. I have specialized in developing methods for training both inexperienced and experienced clinicians.

Over these years, I have become convinced of the necessity of providing the clinician, not only with sound principles, but also with direct examples of how to implement these principles. The clinician needs to see the exact phrases and questions that can transform a sound principle into a sound practice. In the last analysis, mastering medical interviewing is probably not as dependent on knowing what to say than on knowing how, and when, to say it. Thus, as was the case with my previous books, I have tried to pack this text with sample questions, concrete interviewing strategies, and illustrative bits of clinical dialogue that will bring the interviewing techniques alive for the reader.

In closing, it's my wish that the reader thoroughly enjoys the following pages. I certainly enjoyed writing them. I truly believe that, in the last analysis, it is a privilege to be a healer.

As healers, our journey is a rich one. In our efforts to provide relief to our patients, we succeed at times, and, at other times, we fail. No matter what the outcome, we always learn. As we move more deeply into our patient's pains and fears, we encounter the reflections of those pains and fears – their hopes and expectations. Our medications often become symbols of potential cure, and their expectations are that our medications will be the lifelines that lead to that cure. Sometimes they do, sometimes they don't.

It is here, within the chaotic world where suffering and compassion meet and sometimes collide that we move ever more deeply into the souls of our patients. Once there, we have the great privilege, as Albert Schweitzer observed, to suddenly know what it is "to become true human beings." These moments are the moments that define our livelihoods as physicians, nurses, physician assistants, clinical pharmacists, and case managers. This book is about such moments.

Shawn Christopher Shea, MD

Acknowledgments

Let me begin at the true beginning. A deep debt of gratitude goes to my former colleagues on the Continuous Treatment Team – from so many years ago – Denise Gaul, Deb Raab, Barnes Peterson, Linda Vigstedt, Beverly Snow, and Nick Nichols as well as all of the patients they served. I believe I learned more from you regarding the art of talking with patients about their medications than from anybody else in my entire career. You taught me much, and I still miss our work together. It was, indeed, within the clinical work and wisdom of this case management team that the seeds of the MIM were sown.

I would also like to thank the participants in my MIM workshops from around the United States and in Canada. I have learned an immense amount from you that has helped me to help my own patients as well as providing the foundation stones for the development of the MIM. Many of your interviewing tips grace the pages of this book. I hope that I have done justice to your ideas. It is a much better model and a much better book because of your wisdom.

It is a delightful pleasure to thank Peter Gunther, Paulette Thabault, and Suzanne Coble for their belief in the MIM, their enthusiasm for the book, and their valued editorial comments and suggestions.

As with the last book, I owe a great thanks to the wonderful staff of the Susan Colgate Cleveland Library/Learning Center at the Colby-Sawyer College in New London, New Hampshire. In particular, I would like to thank Noelle Bassi and Beth Krajewski for their warm support and laughter that made many a long day shorter.

Concerning the production of the book, I would like to thank Kristina Oberle, my original editor. Kristina's enthusiasm for the book, her rather remarkable patience, and the kindness she showed me during some tough personal times will always be remembered.

And, of course, great thanks to all the members of the editorial, design, and production teams at Wolters Kluwer, who have worked tirelessly to bring this book and the MIM to fruition. Many thanks to my current editor Rebecca Gaertner who picked up the reins with Kristina's departure. Rebecca, your patience, humor, warmth and excellent guidance on the book have been uplifting and greatly appreciated. Alexis (Lexi) Pozonsky, my editorial coordinator, and David Orzechowski, the production manager for the book have bent over backward (and I mean backward) to get the details of the book exactly the way I envisioned, including the handsome cover and layout work created by the talented artists of the Wolters Kluwer design department. A heartfelt thanks to Samson Premkumar and his production team for ably bringing the book to fruition. Finally, many thanks to Rachel Mante Leung, my marketing director. Rachel, it has been a joy to work with you, and I very much look forward to our further collaboration. Your infectious belief in the importance of the book and your imaginative thoughts on how to market it are a treasure.

I could not end without giving my deepest thanks to my wife, Susan, who – as with my previous books – edited every single page of this manuscript, and whose sharp eye and splendid sense of composition have greatly improved it. Susan, my gratitude for your hard work and your sacrifice for our shared mission, go beyond words. I don't think I can say it any better than I did in our last book together, for it is even more true today than it was then . . . You are not only the love of my life, you are the keeper of my soul. Always for good. Always for right.

Shawn Christopher Shea, MD

CONTENTS

PART ONE

When Patients Don't Take Their Medications: Core Principles

CHAPTER 1

"Nonadherence": The Extent of the Problem

"We prescribing clinicians continue to struggle with the most basic of problems: how to get our patients to take the pills that we think they need in the way we think they should. As efficacious as the medications are in research reports and clinical studies, they cannot be effective without moving from the prescription vial to the patient's body."[1]

James M. Ellison, MD, MPH

Introduction

Whether we are medical, nursing, or physician assistant students or graduate students in advanced practice nursing or clinical pharmacy (or perhaps even residents or more experienced clinicians), at some point we have probably heard a favorite attending sharing some sage advice that went along these lines, "The number one cause of treatment failure is not wrong diagnosis, not wrong drug choice, but poor adherence." As far as clinical axioms go, this one is surprisingly valid.

Research has given ample support to these claims for, across many disease states, the number one reason for treatment failure is the fact that the patient's medications are not taken as prescribed or, in many instances, not taken at all. As former Surgeon General C. Everett Koop, MD, ScD, so cogently quipped in his Foreword to the first edition of this book, "No medications work inside a bottle. Period."[2] It is hard to argue with Dr. Koop on this one.

The amount of human suffering – to our patients and to those who love them – caused by this lack of what is traditionally called "medication adherence" is truly disturbing. Whether a patient does not follow through with antihypertensives, oral hypoglycemic medications, antiplatelet medications after a cardiac stent procedure, or antidepressants, the results are often dire (strokes, kidney failure, myocardial infarction, and suicide, respectively). In addition to these potentially life-ending results, the amount of unnecessary suffering, symptoms, and pain caused by medication nonadherence is, quite literally, staggering.

Our journey, in this book, toward addressing this critical topic will be a bit like putting together a jigsaw puzzle. Our first task will be to pull out all the puzzle pieces concerning medication adherence and nonadherence, flipping the pieces over, turning them in our hands to see their nuances and colors, and seeing the extent and drivers of the problem. Our next step will be to put the puzzle pieces together – to find a variety of potential solutions to the problem. Naturally, we will not always be able to find the solution with every patient – occasionally puzzle pieces will be missing – but I wouldn't be writing these pages and you wouldn't be reading them unless we believed that we can have a significant impact on enhancing our patients' interest in, and effective use of, their medications. In short, there is an art to talking with patients about their medications. It is an art in which we share decision making. Moreover, it is an art that is learnable.

Furthermore, as these pages turn, we will find that part of the art of putting the jigsaw puzzle together lies in the fact that we will need to update the process a bit. We will revitalize some age-old rules and terms that, I believe, may have outlived their usefulness. Although we acknowledge the value and wisdom of the traditional approaches, we will forge a more contemporary version of the art.

Specifically, we will eventually, in subsequent chapters, do away with terms such as *adherence* and *compliance,* for they may very well be part of the problem. Instead, we will, as the title of our book implies, help our patients to move away from mere "adherence" to a more genuine understanding, interest, and effective use of their medications. But I am jumping ahead. To continue to do so might take away the intrigue and enjoyment of putting the jigsaw puzzle together. Let us start at the beginning, using the traditional terms, to see the historical context of the problem and how our more contemporary views may help solve it.

Initial Puzzle Pieces: A More Detailed Look at the Evidence Base

The Prevalence of Nonadherence

It has long been known from numerous studies that patients with chronic diseases take their medications as prescribed only about 50% to 60% of the time,[3] a finding supported by more recent research, which also indicates that 20% to 30% of patients never fill their prescriptions.[4,5] The actual number depends on the disease in question, but a glance at earlier work reveals that about one-third of patients comply reasonably well with recommended treatment, about one-third have moderate problems with adherence, and about one-third take their medications poorly or not at all.[6]

More recent work, including data from the World Health Organization, has shown that medication adherence is, shall we say, "robustly bad."[7–9] Whether adhering or not, about one-third of patients with chronic illnesses have strong reservations about the medications they are taking – future examples of discontinuance just waiting to happen.[10]

Statistics aside, many of us don't need to look much farther than the nearest mirror to see the ubiquitous nature of nonadherence; I, for one, know that I have not always taken medications exactly the way I was supposed to take them – and I am not alone. One study showed that only 79% of health care professionals reported good adherence with prescribed therapies.[11] Nor is nonadherence the sole province of any one type of person. From child to grandparent, from high school dropout to Rhodes scholar, from a struggling parent in a welfare line in downtown Detroit to an affluent day trader in a ticket line on Broadway, people from all ages and walks of life are guilty of "playing" with their meds. Nonadherence is everywhere it would seem.

Not only is nonadherence not specific to any single type of person, it is not specific to any single type of disease. The list of diseases in which nonadherence has been tagged as particularly commonplace – diabetes, hypertension, hyperlipidemia, heart failure, epilepsy, cancer, AIDS, depression, and schizophrenia, to name only a few – reads like a veritable "who's who" of crippling diseases.

Closer review of the literature highlights the havoc that nonadherence (or noncompliance as it is still sometimes called)[12] can play in the treatment of specific disease states, such as congestive heart failure (CHF), epilepsy, and diabetes. The authors of one study of more than 7,000 elderly patients who needed daily digoxin found that they refilled their prescriptions enough times to take their medications for only 111 days of the year – 30% of the time![13] One shudders when picturing these patients abruptly stopping, then starting, and then stopping their medications. Easily imaginable are patients madly doubling or tripling any specific dosage when they realize that they have missed some doses and feel a need to catch up – not exactly the safest way to take digoxin.

Another set of researchers found that their epileptic patients managed to take only 76% of their prescribed doses of antiepileptic drugs, with a range of 3% to 100% adherence.[14] In a study by Katon and colleagues, it was found that a whopping 60% of primary care patients discontinued their antidepressants before completing the recommended 6 months of therapy.[15] In a large study coming out of Duke University in 2006, it was found that out of 17,035 US patients prescribed beta-blocker drugs following a heart attack, only 45% reported taking the medications regularly during the first year after leaving the hospital. Perhaps more ominous, the biggest drop occurred during the initial months after the heart attack following discharge, a time ripe for a repeat myocardial infarction (MI).[16]

Putting research aside, any clinician who has been in the clinical trenches for even a few years can attest to any medical or nursing student that nonadherence is not a manufactured problem, but, in the parlance of contemporary slang, "the real thing." As noted earlier, learning the sophisticated interviewing techniques for transforming nonadherence, such as the ones described in this book is, arguably, one of the most important tasks for any medical, nursing, physician assistant, or clinical pharmacist student to undertake. Mastering these techniques and creating new ones are, arguably, two of the most important tasks for any veteran clinician to continue throughout the years, for, as we veteran clinicians know all too well, each patient brings us new challenges and, sometimes, in a refreshing light, new lessons.

The Impact of Nonadherence

Clearly, nonadherence is common, but is it harmful? Do people who fail to take their medications actually become more ill? This is a legitimate question, not just a semantic tease, because not all associated phenomena are causal in relation as we all remember from our undergraduate courses in statistics. Let us see what the data suggest on this point.

To find out, let us return to an older but important study related to beta-blockers post-MI. In the Beta-Blocker Heart Attack Trial of 1990 (a study of post infarction treatment approaches), an important finding was made among the 2,175 patients who were available for a medication adherence analysis. Those patients who took less than 75% of their medications (as measured in pill counts) had a 2.5-fold increase in mortality compared with those patients who took their medications more assiduously.[17] Now that's a finding that will make one reach for the pill bottle more regularly. More recent work has also shown quite significant increases in mortality in the year post-MI, especially if medications such as beta-blockers, aspirin, and statins were all stopped within 1 month of discharge.[18] Such troubling results are common in the field of cardiology[19] but are far from unique to it.

For a moment, let us look at four particularly common diseases that you will encounter on a daily basis whether you eventually find yourself practicing in primary care, internal medicine, cardiology, surgery, or any subspecialty. We will evaluate their relation to adherence by using their rate of hospitalization as a reflection of both patient suffering and financial stress to both individuals and society at large. In looking at diabetes, hypertension, hypercholesterolemia, and CHF, Michael Sokol and colleagues found that hospitalizations were significantly increased with those patients who showed poor adherence.[20] In a similar fashion, in an outstanding review, DiMatteo estimated that over 188 million medical encounters are followed by patient nonadherence every year in the United States with associated costs of up to $300 billion a year.[21]

Data from a study looking at the benefits related to antibiotic adherence show similarly convincing results. For example, a randomized trial of oral antibiotic prophylaxis in patients with cancer showed the following results. Patients who showed good adherence developed fever and infection in only 18% of the cases, in contrast to the development of fever and infection in 54% of those patients with poor adherence.[22]

As one would expect, the field of psychiatry is replete with evidence of the critical role that medication adherence plays in morbidity and mortality in such serious diseases as schizophrenia and bipolar disorder. Valenstein[23] and Weiden[24] have studied the impact of gaps in taking medication based on prescription refill data in large populations of patients. They found that even a gap in medication-taking as short as 10 days resulted in a doubling of the risk of hospitalization. With longer gaps, the risk of readmission to the hospital continues to rise significantly, with gaps of greater than 30 days increasing the risk fourfold.

Indeed, discontinuation of medications can even result in the loss of patients' lives. In a fascinating, yet disturbing, study Herings and Erkens reported on 603 patients with schizophrenia in the Netherlands using a medication-dispensing and hospital discharge database.[25] Adjusting for age and gender, they reported that a 30-day gap in medication treatment increased the relative risk of suicide attempts a stunning 4.2 times. (Thirty-three percent of the patients in their sample had a gap of at least 30 days.)

Improving Adherence Through Language: A Bit of Evidence Base

It appears evident that adherence to medication helps. But can it be improved using specific physician questions and statements – the focus of our book? I'm convinced, from years of training professionals, that it can be improved substantially. But there is also mounting research evidence to support this case.

Let us look at antidepressant adherence because antidepressants are one of the most commonly prescribed of medications in both primary care and psychiatric settings – indeed, primary care physicians prescribe more antidepressants than all psychiatrists combined. Moreover, in a somewhat surprising sense, it has been shown that patients who are depressed, compared with nondepressed patients, have roughly three times greater odds of not using their medications as prescribed for their *nonpsychiatric* medications. Thus, a patient who is not taking his or her antidepressants may have marked problems, including ultimately fatal results, with the treatment outcomes of their concurrent nonpsychiatric diseases such as diabetes, hypertension, or CHF, for the depressive state may lead to nonadherence with the use of the patient's nonpsychiatric medications as well.[26]

A hope-engendering study once again from Katon and colleagues, and spearheaded by Elizabeth Lin of the Group Health Cooperative of Puget Sound, focused on the early adherence rates of primary care patients. I can't convey their results any more concisely than they did in the synopsis of their article, so it is best to let them speak for themselves:

> Approximately 28% of patients stopped taking antidepressants during the first month of therapy, and 44% had stopped taking them by the third month of therapy. Patients who received the following five specific educational messages – 1) take the medication daily; 2) antidepressants must be taken for 2 to 4 weeks for a noticeable effect; 3) continue to take medicine even if feeling better; 4) do not stop taking antidepressant without checking with the physician; and 5) specific instructions regarding what to do to resolve questions regarding antidepressants – were more likely to comply during the first month of antidepressant therapy. Asking about prior experience with antidepressants and discussions about scheduling pleasant activities also were related to early adherence.[27]

The results of the Puget Sound group are highly encouraging, because, in this case, they indicate that specific interviewing statements made during the medication education phase of the appointment can significantly improve adherence.

The Challenge of the Future

An Aging Population

If it were not already the leading problem in nursing and medicine, the problem of medication adherence is destined to present a progressively more ubiquitous threat to our patients' healing in the decades to come. A simple demographic – the age of our patient population – tells us that this is so.

Pressing as the topic of medication adherence is with our typical patient population, it is even more pressing in our care of the older patient. Medication problems take on a new light when the patient is over age 65, as Assumpta Ryan points out in her excellent review article on medication adherence issues in older people, first appearing in the *International Journal of Nursing Studies*.[28] Three key situations complicate the picture with older patients.

First, the physiologic aging process affects absorption, distribution, metabolism, and excretion of medications. The net result is often a narrowing of the therapeutic window with this population. Consequently, smaller errors in adherence can result in bigger problems in care. Inadvertent surges into toxic ranges or precipitous drops out of therapeutic windows can prove to be more frequent outcomes sometimes precipitated by rather modest problems with nonadherence in this age group.

The second confounding factor with a more aged population is the increased frequency of comorbidity. Many of our elderly patients have not only an additional disorder to their primary problem, but also frequently three, four, five, or more disorders. Multisystem disease is so prevalent in this population that the idea of a primary disorder becomes somewhat muted, because such patients frequently have multiple diseases that could kill them if they are not adequately controlled.

Multisystem disorder means multisystem medication regimens. The result is sometimes confusing, not only to the prescribing clinician but also to the patient's own body. More medications mean more possible drug-drug interactions. We begin to run a fine line as to how much of a given medication will interact safely with its fellow residents in the bloodstream and how much is problematic. Once again, medication errors – in this case, the patient taking too much – can prove costly.

Our third confounding factor in this age group is that the use of multiple medications can also prove to be quite confusing, in a psychological sense, to the aging patient. For instance, with failing eyesight, bottle labels become harder to read. Problems with concentration and memory may create ever more treacherous adherence pitfalls, heightened by the fact that the older patient may frequently live alone.

All Is Not as It Seems

At this point, I believe we have made a compelling survey of the extent of the problem of nonadherence, which was the purpose of our chapter. But as we close, it's worth noting that determining the extent of nonadherence itself, especially in a specific patient sitting on a specific exam table in a specific clinic, is not as easy as it may seem at first glance nor as the above studies may suggest.

Many factors make it difficult for patients to share the truth about their actual – versus prescribed – medication use, ranging from poor recall and embarrassment to feeling guilty that they are not doing what they told the clinician they would do or that, somehow, they have become "bad patients." Uncovering the truth about our patients' actual medication practices, outside our offices, has been a persistent challenge in the past and will be an ongoing challenge in the future.

A clever piece of research highlights the elusiveness of uncovering the truth about medication adherence from our patients, for it demonstrates that even the use of blood levels to "get a handle" on whether adherence is happening can be surprisingly misleading. Joyce Kramer and colleagues monitored the adherence of patients taking antiepileptic drugs by having the patients use medication event monitoring system (MEMS) bottles.[29] MEMS bottles contain a microprocessor in their caps that record each opening as a presumptive dose, listing the date and time for later retrieval on a microcomputer. Pretty nifty.

The results were surprising. The patients were monitored during all days between two consecutive clinic visits at least 2 months apart. At each visit, serum blood levels were drawn exactly as they would have been in clinical practice. Not only did adherence drop over time with many patients, but also patients fluctuated on how they took their medications over the course of the 2 months. The 20 patients averaged 88% adherence in the days directly before the first visit to be monitored and 86% adherence in the days directly after the visit. But their adherence dropped to 67% 1 month later. One potentially useful takeaway from this study is that patient adherence may tend to improve with more frequent visits – 2 months being too long in this cohort – as logic would suggest. But there was an even more intriguing finding.

One of the patients showed a problematic pattern of missing more of his medications as the 2 months progressed, but then in the final days before his next scheduled appointment, he took the medications exactly as prescribed. More importantly, by taking the medications correctly in the 4 days immediately before his next office visit, he managed to get the blood level of his carbamazepine into the midrange, almost exactly where it had been at his last visit.

Serum blood levels, whether for digoxin, Tegretol, or lithium, are often valued as reliable reflections of medication adherence. But as seen with this patient, they may convey an illusion of actual medication adherence, a phenomenon cleverly referred to as "white coat adherence" in the literature.[7,30,31]

It is very easy to forget meds or to "just not be bothered with them" on certain days. Especially when patient appointments are spaced far apart, as is common in today's hectic practice, an otherwise conscientious patient who is missing doses rather regularly may return to full medication adherence in the days immediately before an appointment. It would be quite natural to do this because many patients want to appear that they are doing "what is right." Wanting to be viewed by one's doctor as being a reliable patient who "follows doctor's orders" is normal. The subsequent blood level drawn may fall well within acceptable therapeutic range, thus providing the false appearance of good ongoing adherence. It is useful to complement blood levels with direct questions about adherence between visits even if a patient is showing excellent blood levels.

CONCLUSION

With a heightened awareness of the increased ramifications of nonadherence and the surprising difficulties involved in ascertaining the extent of such nonadherence in any given specific patient, we can bring this introductory chapter to a close. The goal of the chapter was to highlight the extent of the nonadherence problem while hinting that there are a number of potential methods for frequently transforming it.

Let us now turn our attention to this transformative process. We saw from Katon's research that sound education about medication use can help patients to improve their medication adherence. In addition, actual counseling techniques such as motivational interviewing and cognitive therapy have, in my opinion, opened the door to even more effective approaches. However, empirical research has demonstrated that the effectiveness of these traditional counseling approaches has been more modest than had been hoped.[32–38] Perhaps the modest results are related to the relatively extensive time required to master such approaches[39] as well as the relatively extensive time it takes to employ them in a hectic medicine clinic.

But what if a different approach was taken? What if one did not borrow from preestablished models of counseling that require ongoing strategies and intensive trainings to master? What if one hunted for single interviewing techniques – easily learned and quickly employed – that seemed to improve medication interest and effective use? And what if one hunted for these interviewing techniques by observing and talking with the frontline physicians, nurses, physician assistants, clinical pharmacists, and case managers who actually prescribe and support patients' use of medications? What would happen then? The next chapter will show us.

In it we will also uncover a hidden truth about healing relationships. In the last analysis, the problem of patient nonadherence inexorably leads to the very core of our understanding of the therapeutic alliance. We will discover that how we resolve the delicate arabesque we call nonadherence is, in many respects, the microcosm to the macrocosm of how we forge our ongoing clinician-patient relationship.

Each clinician-patient relationship is unique, and each clinician-patient relationship must define its own unique set of expectations and methods of joint problem solving. It is often over the issue of "meds" that this definition evolves. The next chapter, as well as the remainder of this book, is an effort to illuminate some of the concrete interviewing techniques that can help clinicians, from all disciplines, to more effectively do their part in defining this potentially powerful alliance – the alliance that helps us to heal when healing is possible and to comfort when it is not.

REFERENCES

1. Ellison JM. Enhancing adherence in the pharmacotherapy treatment relationship. In: Tasman A, Riba M, Silk K, eds. *The Doctor-Patient Relationship in Pharmacotherapy*. New York, NY: Guilford Press; 2000:72.
2. Shea SC. *Improving Medication Adherence: How to Talk with Patients About Their Medications*. 1st ed. Philadelphia, PA: Lippincott Williams & Wilkins; 2006:xviii.
3. Sackett DL, Snow JC. The magnitude of adherence and nonadherence. In: Haynes R, Sackett D, Taylor D, eds. *Adherence in Health Care*. Baltimore, MD: Johns Hopkins University Press; 1979:11–22.

4. Peterson AM, Takiya L, Finley R. Meta-analysis of trials of interventions to improve medication adherence. *Am J Health Syst Pharm* 2003;60:657–665.
5. Haynes RB, Ackloo E, Sahota N, et al. Interventions for enhancing medication adherence. *Cochrane Database Syst Rev* 2008:CD000011.
6. Fedder DO. Managing medication and adherence: physician-pharmacist-patient interaction. *J Am Geriatr Soc* 1982;30:113–117.
7. Osterberg L, Blaschke T. Adherence to medication. *N Engl J Med* 2005;353:487–497.
8. World Health Organization. *Noncommunicable Diseases and Mental Health: Progress Report 2002–2003.* Geneva, Switzerland: World Health Organization; 2003.
9. Viswanathan M, Golin CE, Jones CD, et al. Interventions to improve adherence to self-administered medications for chronic diseases in the United States: a systematic review. *Ann Int Med* 2012;157(11):785–795. doi:10.7326/0003-4819-157-11-201212040-00538.
10. Practice research a potent force for change, says President. *Pharm J* May 30, 1998;260:791–794.
11. Corda RS, Burke HB, Horowitz HW. Adherence to prescription medicines among medical professionals. *South Med J* 2000;93:585–589.
12. Cramer JA, Roy A, Burrell A, et al. Medication compliance and persistence: terminology and definitions. *Value Health* 2008;11(1):44–47.
13. Monane M, Bohn RL, Gurwitz JH, et al. Nonadherence with congestive heart failure therapy in the elderly. *Arch Intern Med* 1994;153:433–437.
14. Cramer JA, Mattson RH, Privy ML, et al. How often is medication taken as prescribed? A novel assessment technique. *JAMA* 1989;261:3273–3277.
15. Katon W, von Korff M, Lin E, et al. Adequacy and duration of antidepressant treatment in primary care. *Med Care* 1992;30:67.
16. Kramer JM, Anstrom K, Fetteroff D, et al. National evaluation of adherence to [beta] blocker therapy for 1 year after acute myocardial infarction in patients with commercial health insurance. *Am Heart J* 2006;152(3):454.e1–454.e8. doi:10.1016/j.ahi.2006.02.030.
17. Horwitz RI, Viscoli CM, Berkman L. Treatment adherence and risk of death after a myocardial infarction. *Lancet* 1990;336:542–545.
18. Ho PM, Sperius JA, Masoudi FA, et al. Impact of medication therapy discontinuation on mortality after myocardial infarction. *Arch Intern Med* 2006;166(17):1842–1847. doi:10.1001/archinte.166.17.1842.
19. Ho PM, Bryson CL, Rumsfeld JS. Medication adherence: its importance in cardiovascular outcomes. *Circulation* 2009;119:3028–3035. doi:10.1161/CIRCULATIONAHA.108.768986.
20. Sokol MC, McGuigan KA, Verbrugge RR, et al. Impact of medication adherence on hospitalization risk and healthcare cost. *Med Care* 2005;43(6):521–530.
21. DeMatteo D. Variations in patients' adherence to medical recommendations: a quantitative review of 50 years of research. *Med Care* 2004;42(3):200–209.
22. Pizzo PA, Robichaud KJ, Edwards BK, et al. Oral antibiotic prophylaxis in patients with cancer: a double-blind randomized placebo-controlled trial. *J Pediatr* 1983;102: 125–133.
23. Valenstein M, Copeland LA, Blow FC, et al. Pharmacy data identify poorly adherent patients with schizophrenia at increased risk for admission. *Med Care* 2002;40:630–639.
24. Weiden P, Rapkin B, Zygmunt A, et al. Post discharge medication compliance of inpatients converted from an oral to a depot neuroleptic regimen. *Psychiatr Serv* 1995;46:1049–1054.

25. Herings RM, Erkens JA. Increased suicide attempt rate among patients interrupting use of atypical antipsychotics. *Pharmacoepidemiol Drug Saf* 2003;12:423–424.
26. DiMatteo MR, Lepper HS, Croghan TW. Depression is a risk factor for noncompliance with medical treatment. *Arch Intern Med* 2000;160(14):2101–2107. doi:10.1001/archinte.160.14.2101.
27. Lin EH, Von Korff M, Katon W, et al. The role of the primary care physician in patients' adherence to antidepressant therapy. *Med Care* 1995;33(1):67–74.
28. Ryan AA. Medication adherence and older people: a review of the literature. *Int J Nurs Stud* 1999;36:153–162.
29. Cramer JA, Scheyer RD, Mattson RH. Adherence declines between clinic visits. *Arch Intern Med* 1990;150:1509–1510.
30. Modi AC, Ingerski LM, Rausch JR, et al. White coat adherence over the first year of therapy in pediatric epilepsy. *J Pediatr* 2012;161(4):695–699. doi:10.1016/j.jpeds.2012.03.059.
31. Feinstein AR. On white coat effects and the electronic monitoring of compliance. *Arch Intern Med* 1990;150:1377–1378.
32. Jackson H. Motivational interviewing and HIV drug adherence. *Nurs Times* 2013;109(41):21–23.
33. Lavoie KL, Moullec G, Lemiere C, et al. Efficacy of brief motivational interviewing to improve adherence to inhaled corticosteroids among adult asthmatics: results from a randomized controlled pilot feasibility trial. *Patient Prefer Adherence* 2014;8:1555–1569.
34. McKenzie K, Chang Y. The effect of nurse-led motivational interviewing on medication adherence in patients with bipolar disorder. *Perspect Psychiatr Care* 2015;51:36–44.
35. Possidente CJ, Bucci KK, McCain WJ. Motivational interviewing: a tool to improve medication adherence? *Am J Health Syst Pharm* 2005;62:1311–1314.
36. Solomon DH, Iversen MD, Avorn J, et al. Osteoporosis telephonic intervention to improve medication adherence (OPTIMA): a large pragmatic randomized controlled trial. *Arch Intern Med* 2012;172(6):477–483. doi:10.1001/archinternmed.2011.1977.
37. Berkowitz SA, Johnson KL. Does motivational interviewing improve outcomes [editorial]? *Arch Intern Med* 2012;172(6):463–464. doi:10.1001/archinternmed.2012.155.
38. Demonceau J, Ruppar T, Kristanto P, et al. Identification and assessment of adherence-enhancing interventions in studies assessing medication adherence through electronically compiled drug dosing histories: a systematic literature review and meta-analysis. *Drugs* 2013;73:545–562. doi:10.1007/s40265-013-0041-3.
39. Miller WR, Rollnick S. *Motivational Interviewing: Helping People Change*. New York, NY: The Guilford Press; 2013:329–330, 354–355.

CHAPTER 2

The Medication Interest Model: What Is It?

"Physicians are confronted by the particular souls of the individuals and families before them . . . People want to know that their opinions and concerns are worthy of interest and response."[1]

Robert Shuman, EdD
FROM THE PSYCHOLOGY OF CHRONIC ILLNESS

THE SPIRIT OF THE MEDICATION INTEREST MODEL

Arguably the most important organizing theme in our book is the idea that the words we use in talking with our patients about their medications is one of the keys to creating genuine medication interest. John Steiner, the director of the Colorado Health Outcomes Program, provocatively captures this fact by reminding us "that our words are as important a part of the pharmacopoeia as the medications themselves."[2]

This specialized linguistic skill set, which is of immediate practical relevance with almost every patient that we see, is important across all medical disciplines. It does not matter whether the reader is a prescriber as seen with physicians, advanced nurse practitioners, and physician assistants or intimately involved with ongoing medication monitoring as with nurses, case managers (whether nurses or social workers), or clinical pharmacists (who in some instances also prescribe), we must talk with our patients about their medications. The Medication Interest Model (MIM) is all about this delicate exchange of ideas.

The MIM has been evolving for over 20 years. It includes roughly 100 behaviorally well-defined interviewing techniques. These interviewing techniques are housed within a conceptual motivational framework – the Choice Triad. The Choice Triad provides a reliable, logical, and simplifying structure for understanding the many complexities of how patients choose to try medications, choose to continue them, or choose to discontinue them. The MIM was designed to be easily learned by medical, nursing, and physician assistant students as well as by residents and graduate students in advanced practice nursing and clinical pharmacy programs. Once understood, clinicians can flexibly employ the interviewing principles and techniques of the MIM throughout their careers. As we shall soon see, in the hectic pace of everyday practice, the Choice Triad provides a practical platform that allows busy clinicians to rapidly and sensitively explore the thought processes and emotional responses patients experience when using medications.

Moreover, enhancing medication interest while gracefully transforming our patients' concerns has a lot more to do with our patients' souls, as our opening epigram hints, than is usually ascribed. By soul, I simply mean "what makes our patients tick" psychologically and spiritually. As health care providers, we reach our patients' souls through the power of our relationships with them as forged by our words and nonverbal communications. Thus, the resolution of the problem of low interest in medication use and poor follow-up with use, to a large extent, ultimately comes down to how we talk with our patients about their medications.

Although the MIM did not directly evolve from any specific model, it was developed in an era filled with pioneering advances in collaborative care and conceptual innovations on how to more successfully forge the therapeutic alliance. It reflects, and indeed is, a prototypic example of patient-centered medicine,[3–5] person-centered medicine,[6–8] and shared decision making.[9–12] The MIM also resonates nicely with the patient-centered medical home.[13–15]

If one were forced to proffer one word that lies at the center of the model, it would be the word "choice." Every single interviewing technique of the MIM is designed to enhance the patient's ability to consider whether the use of medication is the right choice for himself or herself, and, if so, how to choose a particular medication and how to use it most effectively. From the perspective of our model, the practice of "choice" and the issue of "trust" often go hand in hand leading directly to the heart of the therapeutic alliance. The patient's trust of any given clinician is frequently partially, and sometimes substantially, based on the patient's observations of how the clinician discusses the use of medications.

This state of affairs is particularly accentuated if the clinician is expected to make a medication recommendation by the end of the initial appointment as is typical in most primary care environments, as well as in many specialty clinics from endocrinology to neurology and cardiology. Obviously, in such instances, the quality of the therapeutic relationship created during the earlier stages of the initial appointment may greatly determine the likelihood that the patient will be interested in following the clinician's recommendations. But, not so obviously, the reverse may be equally true – the discussion about medications near the end of the initial appointment may determine the robustness of the ensuing therapeutic alliance.

One can argue that concurrent with the development of the overall "therapeutic alliance," a prescribing clinician must also develop a "medication alliance." One can further argue that this "medication alliance" may have a greater impact on the overall "therapeutic alliance" than vice versa. I would argue that the fashion in which a clinician handles the transactions over the potential use of medications may even determine whether the clinician and the patient will ever set eyes on each other again.

Let me be more specific. I am suggesting that the *micro*cosm we call the "medication alliance" may have a profound impact, indeed may represent one of the primary determinants of the *macro*cosm we traditionally, in the fields of nursing and medicine, have called the "therapeutic alliance." The discussion of medications in the initial interview marks the first time that the patient and the clinician must truly arrive at a difficult collaborative decision. In this regard, the *process* of this discussion represents a pivotal database from which the patient will make a formulation of "exactly who *is* this person, often bedecked in a white coat with a stethoscope hanging out of his or her pocket or dangling around his or her neck."

From this initial discussion of medications, the patient will determine whether the clinician is genuinely interested in various ways of approaching symptom relief or is merely a pill pusher. The patient will gauge the clinician's degree of actual concern by how openly the clinician describes the benefits and side effects or adverse reactions of the medication. The patient will pull from the look in the clinician's eyes, and from the tone of his or her voice, whether the clinician is truly registering the patient's concerns about the potential side effects of the medication or is mainly interested in typing on his or her computer or tablet. *Ultimately, the patient will listen to the clinician's recommendations in direct proportion to how well the clinician listens to the patient's recommendations.*

If the patient leaves this first appointment with a positive assessment of these clinician characteristics, a second appointment will be more likely to occur. When such a meeting occurs, one can bet that the patient's evaluation of the clinician will continue. This ongoing evaluation will undoubtedly be greatly based on the dyad's exchanges concerning medications.

In subsequent appointments, the patient will determine the clinician's ability to effectively listen by how carefully the clinician explores the patient's concerns about his or her side effects that have now morphed from abstract possibilities in the first appointment to concrete realities in the days preceding the subsequent appointments. It is one thing to hear about potential problems with sleep. It is entirely a different thing to toss restlessly in one's bed for 2 hours every night before getting to sleep.

The patient will decipher the collaborative proclivities of the nurse practitioner, clinical nurse specialist, or physician by whether the clinician is willing to change his or her medication recommendations (stop a medication, lower its dosage, or switch to another medication or perhaps to an intervention from the field of alternative medicine) on the basis of the patient's input. Put succinctly, exactly as Shuman emphasized in our opening epigram, "people want to know that their opinions and concerns are worthy of interest and response." The MIM is all about this "listening."

Collaborative Exploration: The Transformative Engine of the MIM

"Choice." It is a word to which we will find ourselves repeatedly returning and for good reason. The spirit of the MIM arises with the simple acknowledgment that the decision to put a foreign substance into one's body – sometimes indefinitely – is not an easy choice. Let us be blunt, many people have died from medications, vastly more have been harmed by them. Medications can heal. They can relieve much human suffering. They can literally save lives. But to do so effectively, we must use them wisely. To use them wisely, clinicians must recognize their limitations and risks.

With this note of caution in mind, the MIM views physicians, advanced practice nurses, and other prescribing professionals (as well as those who collaboratively follow medication use such as case managers) not as health professionals whose goal is "to get" a patient to take his or her medications. Instead, their goal is to serve as knowledgeable and compassionate guides, who provide the information that will allow patients the opportunity to make the best possible choice for themselves. Of the prescribing dyad, only the patient puts the medication into his or her mouth. Prescribers don't suffer side effects, patients do.

It is always wise to remind ourselves of the axiom, which can be easily forgotten in everyday practice, that an ideal treatment plan that the patient will not follow is not ideal but foolish. In this regard, treatment algorithms that are solely disease based (e.g., in the sense that "if the patient has such and such a disease then this medication is obviously the correct therapeutic choice from our known evidence base") as opposed to those that are also illness based (e.g., how the patient suffers and experiences his or her symptoms) are prone to foolishness.[16] In helping the patient to choose an intervention, one must also consider contextual factors such as the patient's personal health beliefs, cultural beliefs, spiritual beliefs, and finances all of which can play determining roles in whether a patient even fulfills a prescription.

Added to the list are interpersonal factors such as the beliefs of family, friends, and other patients and concurrent healers (e.g., practitioners of alternative medicine). Truth be told, we don't prescribe medications solely to the patient. We are prescribing them to all those individuals with whom the patient is going to seek opinions about our prescriptions. If the family and friends of the patient would not put our medications in their mouths, it is unlikely our medications will find the mouths of our patients.

It is further complicated by what the patient discovers, both good and bad, accurate or inaccurate, about our medications on the web. Apparently, Dr. Google has become the leading authority on medication use in our wired culture. The choice for patients is truly complex, confusing, and emotionally charged.

For the life of me, I don't know what patients are supposed to think about medications after they are subjected to the barrage of direct-to-consumer ads foisted on them in nearly every commercial break on TV. Inevitably in such commercials, patients are seen dancing "happily about" despite dealing with crippling illnesses. All seems dandy until, near the very end, the viewer hears a litany of serious side effects recited by an off-camera spokesperson who speaks so rapidly as to suggest that the speeding voice might be better suited for an amphetamine-stoked cameo on *Breaking Bad* than as a supposed voice of caution for the unsuspecting consumer. Only a higher power can help unwitting patients if they manage to register anything the mad auctioneer lists, such as the fact that the medication plugged in the commercial – designed to help with breathing – can trigger a potentially fatal asthmatic attack or the featured antidepressant might create suicidal ideation. Meanwhile, as this litany of dangers speeds by the unsuspecting potential consumer, all the patients on the screen continue to smile happily, frolicking and laughing with their families, as cheerful music beams from the TV or smart phone screen.

Moreover, medications are not always the best, nor the only, route for healing. In fact, from the perspective of the MIM, the collaborative exploration does not begin with the question "Which medication should the patient choose?" It begins with the question "Should the first choice be something other than a medication?" Some forms of hypertension and diabetes respond quite well to dietary changes, exercise regimens, meditation, and deep-breathing none of which possess side effects when implemented appropriately. Various approaches from complementary and alternative medicine (CAM) hold promise from acupuncture in pain to Saint John's wort in mild depressions.

In the final analysis, for a patient to trust us, we must always communicate our best possible treatment recommendations, which in many instances are traditional medications. However, if we disagree with the patient's choice, as long as we do not think the nontraditional intervention will cause harm, we can genuinely suggest that the patient should give his or her first choice a try. Indeed, we can enthusiastically do our best to help the nonmedication intervention to succeed in any fashion that we can. If the patient can achieve healing without a medication, so much the better.

If, for some reason, it fails, then the patient will discover for himself or herself that their nontraditional choice did not work, and the patient is more likely to seek out the use of a medication. I am convinced that such a process – allowing the patient to arrive at his or her personal decision that the best intervention is a medication – is frequently, almost always, more likely to result in enhanced interest in ultimately using and sticking with a medication. People want relief from their pain. If they feel that a medication is the best way to get that relief, they will seek it.

The MIM fully recognizes that a truly collaborative exploration of treatment options necessitates an openness from the clinician that the patient is the expert of what the impact of a medication is having on his or her disorder, on his or her body, and on his or her life. Moreover, it is important to carefully listen to what the patient is saying, not merely because it strengthens the therapeutic alliance.

It is important because the patient is frequently right.

In many instances, the dose is too high, the timing of the dose is too rigid to allow for effective use, the medication is not working, the medication's side effects outweigh its benefits, or a different medication might work better (or perhaps an intervention from CAM may be more effective). Thus, the spirit of the MIM is about collaborative listening. It is about learning from the patient. Without question, if we learn from our patients, they are much more likely to learn from us. This listening process – this shared learning – is at the heart of the medication alliance. Bottom line: Few patients will take a medication from a person unless they like that person.

Roots of the MIM

Historical Development

Curiously, the MIM did not begin in the field of general medicine and nursing. It's very first roots arose from the remarkably challenging arena of increasing medication interest and use in patients suffering with severe mental illnesses. The initial insights of the MIM were gained from an "in-the-trenches" case management team that was part of a research study sponsored by the Robert Woods Johnson Foundation and led by Robert Drake from the Psychiatry Department of the Dartmouth Medical School in the late 1980s and early 1990s. These teams were developed to help patients with severe and chronic psychiatric disorders (all of the study patients had poorly controlled schizophrenia, schizoaffective disorder, or bipolar disorder), who were also suffering from concurrent alcohol and/or street drug abuse/dependence – a cohort with traditionally minimal interest in taking medications.[17]

I had the pleasure of developing and directing one of these teams. Our specific team had a high success rate with medication interest and follow-through. By the end of the 4-year study, the team had decreased hospital days on average by 20 days per patient per year (R. E. Drake, personal communication, 1996), a result that seemed to correlate well with higher medication adherence rates. From a concerted effort to tease out the interviewing techniques that seemed to be related to this success (as well as asking our patients why they chose to stay on their medications), the MIM was born and evolved.

The results were so striking that one could not help but wonder "if these interviewing techniques could be such transformative motivators for patients with severe mental illnesses, might they not also be effective in patients with diabetes, cancer, hyperlipidemia, renal disease, congestive heart failure (CHF), and AIDS?" The movement of the MIM from a specialty in psychiatric care to a primary model for use in general medicine and nursing had begun.

This gentle shift in emphasis became a more substantial push from an unexpected circumstance. I began providing a series of over 150 "medication interest" workshops over an 8-year span in the late 1990s and early 2000s across the United States and Canada. Participants representing a wide sampling of disciplines including psychiatrists, psychiatric nurse clinicians/nurses, and other mental health professionals as well as primary care physicians, nurses, and case managers attended.

Of particular note is the fact that a large number of the original workshops were *attended solely by primary care physicians, nurses, physician assistants, clinical pharmacists, and case managers*. The focus in these workshops was not on psychiatric medications. Instead these primary care clinicians discussed and provided a wealth of interviewing techniques – designed to improve adherence when treating illnesses such as hypertension, diabetes, asthma, CHF, cancer, and AIDS. From their input and feedback, it quickly became apparent that the theoretical foundation of the MIM (the Choice Triad) as well as its specific interviewing techniques were equally applicable to both nonpsychiatric illnesses and psychiatric illnesses.

These frontline primary care clinicians were asked to share their best practices regarding interviewing techniques that they had found to be useful in enhancing medication interest and effective follow-through across all disease states. In the subsequent years, and in an ongoing fashion to this day, these workshops continue, with primary care providers and specialists providing interviewing tips that enhance the ever-evolving MIM no matter what disease state a patient is encountering from hypertension to diabetes and lupus.

Pulling on Clinician Wisdom

The MIM was not the first, and hopefully it will not be the last, advance in learning how to improve medication interest and follow-through in primary care and specialty settings. For instance, many readers may be aware of the use of motivational interviewing (as well as cognitive therapy) when applied to medication adherence. In my opinion, motivational interviewing has made significant contributions to helping clinicians better understand and improve medication adherence, and, if unfamiliar with it, I urge the reader to learn more about it. Moreover, the MIM resonates with the general principles of motivational interviewing such as the importance of collaboration, compassion, moving with the patient's concerns, and allowing the patient to discover his or her own personal reasons for motivation.

The MIM, however, did not derive from motivational interviewing. Nor did the roots of the MIM grow from the same soil (borrowing a treatment approach from substance use counseling and adapting its techniques and strategies to a different arena – medication adherence).[18] By contrast, the MIM is rooted directly in the fertile soil provided by tapping the wisdom of the health care providers (physicians, nurses, physician assistants, clinical pharmacists, and case managers) who are routinely prescribing and monitoring the use of medications on a daily basis.

The MIM grew from the belief that although many prescribing clinicians and case managers encounter problems with medication adherence (and to a degree some of the providers may, indeed, lack the necessary interviewing skills to effectively engage patients around the use of medications), many other frontline clinicians and case managers are talented at the process. Moreover, some of these frontline providers are truly gifted at it. Rather than view health care providers as people who need to be taught how to effectively talk with patients about medications, we viewed health care providers as teachers from whom we could learn how to do so more effectively.

Indeed, the earliest work on the MIM arose from the observation and input of the superb set of case managers and nurse clinicians on the original outreach team described above. As the MIM evolved, it was further developed by tapping the wisdom of numerous frontline clinicians by talking and exchanging ideas with the clinicians (ranging from primary care providers to specialists in fields such as cardiology, neurology, endocrinologists, and psychiatry) who participated in the MIM workshops previously described.

As useful interviewing techniques were shared and delineated, an attempt was made to see if a theoretical model of motivation would emerge. It did. The resulting motivational model – the Choice Triad – unlike other frameworks for improving medication interest, such as motivational interviewing and cognitive behavioral therapy, was solely designed for use in enhancing a patient's interest and motivation for using medications. The Choice Triad – which will be described in Chapter 5 – proved to be a unifying and simplifying motivational framework that could be used to clarify and enhance the use of the many interviewing techniques that were being discovered. Thus, the MIM evolved as a "bottom-up model" *derived from the clinicians who were directly prescribing and following medication use with patients on an everyday basis.*

This homegrown development, from those who know the most about how to talk with patients about their medications, and have been doing so for years, would prove to be immensely powerful. It ensured that the techniques would be practical with regard to their application in extremely hectic primary care, mental health, and clinical pharmacy settings, for it was from those settings that the techniques originated. Moreover, since the techniques were developed by clinicians, who prescribed and monitored medications on a daily basis, it enhanced their acceptance by the fellow clinicians who staffed those very same hectic corridors.

Besides the advantage of being developed by listening to the people who actually do the work, in my opinion there is one other defining quality to the MIM, when compared with other interviewing approaches that have been utilized for improving adherence. It is an advantage that will allow readers – from students to experienced clinicians – to gain familiarity and skill in its application quickly and enjoyably. The MIM was born directly from advances that have been made in the exciting field of clinical interviewing and training.[19]

Innovations from the Field of Clinical Interviewing

Interviewing Principles, Techniques, and Strategies: Gateways to Enhanced Learning

An interviewing *principle* is a guiding concept for approaching an interviewing task. Interviewing principles help clinicians to recognize when to use specific techniques, how to flexibly handle new situations, and how to be creative and "think on one's feet" while interviewing.

For instance, I have found the following principle to be of excellent use in day-to-day practice: *Before raising a sensitive or taboo topic (such as missing medication doses, substance abuse, incest, domestic violence, and suicide) metacommunicate to the patient that it is okay to share such material*. This principle clearly provides sound guidance to any interviewer. However, interviewing principles do not show the interviewer, concretely, what words to use. Interviewing principles, because they are abstractions, are by their very nature sometimes unclear to trainees, open to misinterpretation, frequently difficult to learn, and often notoriously difficult to test with regard to trainee competence.

By contrast, an interviewing *technique* (which is a specific attempt to apply an interviewing *principle*) is defined as being a behaviorally defined set of words (often a single statement or a single question) that has been operationalized and tagged with a name. Every interviewing principle can be applied through the use of a single technique chosen from a "toolbox" of numerous interviewing techniques based on the principle in question, flexibly chosen to fit the unique needs of the patient and the clinical task at hand.

Thus, the above interviewing principle can be applied in the real world of a busy clinic via numerous interviewing techniques. With one such technique, called *normalization*, a clinician can sensitively raise the potentially embarrassing topic of missed doses in a way that increases the likelihood that the patient will feel comfortable sharing by saying, "***Some of my patients have told me***, Dave, that when they are taking several medications, especially if they are taking them twice a day like you are, that they find it is easy to miss some doses. Have you found yourself missing a few doses every now and then?" With normalization, the interviewer has metacommunicated that it is safe for the patient to talk about missing doses *because the clinician has heard many other patients describe doing so.* The potentially embarrassing admission has been normalized, hence the name of the technique.

With an alternative interviewing technique, called *shame attenuation*, one could ask, "Dave, with all these different medications on board, and because you have to take them at various times of the day, have you found yourself missing any doses by accident, perhaps because it's just so easy to forget them?" In contrast to normalization, shame attenuation never mentions someone other than the patient. Instead it metacommunicates to the patient that it is safe to share the information about missing doses ***because the interviewer "gets it" in the sense of understanding how easy it would be to do the problematic behavior in question*** (in this case missing a medication dosage). One can see that both *normalization* and *shame attenuation* employ the same principle of metacommunicating safety but they do so in subtly different fashions.

They are only slightly different in the same way that an 8-blade is only slightly different from a 9-blade to a surgeon. But that difference can count in the hands of a gifted surgeon depending on the challenge she meets in her patient's gut. Likewise, as we shall see nicely delineated in a later chapter, some patients may feel more apt to share that they have been missing their doses or are not taking their medications at all when asked with a normalization, whereas others may be more apt to share if the clinician inquires using a shame attenuation.

It is not necessary to understand, at this point, how and when to use these two tools. It is only necessary to notice that as subtle as the difference may be, they are different. That difference can be invaluable in helping a hesitant patient to openly share sensitive material or embarrassing information like missing doses or stopping a medication unilaterally between appointments.

Consequent to their behaviorally specific nature, interviewing *techniques* are less likely to be misunderstood by trainees than interviewing *principles*, are more easily learned, and are quite easy to be objectively tested for competence. If asked to do so, the trainee either does or does not correctly use the interviewing technique – such as normalization or shame attenuation – required by the instructor with a specified patient or a designated role-player or perhaps during an OSCE (Objective Structured Clinical Examination).

Moreover, two or more easily learned interviewing techniques can be sequenced together to form an interviewing strategy. Because interviewing strategies are composed of behaviorally well-defined interviewing techniques they are surprisingly easy to master. The MIM has several short interviewing strategies.

Throughout the remaining pages of this book, in order to provide a guiding framework for effectively talking with patients about their medications, we will explore a variety of interviewing principles, but these principles will always be delineated into specific interviewing techniques. These interviewing techniques will model the exact words that can be used with patients in the exam room immediately enhancing any clinician's ability to effectively implement the interviewing principles being described.

Inquiry Into Lost Dreams: A Prototypic MIM Interviewing Technique

As we wrap up our introduction to the MIM, I thought it would be useful to illustrate a specific interviewing technique from the model. Such an illustration will serve a variety of purposes. It will serve to consolidate our understanding of the difference between interviewing principles and interviewing techniques. It will also demonstrate the fashion in which many of the interviewing techniques of the MIM came into being from the input of frontline clinicians. To boot, it happens to be a technique that I have found to be quite valuable over the years. It is simply known as the "Inquiry into Lost Dreams."

As one would expect, one of the primary factors that motivates a patient toward the use of a medication is the belief that the medication may remove a disturbing symptom. The specific symptom or symptoms will naturally vary from disease to disease. On the simplest level, a patient with strep throat will seek relief from the distressing sore throat that is so common to strep. A patient with benign prostatic hypertrophy may want relief from urinary hesitancy or frequency. On more serious levels, a patient with CHF may seek relief from a disabling dyspnea on exertion or paroxysms of nocturnal coughing.

But some patients are motivated to use their medications effectively by factors that are unrelated to symptom relief directly. These personalized motivators are unique to the patient's worldview and interpersonal situation. They are sometimes surprisingly powerful, indeed sometimes more effective at enhancing adherence than symptom relief per se. Indeed, it has been a long-term tenet of motivational interviewing – and I believe a valid one – that motivators which are determined by the patient are often more powerful than motivators proffered by the clinician. The question becomes, "Are there interviewing techniques that can help patients find such situational motivators?" and "What exactly are the characteristics of such personalized motivators?" For me, these questions were answered through the wisdom of one of my workshop participants.

I was providing a workshop for a group of primary care clinicians from different disciplines. A pediatrician volunteered that he had stumbled on a powerful motivator for enhancing medication adherence in his own practice. He happened to specialize in treating childhood and adolescent asthma.

He went on to describe that many kids and adolescents with asthma resist taking their medications because they don't like the embarrassment of having to use inhalers in front of other kids in gym class or outside during recesses, nor do they like using the accompanying mouthwashes. As with their adult counterparts, kids and adolescents also appropriately complained about various side effects.

In the workshop, he commented that one of the most powerful motivators for some of his adolescent patients was the obvious one: They wanted relief from their acute asthmatic attacks. But he found this to be primarily true if the adolescent was experiencing severe and frightening asthmatic attacks which many of his patients were not. He discovered that with adolescents whose attacks were disruptive but not necessarily frightening in nature, there existed a more powerful motivator for using medications. Curiously, it was not directly related to relief from the asthmatic symptoms themselves. Moreover, it was a motivating factor that he found he could repeatedly tap whenever his adolescents were having tough side effects, even when those side effects were pushing the adolescent toward discontinuation.

What was the secret to generating such tenacious medication interest? What was the personalized motivator so common with kids suffering from asthma? He went on to describe that, more often than not, his patients were not seeking relief from something that the asthma had given them; they wanted back something the asthma had taken from them. They did not so much want relief from episodes of shortness of breath as much as they wanted a chance to play soccer again. They wanted to be normal. They wanted to be able to function again just like the other kids. They wanted to be free of the stigma of "being an asthmatic."

It is no different with our adult patients. In many instances, whether one is talking about diseases from rheumatoid arthritis to chronic obstructive pulmonary disease (COPD) and CHF patients want back their dreams, their livelihoods, their peace of mind, their self-esteem, and the confidence to pursue goals without becoming beset with self-doubts. The desire to recover these lost dreams can often provide powerful motivators that may help patients to tolerate surprisingly unpleasant side effects.

This pediatrician's clinical insight can be extrapolated from a specific disorder (asthma) into a more useful *interviewing principle* that can be applied broadly across many disease states: *The most powerful motivators patients may have for using a medication may be directly related to regaining a lost life activity as opposed to mere symptom relief.*

This process of translating an insight gained with a specific patient into a broader interviewing principle for use with many differing types of patients and disease states is the exact fashion in which the MIM developed. But as useful as this new interviewing principle might be in guiding the interviewer toward a successful hunt for the patient's personal motivator, it is limited by a simple fact. As a principle, it does not show us how to do so. And here is where interviewing techniques become immensely useful.

In this regard, our pediatrician had already developed a specific interviewing technique, which he had found to be useful with many patients over the years. Let us have him describe his technique in his own words as best I remember them from that workshop:

Interviewing Tip Prototype A: Inquiry into Lost Dreams

> I find it useful with my kids with asthma to ask them this question or a variation on it:
>
> "Is there anything that your asthma is keeping you from doing that you really wish you could do again?"
>
> What I find with this age group is that there is often a quick answer to this question, and the answer is often related to a sport – say football or soccer. Another useful thing about this question is that it opens the door for adolescents, who by definition are prone to form oppositional relationships with adults, to tell me what they want me to do for them. They are calling the shots, not me. The opposition seems to dissolve

away. Meanwhile, I gain a deeper insight into their motivation for seeking help from their asthma that goes beyond their desire for symptom relief. I might never have known this powerful motivator had I not asked. I can use this knowledge to enhance the adolescent patient's desire both to start a medication and to stay on it.

Although I never provide false hope, if I feel it is within reason I can use this newly uncovered information immediately to help shape a shared agenda with a comment like:

> "Now I can't promise this, but I have had some very good luck with helping other students, with asthma like yours, to get back into their sports. We have some great medications that can help with that goal. Once again, no promises, but I would like to work with you to see if we might be able to get you back out on that soccer field. How does that sound to you?"

Even the pediatrician's last phrase – "How does that sound to you?" – wisely transfers the power of the decision to even make a decision (to use a medication to get back onto the soccer field) to the adolescent. The Inquiry into Lost Dreams is a wonderful method of translating the principles of shared decision making into actual day-to-day clinical practice that can be easily taught/learned/tested. This pediatrician's simple, yet imminently practical, interviewing technique can be generalized for use across many disease states, "Is there anything your heart condition is stopping you from doing that you really wish you could do again?" or with a patient presenting with a depressive episode in a primary care clinic, "Is there anything that your depression is keeping you from doing that you really wish you could do again?" I think you will find the Inquiry into Lost Dreams to be useful across all age groups and for many diverse illnesses.

Concluding Reflections

We have spent considerable time discussing the Inquiry into Lost Dreams, because it represents a nice prototype for many of the interviewing techniques that will appear in the following pages. Hopefully, it also provides a convincing demonstration of the power of the MIM to generate not only interviewing principles but also specific, easily learned and applied interviewing techniques that may be of immediate use in our everyday practice.

In addition, these interviewing techniques and strategies can be "tagged" and operationally defined. The result is that techniques and strategies can be quantified and empirically studied. Future researchers can design studies in which they train specific cohorts of clinicians in sets of varying MIM interviewing techniques. The rate at which their patients take their medications before and after the training can then be compared as can the ultimate impact of specific MIM interviewing techniques on target goals such as lowered A1Cs, lipid values, and blood pressure readings.

In this fashion, future researchers may be able to demonstrate empirically that some interviewing techniques and strategies work more effectively than others. At that juncture, we will have taken a large step toward developing an evidence-based model on how to talk with patients in ways that are more likely to enhance medication adherence while improving clinical outcomes. (Please see Appendix C, where an article from *Professional Case Management* – describing the ways in which the MIM can generate research – has been replicated in its entirety for the interested reader.)

Having gained a sound understanding of the origins of the MIM, its nature, its distinctive qualities, and its potentialities for advancing our abilities to provide evidence-informed care, we are ready to step into its transformative world in more detail. Our first step is to better understand the nature of medication nonadherence. Why does it arise? How does it resolve?

REFERENCES

1. Shuman R. *The Psychology of Chronic Illness: The Healing Work of Patients, Therapists, and Families.* New York, NY: Basic Books; 1996.
2. Shea SC. *Improving Medication Adherence: How to Talk with Patients About Their Medications.* Philadelphia, PA: Lippincott Williams & Wilkins; 2006. Front-matter quotation from John Steiner.
3. Bardes CL. Defining "patient-centered medicine." *N Engl J Med* 2012;366(9):782–783.
4. Stewart M, Belle Brown J. *Patient-Centered Medicine: Transforming the Clinical Method.* 3rd ed. Boca Raton, Florida: CRC Press; 2013.
5. Fortin AH, Dwamena FC, Frankel RM, et al. *Smith's Patient Centered Interviewing: An Evidence-Based Method.* 3rd ed. New York, NY: McGraw-Hill Education/Medical; 2012.
6. Miles A, Mezzich J. The care of the patient and the soul of the clinic: person-centered medicine as an emergent model of modern practice. *Int J Pers Cent Med* 2011;1(2):207–222. doi:10.5750/ijpcm.v1i2.61.
7. Mezzich JE, Appleyard J, Botbol M, et al. Primary health care and person centered medicine. *Int J Pers Cent Med* 2015;5(2):45–50.
8. Mezzich J, Botbol M, Christodoulou GN, et al. *Person Centered Psychiatry.* New York, NY: Springer; 2017.

9. Elwyn G, Frosch D, Thomson R, et al. Shared decision making: a model for clinical practice. *J Gen Intern Med* 2012;27(10):1361–1367. doi:10.1007/s11606-012-2077-6.
10. Barry MJ, Edgman-Levitan S. Shared decision making – the pinnacle of patient-centered care. *N Engl J Med* 2012;366:780–781. doi:10.1056/NEJMp1109283.
11. Charles C, Gafni A, Whelan T. Shared decision-making in the medical encounter: what does it take? (or it takes at least two to tango). *Soc Sci Med* 1997;44(5):681–692.
12. *Dartmouth–Hitchcock Center for Shared Decision Making*. Available at http://med.dartmouth-hitchcock.org/csdm_toolkits.html. Accessed July 11, 2017.
13. Rosenthal TC. The medical home: growing evidence to support a new approach to primary care. *J Am Board Fam Med* 2008;21(5):427–440. doi:10.3122/jabfm.2008.05.070287.
14. Huang X, Rosenthal MB. Transforming specialty practice – patient-centered medical neighborhood. *N Engl J Med* 2014;370:1376–1379. doi:101056/NEJMp1315416.
15. National Committee for Quality Assurance. *Patient-Centered Medical Home (PCMH) Recognition*. Washington, DC: National Committee for Quality Assurance (NCQA). http://www.ncqa.org/programs/recognition/practices/patient-centered-medical-home-pcmh. Accessed July 11, 2017.
16. Jakovljevic M, Ostojic L. Person-centered medicine and good clinical practice: disease has to be cured, but the patient has to be healed [in Romanian]. *Medicina Academica Mostariensia* 2015;3(1–2):2–5.
17. Drake RE, McHugo GJ, Xie H. Ten-year recovery outcomes for clients with co-occurring schizophrenia and substance use disorders. *Schizophr Bull* 2006;32:464–473.
18. Cheng MKS. New approaches for creating the therapeutic alliance: solution-focused interviewing, motivational interviewing, and the medication interest model. *Psychiatr Clin North Am* 2007;30:157–166.
19. Shea SC. The "medication interest model": an integrative clinical interviewing approach for improving medication adherence – part 2 – implications for teaching and research. *Prof Case Manag* January/February 2009;14(1):6–15.

CHAPTER 3

The Crux of the Problem: The Nature of Medication Nonadherence

"The doctor-patient relationship can be restored. But it will take commitment by people on both sides of the stethoscope."[1]

C. Everett Koop, MD
FORMER U.S. SURGEON GENERAL

Types of Nonadherence: Conundrums Often Come in Twos

The question "Why do patients not take medications as prescribed?" is a query whose answer has many roots. The contributing factors have traditionally been clumped into two main camps: unintentional nonadherence and intentional nonadherence.[2–8]

With regard to the former camp, some patients who *want* to take their medications do not take them because of factors external to their choice. For instance, some patients miss medications because of specific cognitive problems. Such deficits can range from those of a severe nature – dementia – to the not so severe – everyday forgetfulness. Other patients inappropriately take medications because of confusion over the directions or intellectual limitations on their abilities to follow them, an ever-growing problem with the aging of our patient population as mentioned in Chapter 1. Still other patients stop medications because of external limitations – not enough money, no means of transportation to the pharmacy, inconvenient timing of the dosages, late arrival of the medications via mail or an inability to reach the prescriber for refills, etc. These types of interfering factors are often called unintentional nonadherence for obvious reasons. Such patients want to take their medications but factors unrelated to choice get in their way.

On the other hand, a fairly large percentage of patients do not take their medications because they do not want to take them. In short, these patients intentionally *choose* not to take the medications that we recommend, or, if they do take them, they choose to take them in a different fashion than we prescribe them. Of course, some patients may be driven by a combination of both nonintentional and intentional factors.

From an understanding of the two broad types of nonadherence, it only makes sense that two key operational components exist concerning the enhancement of medication adherence. First, the cornerstone of the process consists of collaboratively working with patients so that the individual's personal interest in choosing and staying on a medication is maximized. Once again, we see the overarching theme of patient choice. Second, efforts must be made by all parties involved – not only the patient but by the physicians, nurses, physician assistants, pharmacists, and other health care providers, as well as family members, community support programs, and insurance companies to reduce the numerous external obstacles that can prevent patients from being able to "follow-through" with their interest in taking their medications. We will refer to this second step as the process of "medication follow-through," a term coined by Kim Mueser.[9]

Although recognized in the Medication Interest Model (MIM) as a critical component for enhancing adherence, as well as a rich ground for effective intervention, the MIM does not focus on the process of improving medication follow-through. The reason for this narrowing of focus is simple. The vast bulk of research and intervention (even the very concept of case management itself) has been directed at improving medication adherence by improving medication follow-through. Thus, the reader is referred to the vast literature that has evolved around enhancing medication follow-through.

In this regard, in order to launch the interested reader on their way in this important exploration, you will find a concise introduction in Appendix B to some of the many approaches for improving medication follow-through that have been developed, ranging from improved types of pillboxes to more effective mechanisms for prompting patients to take their medications, to methods of improving patient self-management such as dosage simplification and social skills training. Excellent progress is being made in the arena of improved medication follow-through, and all providers should be aware of the advances available to their patients in this regard. In addition, I believe that we are on the cusp of some major advances in patient "prompting and awareness" as reflected by some of the exciting research being conducted with regard to texting, chat rooms, the use of apps, and other aspects afforded by the web and smart phones.[10–13]

In contrast, the research literature regarding methods for impacting on patient choice has been, in relative comparison, surprisingly small, spearheaded by approaches such as motivational interviewing and cognitive therapy. Consequently, in this book we will focus our attention on the interviewing principles and techniques that can enhance our patients' understanding, interest, and effective use of their medications. For no matter how marked our advances toward improving medication follow-through may become, they don't work if the patient does not want to take the medication in the first place. Period. The most important first step in the process is choice.

What Is Resistance? The Truth No One Told Us About in Medical and Nursing School

From our discussion of the spirit of the MIM in the last chapter, it is clear that the MIM is based on a collaborative model in which the process of decision making is truly a shared endeavor. It is also clear that the MIM represents a style of sensitive listening, collaborative treatment planning, and learning from the patient as opposed to lecturing to the patient. But it is important to understand the origins of these core principles in a more sophisticated manner for they are much more complex than meets the eye at first glance.

One can believe in the axioms just enumerated and one can be fully motivated to employ them, yet neither of these intentions guarantees success. Clinics and inpatient units are tough environments. They are hectic. They are filled with intense emotions, massive expectations, and daunting time limits. Listening carefully, learning from the patient, and shared decision making can often, unintentionally, fall by the wayside – rather rapidly, I might add – once a clinician is in the real world of clinical care.

Yet our evidence base is rock solid: Medication nonadherence is the number one cause of treatment failure. And all of the above processes (sensitive listening, learning from the patient, and shared decision making) appear to be vital components to the transformation of medication nonadherence.

To bring these skills to fruition, three things are needed: (1) An in-depth understanding – not only in the intellect but also in the gut – about why one is using these principles so that their use becomes a primary objective for the clinician despite the rigors and time constraints of clinical care, (2) the development of more *specific* practical principles that can be applied to *specific* patient interactions than the broad generalities of the above axioms, and (3) multiple, concrete interviewing techniques that can be quickly utilized (for time is of the essence in the real world of medicine and nursing) for transforming the complex patient interactions and difficulties that these specific principles were designed to spot and direct our actions.

Parts II and III of this book will provide us with the exact tools needed to accomplish the last two tasks listed above, to maximize our success at transforming medication nonadherence. Consequently, the majority of the pages of this book will be devoted to them. But this clinical practice will not come to fruition – the principles and interviewing techniques of Parts II and III will not be effectively employed – unless we first attend to task number one.

Before proceeding, we must deepen our understanding of what psychological and interpersonal processes lead patients and clinicians to develop seemingly entrenched positions regarding the use of specific medications and how do such positions resolve themselves. To do so, it is useful to develop a more sophisticated understanding of how humans resolve disagreements whether they develop in boardrooms, classrooms, or bedrooms. Without this type of understanding, well beyond "college-taught psychology," we will not be equipped as professionals to meet the needs of our patients and their families. First things first: "What is resistance?" "How is it transformed?"

To understand why our patients choose to not do what we ask – that is, take the medications that we think can help them – it may be useful to look at why any human being does not do what another human being asks. This question brings us face to face with the provocative topic of what is traditionally called "resistance" (a problematic term we will soon abandon), of which medication nonadherence is but one example in health care, for our patients may also be "resistant" to dieting, exercising, or stopping smoking. If we can understand how resistance begins, and, even more importantly, how resistance unfolds, intensifies, and sometimes resolves, we may uncover our first hints as to how to transform medication nonadherence and other such clinical gremlins.

A curious, but, ultimately, very useful place to begin our exploration is through a bit of imaginative play. Picture for a moment that we have hired a cultural anthropologist to help us study and define the nature of "medication noncompliance." Further imagine that we have plopped this anthropologist into one of our primary care or specialty care offices, on a typically hectic day, to watch us interact with those patients who are either refusing medications or not taking them as prescribed.

As clinicians, we know exactly how resistance feels, and if we are really honest with ourselves, most definitions of resistance come down to something rather simple: Resistance occurs when the patient does not do what I want. In some instances, the patient might not take the medications that I suggest. In other instances, he or she may not stop smoking as I suggest. But the bottom line is that the patient is not doing what I have recommended.

At such moments, it is easy for physicians and other providers to become appropriately frustrated because we genuinely care about our patients, and we genuinely feel that our medications can help them – sometimes even save their lives. The question now becomes, would our anthropologist agree with our definition from above of resistance, a definition we based on how it feels when we encounter it?

I believe that the answer is likely to be both "yes" and "no." "Yes," in the sense that the definition is correct as far as it goes, and "no," in the sense that it is does not go far enough. Let us return to our hypothetical anthropologist. We will tell our anthropologist almost nothing about the roles of the two people. We will merely state that in our culture, what is about to occur between the prescribing clinician and the patient is called "resistance," and that we would benefit from a scientific description of exactly what is occurring. We will also ask the anthropologist to watch many different clinician-patient examples of resistance, especially examples of medication nonadherence.

After observing hundreds of "resistant" patient interactions, I believe that our anthropologist would walk out and begin his or her definition of resistance with exactly the same words that we used: "Resistance occurs when the patient does not do what the clinician wants." But I believe that our anthropologist would add "and it occurs when the clinician does not do what the patient wants." This last caveat is not merely a semantic distinction. It is a profound fact of human nature.

It suggests that in many instances, but not all, when our anthropologist found a physician or nurse clinician growing frustrated with a "resistant" patient who did not "get it," there was an equally frustrated patient wondering, "Why doesn't Dr. Shea get it? I don't want to take this drug. It makes me feel bad, and I don't really like taking medications anyway."

From an anthropologic perspective, resistance, and more germane to our topic, medication nonadherence is often a two-way street. *Resistance is not so much a behavior that one person does, as it is an experience that two people share, with both parties experiencing an unpleasant sensation.* Indeed, some patients eventually decide not to come back to a "resistant" physician whom they perceive as always lecturing them to do something that they have no intention of doing, whether it be dieting, exercising, or taking a medication for hypertension that has some rather nasty adverse effects.

I believe that this distinction is the truth that the noted physician and humanitarian Paul Farmer, who also happens to be an anthropologist, meant in a *New Yorker* magazine interview when he provocatively quipped, "Patients are not noncompliant. Physicians are."[14] You see, that is exactly how patients often see the problem. They think we are the problem, and that we are noncompliant with their views. We think they are the problem, and that they are noncompliant with our views. The anthropologist thinks that we are both the problem; it is the anthropologist who may be closest to the truth.

Both Sides of the Stethoscope: Time to Drop the Term "Resistance"

Does this theoretical distinction made by our anthropologist have any real-world practicality for us? Does this distinction suggest any new ways for transforming the problem of medication nonadherence? I suggest that it does, for it suggests that solving the problem via the traditional concept of resistance may be, at best, unproductive, and, at worst, a certifiable red herring.

To understand the problems that arise when clinicians view patients as being resistant – when they are not using medications as prescribed – we must turn our attention to how we, as well as other humans, go about the challenging process of problem solving. Curiously, the words we choose with which to frame a problem often play a major role in whether a problem can ultimately be solved or not. Some words simply point us in the wrong direction. With regard to medication interest and use, the term "resistance," in my opinion, is such a damaging word.

Traditionally, in the fields of medicine and psychotherapy, when a patient disagreed with a clinician, indeed, the word "resistance" was often used to describe the situation. This word carried an implied message: that the patient was the problem. The oppositional roadblock was not viewed as we have just described it above as a conundrum that is experienced jointly by the patient and the clinician, but as a problem that the patient *has*. Consequently, the techniques for resolving resistance focused on how to change the patient's supposedly oppositional thoughts because if one could change the patient's oppositional thinking then that person might change how the patient behaves. The goal was to break through the patient's resistance and to make the noncompliant patient compliant.

Unfortunately, this traditional model is misleading because we have seen above that resistance is a clashing of two worldviews – not necessarily a problem with just one end of the stethoscope as C. Everett Koop so cogently began our chapter. Like the proverbial "one-hand clapping," one person resisting does not exist. Resistance is a dyadic process. Neither party is necessarily at fault. Yet both parties view the other party as being so. Noncompliance is an example of a disagreement. It is not an example of bad behavior.

This insight has immediate and practical ramifications. Indeed, in the fields of mental health, the term "resistance" has been, for the most part, dropped by a variety of schools of thought.[15–19] Patient-centered medicine/nursing have also moved in this direction.

Generally, in these psychotherapy schools of thought, disagreements between therapists and patients are not viewed as examples of "resistance" unless the patient is not doing what is requested because of *unconscious*, problematic defense mechanisms of which the patient literally has no awareness. Instead, therapists have come to realize that they and their patients may be simply having a reasonable disagreement about how to proceed therapeutically, not that the patient is refusing to change or too stupid to understand that change is needed. From this perspective, they may both be playing a role in the problem and, on a more promising note, they may both be able to play a role in its solution. Don't get me wrong, there are indeed some patients who are oppositional (purposely not doing what the therapist wants in order to upset the therapist as seen in some personality disorders) but this is the exception not the rule.

Thus, our first step in learning more effective ways for transforming medication nonadherence will be to drop the term "resistance" when talking about it, for the term propagates the falsehood that the patient is somehow usually to blame for the conundrum. From this point forward, we will simply replace the term "resistance" with the term "disagreement." Naturally disagreements can range from mild ones to strikingly unpleasant ones whether we are looking at a marital spat or a disagreement over medication use between a patient and a provider. In fact, regarding its severity, any disagreement over medication use can be placed on a continuum called the "Agreement Continuum."[20]

In any particular disagreement, from everyday arguments (marital spats, labor negotiations) to clinical differences in opinion (disagreements over the use of surgery, medication, or a naturopathic intervention) the disagreement can be conceptualized as sitting somewhere along this Agreement Continuum from mild (a difference of opinion) to intense (an argument) to really intense (a battle royale). And I should also note that clinical disagreements are not necessarily limited to the patient-clinician dyad. It can be great fun to watch a surgeon and an internist "discuss" the correct approach to back pain during morning rounds as any medical or nursing student can attest.

The Truth of the Matter: Jigsaw Puzzles and Paradoxes

Now that we understand that in the majority of cases of medication nonadherence, we are dealing with an example of a most common human phenomena – a simple disagreement – we can pull on our common-sense knowledge of how disagreements intensify and how they resolve. Our everyday wisdom, based on our years of navigating disagreements in our personal lives, may now provide us with some insights into resolving the one of interest to us in this book – medication nonadherence. Transforming the thorny problem of medication nonadherence is a bit like putting together a jigsaw puzzle. We must first uncover all the puzzle pieces and begin to arrange them by color, content, and form so that we can see how they connect.

The next puzzle piece concerns the question "How do disagreements tend to solidify into rigid stalemates?" How do they move from mere differences in opinion to oppositional walls that separate the patient both from the clinician and from the healing options offered by that very same clinician? Picture an argument you have experienced in your own life. How did it get so nasty? And how did it resolve itself (assuming it did, of course)?

Behavioral experts have come to realize (and I believe our own everyday experience will confirm their realization) that differences in opinion tend to escalate into arguments when *one* of the two participants increases the push on the other, especially when that push includes a personal attack on the other member as opposed to the other member's beliefs. Think politicians. Think Washington, D.C. It is one thing to say,

"I strongly disagree with you." It is an entirely different thing to say, "I strongly disagree with you, but that doesn't surprise me because I've known for a long time that you and every other person in your party is an idiot." Hmmm, this latter approach may not tend to change the other fellow's opinion, methinks. The fight is on. You can bet the attacked member of the dyad is about to unload their own delightfully wicked cannon shot. Note that, generally, not always, *it only takes one of the two people to trigger the oppositional war*.

Curiously, it is the same process at work when oppositional dyads settle themselves. It does not necessarily take two to tango. Anyone who has done marital therapy knows that two people screaming at each other do not spontaneously, at an identical moment, pull back saying, "You know we just need to respect each other's views, for we are both good people." I don't think so.

Oppositional dyads tend to de-escalate when one of the two people pulls back a little. When one of the people decreases the intensity of the attack, when one of the pair softens his or her words, sometimes just a bit, the stalemate often begins to crumble. If one of the people in the couple says with a gentler tone, "You know I still disagree very strongly, but I at least see where you're coming from." Many times, not always, the other member will reciprocate the softening with, "Well, I still feel I'm right, but I get where you are coming from a little better too." At such a moment, frequently the originator of the softening, will soften even more in their next comment, and it too will be reciprocated by the partner with a further softening in his or her tone. In short, angry dyads often de-escalate in a see-sawing fashion. One person softens the attack, the other reciprocates. The first to soften then softens even more, and the partner once again reciprocates until the argument has cooled.

Of most importance to us is the fact that *the de-escalation often is initiated solely by one person backing off*.

Let us now return to the focus of our chapter, transforming medication nonadherence, for it too is a dyadic process. It too is a disagreement. Nonadherence is a roadblock shared by both people, indeed, often partially co-created. It seldom reaches the angry arguments we see from politicians, but it raises its head in much subtler, yet equally damaging ways. Patients often simply don't take their medications or change how they are taking them without telling the clinician. There is no argument, but there is disagreement. And the action taken on that disagreement – the patient discontinues the medication – can have dire, indeed, life-threatening consequences.

We now come to a question whose answer is obvious yet is often overlooked when discussing the transformation of medication nonadherence. As clinicians, whose views do we have the most control over, the patient's or our own? Truth be told we have no ability to force a patient to change his or her personal beliefs about a medication, but we have complete control over our own beliefs and can change them at will. Thus, put bluntly, whose views are we most likely to change quickly and easily regarding a disagreement over medication use (keeping in mind that our model suggests that often times, oppositional dyads resolve after only one party in the dyad begins to "tone it down")? The answer, of course, is our own. Perhaps the best way to motivate patients to take medications lies less on focusing on how to change the patient's beliefs and more on focusing on how to change the clinician's beliefs or *the pressure with which these beliefs are being communicated.*

I should note that in actuality – for instance, with the seriously ill dually diagnosed patients on our outreach treatment team described in Chapter 2 – in many instances we did not change our beliefs. I still felt that a given patient needed a mood stabilizer, an antipsychotic, or an antidepressant. But what I could always change was how I communicated my beliefs. Equally important, *I could always change how I asked my patients about their beliefs.* As the research demonstrated, the results can be impressive.

As clinicians, we have direct control over both our beliefs and how we express them. How we phrase our questions and how we frame our suggestions often result in a complementary change in how patients view our questions and follow our recommendations. Depending upon the words that we use, patients are more or less likely to move from lack of interest to interest, from nonadherence to adherence. What is this change in clinician language? Is it teachable? Is it a skill set like a surgeon has a skill set? Absolutely.

In a clarifying sense, it all comes down to the following interviewing principle. It is a principle that reflects the process – collaborative exploration – that we previously mentioned rests at the very center of the MIM's spirit: *Rather than creating the sensation that we are moving "against them," we want our patients to feel that we are moving "with them" – that we are a team, not opposing armies.*

Moreover, what ultimately determines the intensity of our patients' concerns is not so much that we are, indeed, truly pressuring them, but that their perception is that we are. It is our patient's perceptions of our attitudes that determine whether they feel comfortable with what we are recommending. And it is the words that we choose, and the fashion in which we say them, that determines these perceptions.

The more a patient perceives that we are listening to their concerns about a medication, and moving as much with them as is possible on the Agreement Continuum, the more likely the patient will be to listen to our advice. We can hold opposing views with our patients without being an opponent, depending on the words with which we choose to ask our questions and with which we share our beliefs. Our words, and the tone with which we express them, convey not only meaning. They convey relationship.

In this light, there is one piece missing if we are to complete our jigsaw puzzle: We need a word to talk about patient "nonadherence" that follows our principles and does not set up, by its very connotation, an oppositional feeling toward the patient, an oppositional feeling that the word "nonadherence" and, to an even greater degree, "noncompliance" seem to generate. We have already abandoned the word "resistance." We now need to replace the word "nonadherence" and its kin.

REFERENCES

1. Gordon T, Edwards WS. *Making the Patient Your Partner: Communication Skills for Doctors and Other Caregivers.* Westport, CT: Auburn House; 1997:1.
2. Morisky DE, Green LW, Levine DM. Concurrent and predictive validity of self-reported measure of medication adherence. *Med Care* 1986;24(1):67–74.
3. Horne R, Weinman J. Predicting treatment adherence: an overview of theoretical models. In: Myers LB, Midence K, eds. *Adherence to Treatment in Medical Conditions.* London, UK: Harwood Academic; 1998.
4. Wroe AL. Intentional and unintentional nonadherence: a study of decision making. *J Behav Med* 2002;25:355–372.
5. Lowry KP, Dudley TK, Oddone EZ, et al. Intentional and unintentional nonadherence to antihypertensive medication. *Ann Pharmacother* 2005;39(7–8):1198–1203.
6. Atkins L, Fallowfield L. Intentional and non-intentional non-adherence to medication amongst breast cancer patients. *Eur J Cancer* 2006;42(14):2271–2276.
7. Lehane E, McCarthy G. Intentional and unintentional medication nonadherence: comprehensive framework for clinical research and practice? A discussion paper. *Int J Nurs Stud* 2007;44(8):1468–1477. doi:10.1016/j.ijnurstu.2006.07.010.
8. Weiden PJ. The adherence interview: better information, better alliance. *Psychiatr Ann* 2011;41(5):279–285.
9. Mueser K, Kane J, Shea SC. Improving medication adherence in schizophrenia through innovations in medication follow-through and antipsychotic design. The third installment of a 3-part series entitled "Enhancing medication interest and medication follow-through in the treatment of schizophrenia." *Counseling Points.* Vol. 1(3). Ridgewood, NJ: Delaware Media Group Custom Publishing & Communications, supported by an educational grant from Janssen, L.P; 2008:1–19.
10. Hayakawa M, Uchimura Y, Omae K, et al. A smartphone-based medication self-management system with real-time medication monitoring. *Appl Clin Inform* 2013;4:37–52. doi:10.4338/ACI-2012-10-RA-0045.

11. Patel S, Jacobus-Kantor L, Marshall L, et al. Mobilizing your medications: an automated medication reminder application for mobile phones and hypertension medication adherence in a high-risk urban population. *J Diabetes Sci Technol* 2013;7(3):630–639.
12. Mistry N, Keepanasseril A, Wilczynski NL, et al. Technology-mediated interventions for enhancing medication adherence [review]. *J Am Med Inform Assoc* 2015;22:e177–e193. doi:10.1093/jamia/ocu047.
13. Wald DS, Bestwick JP, Raiman L, et al. Randomized trial of text messaging on adherence to cardiovascular preventive treatment (INTERACT Trial). *PLoS One* 2014;9(12):e114268. doi:10.1371/journal.pone.0114268.
14. Kidder T. The good doctor. *The New Yorker* July 10, 2000:40–57.
15. de Shazer S. *Clues: Investigating Solutions in Brief Therapy*. New York, NY: W.W. Norton Company; 1988.
16. Miller S, Hubble M, Duncan B. *Handbook of Solution-Focused Brief Therapy*. San Francisco, CA: Jossey-Bass; 1996.
17. de Jong P, Berg I. *Interviewing for Solutions*. New York, NY: Brooke and Cole Publishers; 1998.
18. Miller W, Rollnick S. *Motivational Interviewing: Helping People Change*. 3rd ed. New York, NY: Guilford Press; 2013.
19. Cheng MKS. New approaches for creating the therapeutic alliance: solution-focused interviewing, motivational interviewing, and the medication interest model. *Psychiatr Clin North Am* 2007;30:157–166.
20. Shea SC. Transforming anger, confrontation, and other points of disengagement. *Psychiatric Interviewing: The Art of Understanding*. 3rd ed. London, UK: Elsevier; 2016.

CHAPTER 4

Is It Really "Noncompliance"?

"Words make a difference. The terms compliance and adherence should be abandoned because they subtly exaggerate the importance of the clinician, describe behavior inaccurately, and shed little light on motivations."[1]

John Steiner, MD, MPH
Mark Earnest, MD
ANNALS OF INTERNAL MEDICINE, JUNE 2000

The Trouble With the Words "Compliance" and "Adherence"

To solve the puzzle of medication nonadherence, we need a word that will allow clinicians and other caregivers, such as case managers, to acknowledge in a nonpejorative way that the number one cause of treatment failure is that many patients don't take their medications as prescribed. In addition, when they don't, they get sick. From the beginning of our book, we have been emphasizing that one of the critical first steps in increasing medication use is the need to build a collaborative medication alliance with our patients on the "agreement continuum," to create an atmosphere of going with them as allies against their diseases, as opposed to going against them as antagonists to their beliefs. This nonoppositional stance, that resonates so nicely with shared decision making, has been at the very center of the approach described thus far. It is why we eliminated the term "resistance" in the last chapter.

In addition, it would be useful to find a "positive" term for replacing the terms "adherence" and "compliance" (and their corollaries "nonadherence" and "noncompliance") that emphasizes the collaborative spirit of the alliance, not just between the patient and the prescriber but also among all the parties involved in the battle against the patient's disease. Today, this treatment alliance may include a surprising number of diverse members including the patient, his or her family members, and the prescribing clinician (whether this be a physician, advanced practice nurse such as a nurse practitioner or a clinical nurse specialist, physician assistant, or clinical pharmacist). It will also include other health care professionals such as registered and licensed practical nurses, medical social workers, and retail pharmacists who may interface with the patient during ongoing care. Last, but certainly not least, it will also include the outpatient case managers directly assigned to the patient's wrap-around care (who may be nurses, social workers, or nondegreed health care providers).

I believe that this last group – case managers (some providers prefer the term "care mangers") – are pivotal members of the treatment team for enhancing ongoing medication use in patients with diseases as diverse as AIDS, CHF, asthma, diabetes, cancer, and schizophrenia. Not infrequently, case managers can meet with their patients considerably more often than prescribers and, consequently, may have an equal, if not more powerful impact on the potential *interest* of their patients in taking a medication than prescribing clinicians can muster.

As illustrated by the preceding sentence, the word that was ultimately chosen to replace terms such as "adherence" and "compliance" sits at the very center of the name of the Medication *Interest* Model (MIM). The concept of "medication interest" is not merely a politically correct coinage. It represents a genuine change in conceptualizing why patients don't take medications and how prescribers, as well as those allied health professionals who monitor ongoing medication use, go about the business of increasing the effective use of medications. Consequently, to better understand how to utilize the interviewing strategies and techniques of the MIM, it is well worth our while to examine historically how the concept of "medication interest" evolved.

As John Steiner and Mark Earnest note in our opening epigram, the most commonly used terms "compliance"/"noncompliance" and "adherence"/"nonadherence" don't seem to fit the criteria we have listed in the first two paragraphs of this chapter. Not only do these terms tend to set the stage for an oppositional field of communication, but they also have other inherent problems, as Steiner and Earnest succinctly state.

There appears to be a long tradition of labeling patients, as opposed to their behaviors, as problematic. As Steiner and Earnest pointed out in their provocative article, "The Language of Medication Taking,"[2] in pre-1960 research studies that focused on patients, who were not taking their medications as prescribed, such patients were described as "faithless"[3] to the treatment programs or as "untrustworthy" and "unreliable."[4] Near this time frame, the term "compliance" and its corollary "noncompliance" came into vogue, and they have set an oppositional tone ever since. Although a good deal less castigating than *faithless,* these terms are hardly value-free.

One of the major problems with the term "compliance" is that it seems to imply that physicians and nurses are the ones who make decisions on treatment. Patients are merely supposed to *comply* with these recommendations. Once again, we can see the power of language to set up, insidiously, the feeling of going against as opposed to going with our patients. But there is more to the problem because these words also suggest that physicians and other prescribers and case managers have more control over medication use than they really do in actual clinical practice.

For example, the term "compliance" seems to suggest that prescribers choose the medication. But, as we saw in Chapters 2 and 3, although prescribers may limit the field of medications available to a patient, prescribers do not choose medications; patients do. They are the ultimate deciders as to whether they want to try a medication or they don't. Also, as the sociologist Peter Conrad[5] pointed out, not only do patients choose which medications they want to take, they also decide exactly how they are going to take them, a process Conrad aptly calls the patient's "medication practice." In the end, he points out that the only medication practices that count are those practices that patients choose to do, not the medication practices that prescribers tell them to do.

The only time that a clinician indirectly controls medication practice is if the clinician literally hands the medication to the patient and watches the patient swallow it, as might occur on an inpatient unit. The only time the clinician directly controls both medication choice and practice is through the forced administration of medications via an involuntary commitment. Otherwise – concerning medication choice and dosing – the patient holds the cards. Before the patient walks out of our offices, it is to our advantage to see how he or she intends to play them. The term "compliance," with its misleading suggestion of clinician power, makes this simple truth too easily forgotten.

Another problem with the term "noncompliance" is that it is too generic, often yielding an inaccurate picture as to why the patient is not taking a medication. As we have seen, *noncompliance* has a not-so-subtle pejorative tone, yet it is often casually applied, not only to that small percentage of patients who may be purposefully oppositional – perhaps as the result of a personality disorder – but also to patients who forget easily, do not have enough money for the medication, are genuinely afraid of the medication, or simply do not think that there is anything seriously wrong with them or, if they do, do not feel that the pros of taking the medication outweigh the cons. Similarly, patients who miss a dose twice a week are often grouped together as being "noncompliant" with patients who almost never take their medication.

According to sociologist James Trostle,[6] in his pioneering article, "Medical Compliance as an Ideology," various alternative terms have been suggested to replace *noncompliance,* such as *nonadherence, defaulting, self-regulation,* and *self-management.* Others have suggested distinguishing those situations in which the patient has decided against medications because of genuine personal beliefs against the use of a medication (*intelligent noncompliance*) versus those patients who refuse medications solely for oppositional reasons (*capricious noncompliance*).

More recently, researchers have tried to more cleanly define terms such as "compliance," "adherence," "concordance," and relative newcomers such as "persistence" and "reconciliation," striving to arrive at uniform definitions across fields. Despite these efforts, some disagreement and variations in the use of these terms still exists.[7–9]

As an example of a more recent classification system, in trying to standardize terminology for use in research that employs electronic medical records, Marsha Raebel and her colleagues adopted the following definitions from their literature review: "Adherence connotes the degree or extent to which the patient conforms to the medication use recommendations specified by the prescriber (e.g., frequency/interval of administration, time of day ingested, strength of dosage). In contrast, persistence encompasses the time over which a patient continues treatment or continues to refill the prescription, from starting to stopping therapy."[10] Generally speaking, the terms "compliance" and "adherence" are used interchangeably as synonyms. Other writers feel that the term "compliance" indicates a more passive following of the prescriber's orders by the patient.

In my opinion, although of promising use in research settings, none of these terms seems to have caught on with busy frontline clinicians, whether in primary care or specialist settings. Even more recent terms, such as "reconciliation," seem to metacommunicate that the patient and the clinician began at opposite ends of the agreement continuum but have managed to somehow reconcile their differences.

Perhaps the best of the lot, *adherence* is generally the most commonly used in the parlance of today. At one level, *adherence* (whether it is the best of the lot or not) is certainly less oppositional sounding than *compliance*. But it still seems to lack appeal to many clinicians perhaps because it sounds more like we are discussing the qualities of a roll of scotch tape than the intricacies of a therapeutic alliance. For many clinicians, *adherence* simply sounds sterile, cold, and uninviting.

Ideally, I think the goal is to find a term that frontline clinicians in fields such as medicine and nursing find highlights not the oppositional beliefs that can arise between health care providers and the patient, but the shared goals that they both embrace – finding symptom relief and, if possible, a cure for the disease. It should be a term that emphasizes that the goal of the provider is not to choose the medication for the patient but to help the patient to make a wise choice, which, as we discussed earlier, might even include the choice to not take the medication in the first place. Otherwise, we risk making our patients feel that they are being pressured to take *our* medications, not guided to choose *their* medications.

As one can imagine, in the years preceding the first edition of this book in 2006, I spent more than a little time trying to find a word that effectively captured the above principles. I should admit up front that I was not originally successful in this quest. For instance, years ago, I had the brilliant idea to capture the model not with a single word but with a more comprehensive catchphrase because there seemed to be so many important facets to the approach. The result read like this: *Non-Oppositional Nonadherence Strategies: Empathy, Nonjudgment, Sensitivity, and Engagement*.

At first glance, I was rather pleased with this catchphrase because it seemed to summarize my key points while satisfying my more-than-ample obsessive psychological needs. However, when I shared it with my wife, who astutely edits my work, I could tell by her frown that she was not overly impressed. She commented, "I don't like it for three reasons: (1) It's too wordy, (2) It doesn't exactly roll off the tip of the tongue, and (3) Its acronym is the word NONSENSE."

Hmm. Good points.

Fortunately, a better term can be used to address the traditional problems housed under the labels of *compliance* and *adherence*. To find it, we simply must return to the bottom line. Either a patient is interested or not interested in taking a medication.

The Missing Piece of the Puzzle Found

The terms "medication adherence" and "medication compliance" can easily be replaced with the term "medication interest." In this light, the principles that we have been describing in this book have come to be known simply as the *medication interest* philosophy, and their clinical application appears in the clinical literature as the Medication Interest Model (MIM) as reflected in the title of our book.

In my workshops provided over the past 18 years, for audiences composed of experienced physicians, nurses, and other health care professionals, the participants have given a warm reception to the term "medication interest." Perhaps the positive nature of its reception results from its name metacommunicating a point – well acknowledged by veteran clinicians – that one of the main skills of a successful clinician is the ability to teach. Teaching is ultimately about generating interest whether in a pupil or a patient. Bottom line, we clinicians are all teachers; we are motivators. Our successes depend directly on our ability to find an effective medication (or an effective nonpharmacologic treatment) and then to motivate the patient to try it. Our treatment failures arise from our failure to do so.

With a sense of shared exploration and decision making, we help our patients achieve an understanding that there is something wrong and identify what it is, motivate them to try a medication to help relieve what is wrong, and help them to weigh the complex pros and cons of the specific medication in question. After they have carefully weighed the pros and cons, the MIM views patients as capable partners, who, if their interest becomes high enough, will, ultimately, cross a threshold of interest that leads them to try the medication that we are suggesting, not because we tell them to, but because they believe in it – and in us. The term "medication interest" emphasizes that the real goal of prescribing clinicians, no matter what their discipline, is to increase understanding and motivation.

On the original case management team in the study from which the MIM evolved, that was described in Chapter 2 (you will recall we were working with patients with severe schizophrenia or bipolar disorder and concurrent alcohol/substance abuse), we found that we could completely eliminate the use of the terms "compliance"/"noncompliance" and "adherence"/"nonadherence" as well as the term "resistance," exactly as Steiner and Earnest suggested in our opening quotation, by simply referring to the patient's level of medication interest.

Instead of using oppositional terms, such as "compliance" and "adherence" (as in the question, "Is Jim complying with his meds?"), we would ask each other questions such as the following:

1. How interested is Jim in taking his medication (followed up with a question that provides a more concrete idea of the level of interest, such as, "What percentage of the doses do you think he is actually taking?")?
2. If he were here, how would he list the pros and cons that have led to his low interest?
3. Does anybody have any ideas how we could increase his interest?
4. How interested is his family in his taking the med?

In addition to asking questions, we also found that during our treatment team meetings, the word "interest" was effective in helping us phrase our answers to those questions in a nonjudgmental fashion with statements such as, "I think he is reasonably interested, but he is genuinely having trouble remembering the nighttime dose," "At one level he is clearly interested, but the bottom line is that he is simply frightened of the orthostatic dizziness. He is really worried that he'll fall and break his hip, which, at one level, is a reasonable worry," and "I think the problem with the interest here is a lack of money, and it's a genuine problem."

Moreover, in sharp contrast to my first shot at a catchphrase for our model (Non-Oppositional Nonadherence Strategies: Empathy, Nonjudgment, Sensitivity, and Engagement), *medication interest* seems to roll off the tongue rather nicely. It also allows us to discuss openly and frankly the main roadblock (i.e., not taking medications) to our patients' healing in a fashion that has no pejorative quality or oppositional bias to it.

From this point forward, we will no longer use the terms "resistance," "adherence"/"nonadherence," or "compliance"/"noncompliance." Instead, we will always talk about our patient's level of interest in taking or not taking a medication. The only exception will be in emphasizing the outmoded nature of the above terms in which case they will always appear between quotation marks, as with "compliance" or "adherence." (As mentioned in Chapter 3, the phrase "medication follow-through" replaces these terms when we are addressing the patient's success in overcoming external obstacles to effective use.)

It appears that we have found our final piece to the puzzle – a reasonable replacement for the words "adherence" and "compliance" when describing the first stage of effective medication use (patient choice). In the process, we have discovered the origin of the title for our model. We are now ready to put this model to the acid test, but before we can do so, we have one last process to examine. It is a process that is complex, sometimes puzzling, and always pivotal in determining the success of our treatments. We need an answer to the question: "How do patients choose to take a medication?"

REFERENCES

1. Steiner JF, Earnest MA. Lingua medica: the language of medication-taking. *Ann Intern Med* 2000;132(11):928.
2. Steiner JF, Earnest MA. Lingua medica: the language of medication-taking. *Ann Intern Med* 2000;132(11):926–930.
3. Jenkins BW. Are patients true to t.i.d. and q.i.d. doses? *Gen Pract* 1954;9:66–69.
4. Dixon WM, Stradling P, Wootton ID. Outpatient P.A.S. therapy. *Lancet* 1957;2:871–872.
5. Conrad P. The meaning of medications: another look at compliance. *Soc Sci Med* 1985;20(1):29–37.
6. Trostle J. Medical compliance as an ideology. *Soc Sci Med* 1988;27(12):1299–1308.
7. Cramer JA, Roy AR, Burell A, et al. Medication compliance and persistence: terminology and definitions. *Value Health* 2008;11(1):44–47. doi:10.1111/vhe.2008.11.issue-1/issuetoc.
8. Horne R, Weinman J, Barber N, et al. Concordance, adherence and compliance in medicine taking. Report compiled by the *National Co-ordinating Centre for NHS Service Delivery and Organization R & D*. London: NCCSDO; 2005:12.
9. Agency for Healthcare Research and Quality. *"What is Medication Adherence?"* Rockville, MD. http://www.effectivehealthcare.ahrq.gov/ehc/products/296/1248/EvidenceReport208_CQGMedAdherence_FinalReport_20120905.pdf.
10. Raebel MA, Schmittdiel J, Karter A, et al. Standardizing terminology and definitions of medication adherence and persistence in research employing electronic databases. *Med Care* 2013;51:S11–S12. doi:10.1097/MLR.0b013e31829b1d2a.

CHAPTER 5

The Choice Triad: How Do Patients Choose to Take a Medication?

"To desire to take medicine is perhaps the greatest feature which distinguishes man from animals."[1]

Sir William Osler, MD
RENOWNED PHYSICIAN (1849–1919)

I firmly believe that if the whole materia medica as now used could be sunk to the bottom of the sea, it would be all the better for mankind – and all the worse for the fishes.[2]

Oliver Wendell Holmes, Sr.
RENOWNED PHYSICIAN (1809–1894)

THE "GREAT DEBATE" IN THEORY

Inside each patient contemplating taking a medication or deciding to stay on it, a debate is waged. For patients who feel most comfortable passively accepting the recommendations of their physician, advanced practice nurse, physician assistant, or clinical pharmacist, it is a relatively quiet matter, without much ado. For patients who feel more comfortable aggressively evaluating their prescriber's recommendations, it can be a rather raucous affair, sometimes with much ado about everything. Most patients have a healthy admixture of both perspectives, which enhances their likelihood of being well-informed consumers. But the process of choosing to put a foreign substance into one's body is always a complex one.

The process is as if there were dueling lawyers inside the courtroom of each patient's mind. One lawyer sees only the very real benefits of medications and taps into the deep leanings of the human spirit for almost magical relief as Sir William Osler describes in the opening epigram of the chapter. The other sees only the very real dangers of medications and taps into the equally deep doubts of the human psyche, as Oliver Wendell Holmes, Sr., so acerbically attests. Across this wide spectrum, the bottom line remains the same for all patients, that is, ultimately, they have to make a choice.

It is not an easy choice. The datum is sometimes conflicting. Weighing the potential impact of side effects and serious adverse reactions versus the benefits of a medication (risk/benefit analysis) is not as cut-and-dry a question as it may first appear. Determining whether the advice of the prescriber is biased or unbiased can also pose a problem for the patient especially when meeting the prescriber for the first time. To return to our courtroom analogy, is this expert witness a "hired gun" or a "stalwart advocate" for truth? How is a patient to know for sure?

Moreover, it is not so much that physicians, advanced practice nurses, and other prescribers are hired guns than I think it is the fact that in a busy clinic or hospital atmosphere, it can be surprisingly easy to underestimate the severity of the impact of a side effect from the patient's perspective. I certainly have misjudged this severity on numerous occasions over the years. Each patient is different. Each patient will have differing opinions on how tolerable or intolerable a given side effect is perceived.

The variable quality of interpretation given to side effects by patients, in some respects, is mirrored by the vagaries of how clinicians and researchers define the phenomena, specifically how the terms "side effect" and "adverse reaction" are used in the literature and on clinical rounds. Technically, these terms vary, although they are often used interchangeably. Consequently, I should clarify their use in this book (no claim is made that this use is the correct format, but it is merely presented to avoid confusion for the reader). The World Health Organization (WHO) makes the following distinctions: (1) adverse drug reaction – a response to a medicine that is noxious and unintended, and that occurs at doses normally used in a patient, and (2) side effect – any unintended effect of a pharmaceutical product occurring at doses normally used by a patient, which is related to the pharmacologic properties of the drug.[3]

Note that in the WHO definition, a side effect can be either noxious or not. Also, note that a side effect is caused directly by the pharmacologic properties of the drug *not* by the patient's unique or allergic response to the drug. By way of example, the sleepiness induced by an antihistamine is a classic side effect. For some people, it is unwanted (daytime drowsiness at work) and for others, it may be wanted – or even prescribed – for its side effect (helping to induce sleep for a person with insomnia). In either instance, the sleepiness is a direct result of the antihistamine's normal pharmacologic actions. Side effects are often common, transient, and can be mild to severe in nature.

By contrast, an adverse reaction is always unwanted and noxious. It is not necessarily related to the pharmacologic properties of the drug. Adverse reactions can also range from mild to severe, but the term (depending on who is using it) is sometimes limited to serious complications (such as life-threatening/fatal, permanent/significantly disabling, requiring prolonged hospitalization, or a causing congenital anomaly). Such serious adverse reactions require interventions such as decreasing dosage or discontinuation of the drug or permanent damage may ensue.

As I said, some book authors, clinicians, researchers, and grant providers use the terms interchangeably or generally note a distinction between serious adverse reactions, as delineated above, and the category of "other adverse reactions" that are not serious in nature. In this book, you will see me using the terms essentially as described by the WHO definition with the following caveat. Although, occasionally, side effects can be quite serious in nature, I will generally use the term "side effects" when discussing the more mundane, common, and often transient effects of a drug caused by its natural pharmacologic actions (keeping in mind that these can be very disturbing to patients and appropriately warrant trying a different medication). Although the term "adverse reaction" can be legitimately used for *mild* and *moderate* noxious effects, to avoid confusion, I will limit my use of the term for those unwanted and unintended responses to the drug (not caused directly by the intended pharmacologic actions of the drug) that are more serious in nature, using the term "serious adverse reaction."

I personally find it useful to remind myself of something that is probably not discussed enough during the training of medical, nursing, physician assistant, and clinical pharmacy students: side effects and adverse reactions are diseases, mild in the former, more severe in the latter. To affirm my point, according to *Merriam-Webster's Dictionary*, a disease is a condition of a living organism in which there is impairment of "normal functioning and is typically manifested by distinguishing signs and symptoms."[4] Even common side effects such as nausea, diarrhea, orthostatic hypotension, and sleep disruption certainly are examples of abnormal functioning, caused by pathophysiology, thus satisfying *Webster's* definition of a disease. Although there is a large list of possible etiologic agents triggering diseases, a goodly number are caused by environmental toxins. It does not matter if the toxin is a naturally occurring one (lung cancer from carcinogens in tobacco) or one concocted by science (a medication-induced side effect or adverse reaction).

When we prescribe a medication that causes a side effect or serious adverse reaction, in essence, we are asking a patient to swap diseases. *I don't use such phrasing with a patient, for I feel it can be easily misunderstood and overly frightening when taken out of context.* But I do use it with myself and with my trainees. It is easy to recognize an adverse reaction such as Stevens-Johnson as a disease, but one might need to remind oneself that a side effect like dry mouth or sexual dysfunction is a disease, albeit a reversible one. Side effects may not be life threatening as one might see with an adverse reaction, but they can be, nevertheless, quite disturbing to a patient. No one likes to be given a new disease even if it is merely an annoying one or transient in nature.

As we shall see in our later chapters, it is also important to keep in mind that side effects and adverse reactions are only one of the many factors (ranging from the cost of the medication to the convenience of their use to the opinions of family and friends as to the advisability of their ingestion) that will influence whether a patient will choose to start and/or continue with a specific medication. Obviously, it is to our benefit to spend considerable time addressing the question that lies at the very center of the patient's internal courtroom: "How do patients choose to take a medication?"

Curiously, one of the very best ways to most directly answer this question is to ask the question of the patients whom we, as health care professionals, know best – ourselves. Each of us has been a patient who, at one time or another, has had to decide whether to start a medication. We may be professional providers, but all of us have been on the other side of Koop's stethoscope as well. All of us have taken medications at some time from antibiotics and cold capsules to antidepressants, antihypertensives, and oral hypoglycemic agents.

In addition, most of us have been asked by friends or relatives what we think of certain medications, and many of us have had to decide whether one of our children should take a medication. Thus, we have a vast reservoir of direct personal knowledge about how humans, of sound mind and reasonable intellect, choose whether to take any given medication. Our question is thus perhaps best reworded as, "How do we, personally, decide to take a medication?"

THE "CHOICE TRIAD"

In my workshops for primary care physicians, specialists, and mental health professionals, I have had the rare opportunity to ask the members of my audience this exact question. When doing so, I always remind my audience, "As you answer this question, forget about your own patients. I want to know how you personally decide to take a medication. Please start your answers with the first-person word 'I' as in 'I take a medication because . . .'" The results have been remarkably similar. Physicians, nurses, and providers of all disciplines, both nationally and internationally, tell me that they take medications for themselves if the following three criteria are met:

1. They feel that there is something wrong with them from which they personally want relief.
2. They feel motivated to try a medication because they believe it has the potential to bring them relief from their perceived problem (or perhaps prevent a serious future problem as with a vaccine).
3. They believe that the pros of taking the medication outweigh the cons.

Nothing startling here. In all of the workshops I've given, I have never met a physician, nurse, physician assistant, clinical pharmacist, or case manager who would ever take a medication (outside of "meds" such as vitamins or vaccines), unless they thought that there was something wrong, and they felt motivated to get help with the problem via the use of a medication. I have also never met a clinician from one of my workshops who would ever take a medication in which he or she thought the cons outweighed the pros. Why would any intelligent person do so? And so it is with our patients. I am reminded of a wise insight by the researcher Colleen McHorney, "Non-adherence is rational behavior – it is driven by patient beliefs about their treatment, disease, and prognosis as well as their objective experience with their treatment and disease."[5]

For ease of discussion, we will refer to the three steps that a patient must navigate before trying a new medication (as well as staying on an old one) as the "Choice Triad." We will find ourselves repeatedly returning to this Choice Triad as a theory of motivation because an understanding of its nuances will provide a rich soil from which to transform our patients' hesitancies and fears about medications. Although not its original purpose, I think you will also find that the Choice Triad can be effectively applied to many motivational situations outside of medication use such as undertaking a diet regimen, an exercise program, a drug-and-alcohol-rehab approach, or deciding whether to undergo a diagnostic procedure or surgery.

THE "GREAT DEBATE" IN ACTUAL PRACTICE

Now let us take a look at two very real patients in two very real settings with two very real, yet different, diseases. Despite their differences, we will find that the Choice Triad will prove to be a valid compass for determining their degree of motivation. To begin our discussion, I will pull from my own field of practice. Our first patient will be from the field of psychiatry.

A typical 16-year-old male high school student experiencing his first break of schizophrenia seldom believes that there is something wrong with him (he does not accept the first step of the Choice Triad). If a clinician suggests taking an antipsychotic for an illness that this 16-year-old does not believe he is experiencing, it would be rather odd for the student to agree, would it not? Any dutiful clinician must also alert the student that this particular medication might make his tongue dart in and out like a lizard's tongue for the rest of his life with the additional admonition, "I might be able to reverse this but I might not." I believe it would be odd indeed to expect a student to reply, "Awesome Dude. Who wouldn't want to be permanently disfigured by a drug you want me to take for an illness I don't even have. Sweet. Let's do it."

I don't see why one would expect such an answer, for this student genuinely does not believe that there is anything wrong with him. Exactly like ourselves, if we did not feel that there was anything wrong (Step 1 of the Choice Triad), none of us would take a medication. In this instance, refusing medications is not so much evidence of a person being illogical, as it is evidence of a person being smart. If indeed he or she thinks that there is nothing wrong it is quite illogical to take a medication of any kind little lone a medication that can cause serious adverse drug reactions like tardive dyskinesia (TD) or the neuroleptic malignant syndrome. *The student is making the exact same choice that I would make if I shared the same belief.* It just so happens that in this case, I don't.

Let us return to our 16-year-old for a moment for yet another nuance. Imagine that the prescriber, with all good intentions, pushed the student to take the antipsychotic in that first session, I would not be surprised to hear our patient eventually react saying something to the effect of, "Look, I don't need your medication. I don't want your medication. I'm not going to take your medication. And I'm about to tell you where you can stuff your medication (and he is not referring to a medicine cabinet here)."

I believe it would be a mistake to view such an apparently antagonistic statement as an example of oppositional behavior. I believe that the student is simply angrily responding to what he perceives as intense interpersonal pressure to take a medication that he feels is patently inappropriate for him to take – for there is nothing wrong with him – therefore it cannot help him. To add insult to injury, the proposed medicine has remarkably dangerous potential adverse effects. No wonder he is angry. Moreover, if this is the first meeting of the patient with this prescriber, he will most likely see little reason to trust this person in future meetings, if indeed there ever is a future meeting.

Now let us take a look at our second patient, who represents a situation much closer to home for the typical primary care physician or specialist functioning in a hectic clinic or hospital setting. Let us look not at a patient with schizophrenia – patients well known for refusing medications – but to a patient with early onset diabetes.

We will look at a middle-aged woman, who is relatively symptom free, except for unusually frequent daytime urination, nighttime awakening with trips to the bathroom, and the recent onset of a sensation of feeling weary. Moderately overweight and out of condition, the level of her blood sugar suggests not only the need of behavioral interventions such as diet and exercise but also the use of an oral hypoglycemic agent.

How many of these early diabetic patients – starting on a long-term medication ripe with many potential side effects and some possible adverse effects as well – truly believe in their gut that they have a serious disease on board, one that can have crippling consequences and even have death as an end point? Once again, I have had the luxury of asking many hundreds of primary care clinicians and specialists (including endocrinologists) this exact question during my workshops. Even as I am phrasing the question, I frequently see many clinicians nodding their heads in agreement with the anticipated point because they quickly recognize that the answer is similar to the one that we observed in our patient suffering from schizophrenia – that is, not many.

Indeed, patients whose diseases show minimal symptoms at first, such as early diabetes or hyperlipidemia, are notorious for low medication interest and poor follow-through. Early hypertension, where only an abnormal number magically culled from a blood pressure cuff is evidence of disease, may be the king of problems in this regard. For such patients, they may very well have a disease, but their disease has yet to manifest as an illness.

Sometimes, in my workshops, after the previous point has been made by a member of the audience, a silence follows, and then a physician or nurse will animatedly raise a hand, commenting, "I have a caveat to that, though. The one set of my patients with early diabetes who fairly frequently do stay on their meds are those patients who have a parent with severe diabetes or a friend with it. You know, if their mom doesn't have a leg from the knee down or their uncle has a pipe in his arm from dialysis, those patients get it. They take the meds, and they often stay on them almost religiously."

Thus, our point is made.

Exactly as the Choice Triad would predict, these patients choose to start their medication because they believe there is really something wrong with them. They have a vivid picture of what could happen to them that motivates them to try the medication, and they project that whatever the cons of this medication may be, it is probably not as bad as the potential cons of their disease – renal dialysis, stroke, blindness.

The issue is not that these patients are smarter or less "oppositional" than our more typical patients with early diabetes, who refuse medications or who, more commonly, use them sporadically. Simply, these patients truly believe there is something wrong. If they did not, they would not agree to taking the medication.

More importantly, if our supposedly "resistant" patients could be led to understand that there is something seriously wrong (i.e., they come to believe in the first step of the Choice Triad), there is a good chance that a large chunk of them will take us up on our recommendation for an oral hypoglycemic agent. They will have developed a sincere interest in the medication because of their personal belief (as opposed to our professional belief) that it could stave off serious problems. Patients take medications because of their beliefs, not ours.

Once this insight is understood by prescribing clinicians, it follows suit that they develop a newfound respect for the patient's decision-making *process* – for it is the same logical process as their own – while not necessarily agreeing with the patient's database from which the decision was made or the decision itself for that matter. Indeed, there exists a shared decision making in which we provide the best information that we can about a medication and the patient chooses whether to try it on the basis of their health beliefs, cultural influences, and where he or she logically stands in relation to the Choice Triad. As we delineated in our section on the spirit of the MIM, our role becomes not one of making a so-called "resistant" patient become "compliant," but of helping a patient with poor information become more informed. We become teachers as we emphasized in the last chapter.

Our goal is to increase our patients' genuine ability to decide whether a medication is a good idea for them or not, and, if they try a medication to effectively use it. It has been my experience that once patients decide for themselves that there is something wrong that they want help with, that a medication might provide them that help, and that the pros of the medication outweigh the cons, they are often highly interested in taking medications. People don't like to be in pain or to be frightened. They will gravitate to whatever they feel will effectively end their pain and/or relieve their fears.

Over the years, I have found that once medical students, nursing students, and residents of any discipline, as well as other health care professionals in training truly understand the surprisingly simple yet elusive fact – *that patients refusing meds are often making the same decision we would make if we shared the same belief set* – it is rather remarkable how deeply it changes their attitudes toward so-called "resistant" patients. More importantly, it changes how clinicians "come across" to their patients, often disrupting a troublesome atmosphere of potential patient/clinician opposition before it can become a problem. The negative feelings of frustration within the clinician that if communicated to the patient could worsen or even trigger a decrease in medication interest and use seem to melt away because the clinician realizes that the patient is making the wisest decision possible given the belief set that the patient has at the time. Instead, this potentially oppositional dynamic is replaced with a process of collaborative problem solving from which the clinician-patient medication alliance will evolve.

It is of note to our argument that a pioneering piece of research by Colleen McHorney, who I quoted earlier in this chapter, retrospectively provided support for key elements of the Choice Triad as we have described it. In examining the reasons that 1,072 patients stayed on medications or stopped them, McHorney found that the three top reasons were as follows: (1) the patient was convinced or not convinced of the importance of the medication (first and second steps of the Choice Triad), (2) the patient worried that the medication would do more harm than good (third step of the Choice Triad), and (3) it costs too much (one of the specific elements of the third step of the Choice Triad).[5] As our case management team had discovered in the 1990s through clinical interviewing, McHorney confirmed through research in the 2000s that the decision to refuse a medication is often a logical choice made by a logical consumer.

From Theory to Practice

The Trapdoor Question: The Choice Triad Put to the Test

Now that we have developed a better theoretical understanding – through the concept of the Choice Triad – of how patients go about the complicated business of choosing to start and/or stay on a medication, I feel it is useful to provide a foretaste of how our theories may actually be put into practice. To do so, I'd like to share another technique that will serve as a prototype of the types of techniques we will be exploring in the rest of our book, much as we did in Chapter 2, when we looked at the Inquiry into Lost Dreams.

Let us look at the third step of the Choice Triad: the patient must feel the pros of the medication outweigh the cons. We will examine an interviewing technique, the "Trapdoor Question," designed specifically to help clinicians explore this delicate balancing act, a balancing act that will ultimately determine whether the patient chooses to stay or not to stay on a prescribed medication. In Chapter 9, we will pursue a more in-depth look at the practical application of the Trapdoor Question, as well as a variety of other techniques that can help us to explore our patients' weighing of the pros and cons.

In this chapter, our goal is to merely get a hint of how such techniques can be used to significantly increase a patient's trust in his or her clinician and consequent interest in trying the clinician's medication recommendations. It is not a given that a medication that is effective at symptom relief is necessarily good or bad. It *is* a given that the clinician is going to help the patient to see if – from the patient's personal perspective – the "good" of the medication is worth the "bad."

You may recall from the epigram to Chapter 2 that Robert Shuman had poignantly commented that when working with physicians, nurses, and other health care providers, "People want to know that their opinions and concerns are worthy of interest and response." Put more bluntly, patients want to know if we are truly listening to them or just typing away on our laptop or tablet. Undoubtedly, one of the most important opinions that patients want heard, loud and clear, is their views as to whether the dosage of their medication is too high. But all sorts of things can get in the way of this opinion being voiced or heard. The barriers arise from both sides of the stethoscope.

From the patients' end of the stethoscope, he or she may have the misperception that the prescriber will be upset if the patient does not like the current medication dosage (usually the patient is feeling something like, "I'm on too much of this thing."). In other cases, patients may lack the communication skills or assertiveness to spontaneously describe their hesitancies about the dose of the medication.

From the clinician's side of the stethoscope, the problems are no less significant. One problem is truly daunting – time – not enough of it. In the hectic rush of a clinic or inpatient unit, it is easy, in fact, tempting, not to take the time necessary to sort out the patient's opinions, even when those opinions are as important as hearing the patient's views on current dosage. Frequently, this key point is not addressed unless the patient spontaneously raises it. And, if we are honest with ourselves, unconsciously we might not want to hear it anyway, because if a patient does not want to advance a dose and is still sick, new interventions will need to be found and discussed. All of this takes time. It is so much simpler when the patient is thrilled with the medication and its dosage!

Along these lines, one of the most likely periods for a patient to consider stopping a medication unfolds when a prescribing provider – focusing on inadequate relief of target symptoms – suggests increasing the dosage of a medication to a patient who already feels that he or she is on too high of a dose but does not *spontaneously* voice that concern to the provider. If the provider then suggests the increased dosage – and the patient does not bring up his or her concerns for fear of being viewed as a "bad patient" – I believe that a large portion of such patients will likely have lowered or stopped the medication by the next session.

This phenomenon – patients not informing clinicians that they are displeased with a dosage increase and subsequently stopping the medication in the days or weeks after such an increase has been made – is so common that it warrants a name, the "trapdoor effect." The name comes from the fact that when this situation arises, the patient's interest in taking a medication seems to disappear as if a trapdoor had opened beneath it resulting in medication discontinuation.

From these considerations, a new interviewing principle has emerged: *Before making a recommendation to increase the dosage of a medication, take the time to ask the patient his or her opinion regarding the current dosage – as opposed to assuming one knows it.* The question now becomes, "How?" There could be various ways of doing so. Let me share a specific technique that I have found to do so quite effectively.

Interviewing Tip Prototype B: The Trapdoor Question

> "At this point in time, in your own opinion, do you feel that you are on too little, too much, or just the right amount of this medication?"

The Trapdoor Question directly opens the door into the third step of the Choice Triad (the patient's weighing of the pros and cons). It is important to remember that sometimes, in fact not infrequently, this door will remain hidden unless one asks directly with questions such as the Trapdoor Question. Unopened, clinicians will have no idea that the patient is losing his or her medication interest because of fears that the current dosage is too high. Increasing the dosage with such patients will often result in a precipitous drop in medication interest frequently followed by unilateral discontinuance of the medication.

One of the strong points of the Trapdoor Question is that it inquires along a continuum. Thus, it does not bias the patient in any specific direction. The important point is to *routinely* ask for the patient's opinion about the current dosage before suggesting an increase in dosage—once again, assuming nothing.

Another strong point of the Trapdoor Question is that it allows the clinician to utilize the patient's nonverbal communications to ferret out the truth. I have found in actual practice that even a slight hesitation by a patient in answering positively to this question almost always indicates that the patient has a concern about the current dosage. At such a moment, even if the patient answered with a positive answer such as, "I guess it's okay," it is useful to make a comment such as, "You know, you don't look too sure of that answer, is there something about the medication or its dosage that is concerning you. I really want to know anything that might be concerning you."

If the patient responds to the Trapdoor Question by sharing hesitancies or fears about the current dose either indirectly (nonverbally) or directly (e.g., "Yeah, I think I'm on too much of this thing"), the interviewer has an opportunity to address these concerns before proceeding with any suggestions for an increase in dosage. Sometimes you will discover that your patient was already considering stopping the medication without telling you. Indeed, sometimes the patient is correct and this is not the right medication for him or her.

At other times, the Trapdoor Question also uncovers a particularly problematic side effect, which, secondary to stigmatization, the patient had never shared with the clinician *even if the clinician had previously asked directly about the side effect*. I have found sexual dysfunction (as seen with statins, some antihypertensives including diuretics, beta-blockers, and alpha-blockers, H_2-receptor antagonists, antidepressants, and antipsychotics) to be just such a hidden side effect. Once uncovered through the sensitive use of the Trapdoor Question, the clinician can take actions to alleviate the side effect or may find it expedient to switch medications. I often find that patients know they are on the wrong medication before I do, and the Trapdoor Question sometimes helps me to find out.

THE PUZZLE COMPLETED: AN INVITATION OF SORTS

We have now completed our jigsaw puzzle regarding the practical theory of the MIM and its potential solutions to the troubling problems that follow when patients discontinue medications or choose not to start them in the first place. As we finish Part I of our book, the core processes driving patients toward decreased medication interest and use have been brought into a clarifying light. Indeed, we have already begun to move from theory to practice. The power of our model is already beginning to emerge.

REFERENCES

1. Cushing H. *Life of Sir William Osler.* Oxford, England: Clarendon Press; 1925.
2. Holmes OW Sr. From address to the Massachusetts Medical Society. 1860.
3. World Health Organization (WHO). *Safety of Medications: A Guide to Detecting and Reporting Adverse Drug Reactions.* 2002. Geneva, Switzerland: World Health Organization. http://apps.who.int/iris/bitstream/10665/67378/1/WHO_EDM_QSM_2002.2.pdf. Accessed July 19, 2017.
4. *Merriam-Webster's Collegiate Dictionary.* 11th ed. Springfield, MA: Merriam-Webster Inc; 2012.
5. McHorney CA. The adherence estimator: a brief, proximal screener for patient propensity to adhere to prescription medications for chronic disease. *Curr Med Res Opin.* 2009;25(1):215–238.

PART TWO

Interviewing Techniques and Strategies: The Real World of Clinical Application

CHAPTER 6

The First Script

"It may be argued that the ongoing personal relationship with each patient is the . . . tool of the trade for the primary care physician. The primary care physician's approach to the patient's problem is grounded in the way the patient defines the problem."[1]

Howard Brody, MD
From THE HEALER'S POWER

Before We Begin: Introduction to Part 2

In Part 2, we will explore a wide variety of interviewing techniques for enhancing medication interest. We will examine the tools, implied by Howard Brody's passage above, that will allow us to address the individualized needs of our patients whether we are meeting them in a hectic clinic setting or on an equally hectic inpatient unit. From this survey, the reader will be able to develop a set of diverse interviewing techniques with which he or she is personally comfortable. The diversity in the nuance of their wording and application will allow both students (from medical, nursing, physician assistant, and clinical pharmacy schools) and experienced physicians, nurses, and other providers – whatever their disciplines from family medicine, internal medicine, and surgery to specialties such as nephrology, pulmonology, and psychiatry – to develop a sophisticated understanding of the array of flexible interviewing techniques and strategies that are available for transforming the roadblocks to medication interest that complicate everyday practice.

In this chapter, as well as in the subsequent chapters of Part 2, I invite you, the reader, to pick and choose from the following techniques. Pick those techniques that appeal to you and discard those that don't. It is my hope that the principles outlined will even prompt the reader to create new interviewing techniques not described in these pages. There is no "right way" to talk with patients about their medications. But the Medication Interest Model (MIM) provides an avenue on which each clinician can create his or her own way. The MIM allows the interviewer to move from a merely habitual method of discussing medications with patients to the intentional style of collaborative interviewing that lies at the heart of the MIM, a shared decision making, that can transform lives and sometimes even save them.

With the intense time limits of contemporary practice, to effectively utilize specific interviewing techniques for enhancing medication interest, it becomes critical that interviewers possess a flexible framework for recognizing when to use such techniques. Time is of the essence. The Choice Triad, delineated in Chapter 5, will provide us with an excellent method for spotting "where the patient is at" regarding medication interest and choice. It provides a reliable system for alerting clinicians as to when a psychological need or concern of a patient is present and is about to result in refusal or discontinuance of a medication. This sophisticated understanding offers the clinician an opportunity to either transform the discontinuance before it damages the patient or, perhaps, to discover that the patient is correct in his or her concerns. The latter – not infrequent situation – may suggest that a different medication may be worth trying or, perhaps, no medication at all.

To build on the metaphor suggested by Howard Brody's opening epigram, we are not unlike skilled woodworkers and artisans who have, over the years, created toolboxes filled with a wide variety of well-tested tools, each of which has its specific purposes and advantages/disadvantages. Depending on the type of wood, or the type of structure the artisan is creating, he or she selects the most effective tools for the purpose, always working with the wood and never forcing an ill-conceived approach that goes against the grain of the wood.

We too have an artistic medium, but unlike our master craftsman, our art is a living art. Our toolboxes are not filled with woodworking tools but interviewing principles, techniques, and strategies. Our art does not create sculptures, furniture, and houses but relieves the suffering and pain of those who appreciate those sculptures, sit on those pieces of furniture, and live in those houses.

In the remaining pages of this book, we will find that there are "core interviewing toolboxes" comprising specific interviewing techniques for each step of the Choice Triad. In addition, there are a variety of other "specialty toolboxes" designed for specific clinical situations. In this chapter we will look at one of these specialty toolboxes – how does one introduce the very first medication to a new patient.

As a point of emphasis, it is important to remember that, with any given patient, depending on time constraints and clinical context, the interviewer will use only a relatively small number of the following tips described in Part II – *frequently only one or two* – in a given appointment with a patient. Other techniques can be used in subsequent appointments as deemed useful and as time permits. The beauty of the MIM is that even a single technique can help create a collaborative medication alliance that may improve medication interest and use. Flexible, ongoing use of various techniques can create an ever-deepening medication alliance on the basis of genuine respect and shared decision making.

It is also important to remember that the MIM techniques are not used in a solid, specified block of time during the interview. The individual interviewing techniques are utilized throughout the initial appointment – and subsequent medication checks – as needed and where the individual interviewing techniques most naturalistically fit for the patient. For instance, the specialty toolbox on understanding the patient's general attitudes about medications and past experiences with medications is often, although not always, used somewhere near the middle of an initial appointment when taking the patient's history of medical treatment. In contrast, the techniques designed to help clinicians introduce their personal approach to medication use will fall much later in the initial appointment, after the H&P has been completed and the conversation has turned to treatment planning.

With these caveats in mind, we are ready to enter Part 2 and begin the fascinating process of assembling our toolboxes. In this chapter, we will begin with a study of the very first prescription in a first appointment with a new patient (although some of the principles and techniques may be of value when prescribing a new medication during subsequent treatment). It is with this "first script" that the medication alliance is first created. As discussed earlier, it will be the success of this birthing that will determine the fate of much of the subsequent therapeutic alliance for good or for bad.

TOOLBOX FOR THE FIRST PRESCRIPTION

The act of writing (or typing an e-script) for the first prescription is an act of immense import to our patients. It is an act of trust with an almost total stranger. Whether the patient will follow through with what we write or type is not known. Indeed, the patient's subsequent, and ultimate, perception of the value of that first prescription may be the determining factor as to whether there is a return visit.

Whether a prescriber, from whatever discipline, decides to provide a prescription at the end of the first appointment will be determined by a variety of factors including the proclivities of the prescriber, administrative pressures to do so, and time pressures within the clinical setting itself. It should also be related, indeed, determined, by whether the prescriber feels that the therapeutic alliance is strong enough that this particular patient is open to the idea of using the medication that will be waiting for him or her at the pharmacy.

If, as the initial appointment proceeds, the clinician intuits that the patient has little or no interest in the use of a potentially helpful medication, it is generally folly to push the issue by writing a prescription, for the nascent therapeutic alliance may suffer irreparable harm by such an oppositional push against the Agreement Continuum. Such an ill-advised push may result in there being no second appointment. Instead, the clinician can opt to recommend the medication in the next or a later appointment once the therapeutic alliance has been strengthened and the patient is in agreement with the medication choice. (Note that in subsequent chapters we will address interviewing techniques that can be used in the relatively infrequent situations where the seriousness of the patient's medical state in the initial outpatient appointment suggests that it is very important that the patient begin the medication immediately, if at all possible).

The following toolbox is designed to minimize the likelihood of precipitating the type of dismal initial outcome caused by premature prescribing. Indeed, in a more positive sense, the chapter is designed to maximize both the patient's medication interest and the power of the therapeutic alliance in the fastest possible fashion. Directly concerning medication use, other than eliciting an accurate medication history, there exist three tasks during the first appointment: (1) uncovering the patient's views on his or her current medications (as well as the concept of taking medications at all), (2) introducing your personal approach as a prescriber to the use of medications, and (3) if one feels that a new medication may be indicated, providing an ample introduction to its pros and cons, collaboratively arriving at a decision as to its use, and delineating directions for its use while checking to make sure the patient understands these directions.

Later in the book, we will be examining many useful techniques for the sound implementation of the multitiered third step above, but in this chapter our focus will be on the first and second steps – (1) uncovering the patient's feelings about his or her medications and (2) introducing our personal philosophy of how we approach the use of medications. As hinted above, without a successful navigation of these first two steps, Step 3 is often doomed for failure.

Eliciting the Patient's Views on Current Medications: The Medication Passport

Many of the patients entering our offices, or appearing on our inpatient units, have been on a long journey regarding the medications that they have taken for illnesses ranging from the common (diabetes, hypertension, and depression) to the less frequent (multiple sclerosis, rheumatoid arthritis, and epilepsy) to the infrequent or rare (carcinoid syndrome and amoebic meningoencephalitis). Many patients have seen many clinicians, many offices, and, in some instances, many inpatient units.

Our elderly patients are often walking pharmacies with 10 or more medications on board. Indeed, a survey of 17,000 Medicare patients demonstrated that two out of every five patients reported taking five or more medications.[2] In a Canadian study with patients averaging 81 years of age, the patients were juggling a disturbing 15 medications daily (range 6 to 28).[3] Except for the young, many patients have had a long list of encounters with physicians, nurses, physician assistants, clinical pharmacists, and case managers.

Some of these encounters have been good and some not so good. Thus, patients enter our offices with preconceptions, expectations, and fears of what and whom they are about to encounter behind the exam room door. Sometimes they have every right to be worried, for our patients have encountered pill-pushers who have had little interest in what they want or believe. Other times they have been fortunate to have met talented clinicians, who have listened carefully and shared decision making with them. So much the better for us, for these patients are anticipating good care. Nevertheless, all patients have a track record with prescribers and the medications they prescribe. Each patient arrives at our office for a first appointment with a certain degree of anticipatory "baggage" in tow. This baggage will often shape the patient's level of interest in our first prescription.

One can view this treatment journey, sometimes decades in length, as being recorded in a psychological "medication passport" of sorts. It is useful, I would argue – critical – to get a look at this passport before recommending a new medication or a change of medications during the first or subsequent meeting. *A good understanding of how the patient views medications can greatly alter how we first suggest their use and even whether it is wise to suggest their use as an initial line of intervention in the first place.* Whether one is a prescriber (physician, advanced practice nurse, etc.) or following the patient's subsequent care (nurse or case manager), the principles in this chapter can help to forge a powerful and honest medication alliance, not only during the initial appointment, but in ongoing care as well. We will find that it is not enough to just take a patient's medication history, for it is important to find out not only what medications a patient has taken but also to uncover what the patient thought about those medications when taking them.

Requesting the Passport

We have arrived at our first interviewing principle. It is simple in theory and powerful in practice. *Before prescribing a first medication, review the patient's personal views on his or her current medications and/or past medications*. It is also a bit trickier to do effectively than first meets the eye. Time remains problematic, especially in an initial appointment that will include an H&P. Indeed, as we shall soon see, it will be next to impossible to review the patient's full medication passport in the first meeting, especially if the patient is elderly and enters our offices with a suitcase of medications. Prioritizing will have to be done.

One of our first practical questions might be, "When do I address the patient's views on his or her medications?" The answer can vary, depending on the clinician's personal proclivities as well as the unique unfolding of the relationship with the patient in the first encounter or those that follow. You may find that you prefer to elicit this information when taking the patient's medication history or while immediately eliciting the patient's list of current medications. Or you may decide that you prefer to elicit the patient's views on current medications after you have introduced the patient to your own approach to using medications. There is no right or wrong way as long as the task is completed before the patient departs with prescription in hand or the e-script has been sent. In this chapter, you will have a chance to see various approaches.

No matter when in the initial appointment you decide to uncover the patient's medication passport, I have found that the easiest way to do so is to simply ask as with the following inquiry, our very first interviewing technique:

> **TIP 1 Medication Passport Question**
>
> "How do you feel about the current medication(s) that you are on for your diabetes?"

I think that you will discover that the patients' responses to the Medication Passport Question can range from a short, "They're okay" to a spirited discussion in which the patient relays significant concerns, and may even openly share what – without our inquiry – might otherwise have been a withheld secret such as, "but I don't take that medication the way the doctor wanted anyway." By the way, if the patient is not on any medications, the Medication Passport Question looks like this:

"What are your feelings about taking medications in general?"

Patients with a strong leaning toward complementary and alternative medicine (CAM) may have antagonistic or ambivalent opinions about medications. It is best to have these feelings out on the table for shared discussion as opposed to having no idea they exist. Indeed, a CAM intervention may be an excellent first choice.

In any case, I have found that many patients seem to appreciate that the prescriber is asking for their opinions. Apparently, not every previous clinician may have shown such spontaneous interest. In a similar vein, some patients may have a preconceived notion that all that doctors like to do is to prescribe medications, and that the role of the doctor is to make sure the patient stays on his or her medications. Naturally, such a preconception predisposes to the creation of an oppositional alliance as described in Part I. Despite its simplicity, the Medication Passport Question can go a surprisingly long way toward dispelling this potentially damaging preconception.

A physician at one of my Arizona MIM workshops, Harold Meyerowitz, shared some questions for use after asking the Medication Passport Question that he has found useful for more effectively undercutting such an unproductive preconception before it can even raise its head. With the use of these follow-up questions, the prescriber openly acknowledges the possibility that the current medications may or may not be totally pleasing to the patient, thus metacommunicating a genuine interest in the patient's end of the stethoscope.

A more detailed inquiry – utilizing some of the following questions – will often need to be undertaken in later sessions because of the extremely tight time constraints in an initial appointment. Even in subsequent sessions, these very same time demands will generally necessitate that only a few of the questions on the list can be discussed. Fortunately, through familiarization with the following types of questions the reader can make a well-informed selection of which questions, if any, may be of particular importance with a given patient, thus ensuring that a shortened exploration does not become an inadequate one:

TIP 2 Medication Passport Follow-Up Package

a. "What is your understanding of what this medication is supposed to do for you (provide the name of one of the patient's specific medications, and subsequently do so for each medication)?"
b. "Do you think it helps you?"
c. "Do some of your medications seem to help better than others?"
d. "Do you like your medications?"
e. "Were you interested in making any changes in any of them?"
f. "Do you think that you need to be on medications?"
g. "Have you ever thought of alternative treatments in addition to your medications or perhaps instead of them?"

Note the importance of first uncovering the patient's understanding of the purposes of his or her medications. I have found that many patients do not understand the reasoning behind their medications and, hence, do not understand their importance. It is particularly important to make sure that a patient understands the reasoning behind the use of any medications that are critical to his or her recovery or relief. *Without such knowledge about crucial medications (and not all medications are crucial), an elderly patient on 15 medications who grows tired of their use may choose to stop or lower the dose of a critical medication thinking that all of his or her medications are of equal importance*. To do so would be quite natural. It could also be quite dangerous.

The fashion in which your patients respond to the above questions can also shed light on various useful bits of information, including your patients' intelligence, memory retention, ability to express themselves, and ability to effectively assert their viewpoints. Patients' answers may also provide indirect information on the quality of the previous patient-prescriber alliance and the quality of previous provider education regarding medication use. For a small number of questions, the Medication Passport Follow-Up Package goes a long way toward fostering a nonoppositional partnership, while yielding surprisingly useful information.

Depending on your practice, it should be noted that your patient's medication passport may be held in small hands. In another MIM workshop, a pediatric social worker, Kay McAuliffe, pointed out that with children below age 10, it is often still important to uncover their personal views (as opposed to relying solely on their parents' views) as to "what this pill business is all about."

Despite the fact that the child's parents are distributing the medication – ensuring that the medication is being taken – important psychological concerns can arise in a child ingesting a pill that may warrant attention. Medications can be extraordinarily confusing to kids, and they may develop untrue and potentially worrisome distortions about their medications, even medications as "simple" as antibiotics. She further points out that, although the clinician is basically exploring the same material as with adults, there are some subtle changes in the wording that can make the inquiries more effective at getting a child's true opinions. Such questions are encapsulated in her following technique, which is employed selectively as indicated by the child's level of intellectual development:

TIP 3 Medication Passport for Small Hands

a. "Why do you think you are taking this pill?"
b. "How is it supposed to help you?"
c. "Do you want to be taking it?"

Besides immediately allaying the fears of a child regarding his or her medications, it should also be noted that any person's subsequent adult views on medications may have first been forged – and rather permanently forged at that – by his or her interactions with those who prescribed medications to him or her as a child, a fact of which talented pediatricians are often well aware.

The Medication Passport Question alone – even without the Medication Passport Follow-Up Package – can uncover a rich database for understanding the patient's feelings about medications, immediately suggesting avenues for discussing medication recommendations later in the initial appointment as well as in future appointments. Consequently, I always try to fit this question into a first meeting with a patient. I then use as much of the Medication Passport Follow-Up Package as time permits. There is one more question that I recommend trying to ask in the first meeting as part of the patient's medication passport, if at all possible.

Directly Exploring for Perceived Medication Sensitivity

The question in question was developed in response to the simple recognition that few encounters are more critical in establishing alliances with our patients than our first meetings, and few moments are more treacherous to their development. The success of the first encounter can be more assured if we keep in mind that two opinions exist about every medication prescribed: the prescriber's and the patient's. With regard to whether the medication ever leaves the bottle, in the final analysis, only the latter opinion counts.

In this light, it can be argued that one of the most important questions to ask during a medication history is, "Do you take your medications as prescribed?" because the answer undoubtedly determines whether the medications that we are about to suggest will be given a fair chance to help (or even be tried in the first place). The art is how to ask this question in such a manner that it is engaging, not challenging, in nature.

Let us see whether the MIM can provide some guidance on how to proceed. Keeping in mind that we want to minimize any phrasing that causes even subtle hints of opposition, the above question may be too socially blunt, almost accusatory in tone. It is probably ill advised. To figure out how to phrase the question in a less oppositional manner, it may be useful to examine the patient's perspective on it, for our question – "Do you take your medications as prescribed?" – is often mirrored by a quite different question on the patient's side of the stethoscope: "Is this guy going to overmedicate me?"

The latter question frequently arises from an ingrained opinion that previous prescribers have "overmedicated me because they just don't get how sensitive I am to medications." It is an opinion that, for many patients, is a deeply held belief. In fact, it is often an entrenched conviction garnered from decades of legitimately bad experiences with prescribing clinicians.

Furthermore, from the perspective of the MIM, it is a smart question for patients to ask because it allows them to address the third step of the Choice Triad directly. If the medication is given at too high a dose for their bodies, disturbing side effects or serious adverse reactions may indeed occur. The cons will outweigh the pros. From an intelligent consumer's perspective, it would make good sense to consider not filling such a prescription or, if filled, to take the medication at a lower dose than recommended.

In short, if patients feel that the answer to their question is "yes" – we are going to overmedicate them – they are primed to have little interest in our medication recommendations from the get-go. Very few of our patients directly ask this critical question because, like our own question ("Do you take your medications as prescribed?"), it is socially awkward. Consequently, they are forced to intuit whether we might overmedicate them, which is not a good state of affairs, for their intuition, perhaps primed by their bad experiences with previous prescribers, may be very wrong indeed. An effective and reliable way exists to get around this potentially fatal trap to engagement.

The spirit of the MIM suggests that, paradoxically, the key to uncovering valid answers to our question, "Do you take meds as prescribed?" may well be to first answer (directly or indirectly) the patient's question, "Do you overmedicate?" Only after the patient feels safe about this issue are we likely to get valid answers to our question or, for that matter, to trigger interest from the patient in our medication recommendations. Specifically, we want to demonstrate that we possess a keen interest in their concerns about side effects and, even more particularly, their views as to their medication sensitivity. The question becomes, "How?"

I have found that one practical, and surprisingly effective, answer to the dilemma lies in a simple question that can be asked when exploring the patient's medication passport. It is a question that indirectly metacommunicates that, not only am I not a stereotypic overmedicator, I am actually a person who is quite concerned about the potential for overmedication. Note that I often personalize it by using the patient's name. See what you think:

TIP 4 Medication Sensitivity Inquiry

"Mrs. Jenkins, do you think that you are particularly sensitive to medications?"

. . . or a slightly different variation is worded as follows:

"Do you feel that you tend to get bad side effects from medications?"

The answers are occasionally fascinating and, almost always, useful. If the patient quickly answers, "No, not particularly," then we have a "green light" to proceed with our initial medication recommendations. But, if the patient answers "yes" or indicates nonverbally through broken eye contact, tone of voice, or a pause before answering, then we have a "red light."

The light will not turn green until we sensitively uncover the patient's concerns and address those concerns, a process that, in itself, will convincingly demonstrate that we have no intention of overmedicating him or her. Paradoxically, we will have answered the patient's question "Is this guy going to overmedicate me?" by asking one.

If the patient says that he or she is very sensitive to medications (and a good number of my patients emphasize, "I'm *very* sensitive to medications"), then it is common sense to follow up with an exploration of that patient's potential sensitivity with an open-ended question such as, "What types of bad experiences have you had?" or "What are some of the things you've encountered that have shown you that you are overly sensitive to medications?"

Not only does such a question convey the clinician's genuine concern, but it can also dig up all sorts of interesting information. In some instances, we discover that the patient does indeed seem to experience an overabundance of side effects, perhaps suggesting that the patient is a slow metabolizer. This information is invaluable in setting an appropriate initial dose to minimize side effects while maximizing medication interest and safety.

However, as I am sure you have seen in your own practices, or will see in your future practices, we sometimes discover that some patients who view themselves as particularly sensitive to medications are, in truth, not so. They simply encounter the typical side effects seen with medications of the class in question and, mistakenly, view themselves as being more side-effect prone than are other people.

Obviously, with such patients, their inaccurate view of being "unusually sensitive" to medications will cast a considerable damper on their medication interest. In the past, I saw the uncovering of this unwarranted bias as an opportunity to provide some productive education to counter my patient's misinformation. I might say something like, "Mrs. Jenkins, I have some good news for you. In actuality, you aren't really overly sensitive to medications. You are simply getting some of the very common side effects we see with those types of medications. Thus, we can try some other medications, and you may not get many side effects at all."

My hope was that by clearing up Mrs. Jenkins's misperception of being biologically overly sensitive, I would increase her interest in trying subsequent medications. Sometimes this happened, but many times, it did not.

To my puzzlement, the "Mr. or Mrs. Jenkinses of the world" did not seem overly impressed by my well-intentioned educational foray, and, if their frowns were any indication, they were not particularly pleased with it.

Here is where the MIM suggests not only what to say, but also what might be best not to say. Keep in mind that we are discussing our first encounter with a patient. According to the MIM, the single most important thing to achieve by the end of the interview is that the patient feels allied with us. Any feelings of lingering opposition as the patient walks out the door may be fatal to the filling of our first prescription and may undercut the likelihood of a return visit as well.

With these ideas in mind, let us look at what – beneath all my well-intentioned verbiage and intentions – Mrs. Jenkins may be actually "hearing" as I provide the educational information described above:

Clin.: Mrs. Jenkins, do you think that you are particularly sensitive to medications?

Pt.: Yes, definitely.

Clin.: Well, I don't (patient's eyes get big). In fact, I have all sorts of other medications I'd like to try on you (eyes getting even bigger).

Pt.: Okay (patient thinking, God help me! He's going to overmedicate me like all the other idiots).

If we are honest, this is exactly what some of our patients are thinking at the time and "it doesn't bode well" for medication interest. From the perspective of Mrs. Jenkins, I have asked for her opinion. She gave it. I ignored it. And I have assured her that I intend to continue to ignore it.

Hmm. I think I might be in a bit of trouble here.

Our model clearly suggests that this may not be the most effective direction to be taking in an initial appointment unless we want it to be the patient's last appointment, in which case it is very effective. But what direction might be better, keeping in mind that Mrs. Jenkins may be convinced by years of bad experiences with medications that she is overly sensitive?

What to Do If Patients Perceive Themselves to Be Overly Sensitive to Medications

If it is clear that the patient is, indeed, sensitive to medications (each person's body handles medications differently and genetic variations can significantly alter blood levels at similar doses) or if the patient perceives himself or herself to be overly sensitive (when he or she may not be), it makes no difference in how we approach the first prescription. In either case, it should be approached with great caution and with appropriate deference to the patient's concerns. The patient's perception of sensitivity (whether accurate or not) is the key to the patient's subsequent interest in taking the medication. We are once again reminded of the wisdom of our opening epigram, "The primary care physician's approach to the patient's problem is grounded in the way the patient defines the problem."

For a moment, imagine that I simply acknowledge her opinion that she is overly sensitive to medications (noting to myself that in future sessions, once we have developed a stronger alliance, I might be in a better position to transform it). Further imagine that near the end of the first appointment (if it is medically appropriate and safe), after I have written the name of the medication on my first script or typed it up on my computer as I prepare an e-script, I pause, look up at Mrs. Jenkins and say something like:

TIP 5 Mini-Dose Recommendation

"Mrs. Jenkins, would it be okay with you if I start you off at one half of the recommended starting dose for this medication because of your history of being sensitive to meds? I think this would be a smart way to start you off. I call this a mini-dose, and I think it is a very gentle way to begin medications. This way, your body can get a feel for the medication first before we give you much of a dose. Any side effects, and there might not be any with this little of a dose, will probably be much smaller in nature. Then if you are feeling comfortable on the medication, we can slowly increase it to get you feeling better and better. By the way at this tiny dose you might not get any benefits from the medication but I just think it is a smart way to start because of your sensitivity. What do you think?"

This looks good on paper, and, in practice, I have been pleasantly surprised just how effective the above pair of interviewing techniques – Medication Sensitivity Question and the Mini-Dose Recommendation – can be in both spotting patients who have concerns about medications and in allaying those concerns before the first encounter ends. A patient, such as Mrs. Jenkins, who enters my office having been wary of prescribers for years, may now leave my office feeling that she is in safe hands.

One can easily picture on her return home, Mr. Jenkins asking his wife, "What did you think of Dr. Shea?" and his wife replying with an unexpected,

"You know, he's the first damn doctor who ever listened to me." Here we have a nice example of a set of behaviorally defined interviewing *techniques* that have been woven together into an effective interviewing *strategy* for enhancing the medication alliance while increasing medication interest.

For the Mini-Dose Recommendation to work effectively, several things are worth noting. It seems to be important to "ask permission" at the end of the technique, as reflected by my words, "What do you think?" because such a question further reenforces our desire to work as a collaborative team. Telling patients why we are recommending a low dose (as a response to their concerns about being overly sensitive) is also important because it conveys that we are not only carefully listening to the patient's input but also demonstrates that we are willing to act on it, a point not missed by the patient.

In the above approach, we have seen our first example of a sequential interviewing *strategy*. As you will recall from Chapter 2, interviewing strategies occur when two or more specific interviewing *techniques* are serially connected to achieve a set clinical goal. More specifically, if two or more interviewing techniques can be used sequentially to achieve a specific therapeutic goal more effectively, their order can be operationalized and the sequence is given a name for ease of teaching and employment in clinical practice (in this case, the pairing of the two interviewing techniques – the Medication Sensitivity Inquiry and the Mini-Dose Recommendation – is simply called the **Medication "Wary" Engagement Strategy**). I believe that you may find the Medication "Wary" Engagement Strategy to be one of your most effective strategies during an initial appointment for improving medication interest and follow-through with your first new prescription.

I vividly remember a woman who had been suffering with a major depressive episode for years, who had discontinued five consecutive antidepressants "because I have had horrible side effects on those damn things." She had also been in ongoing psychotherapy with little relief. After having applied the first technique (the Medication Sensitivity Inquiry) of the Medication "Wary" Engagement Strategy, I employed the second technique, the Mini-Dose Recommendation (in this instance, at one-fourth the typical starting dose). We gradually increased the dose over several months at tiny amounts, and at her own pace, till we arrived at a therapeutic dosing. Her depression went into a complete remission. Note that, even with patients viewing themselves as overly sensitive to medications, with some serious conditions it may be advantageous to start a medication at a typical or higher-than-typical dose (Effective MIM approaches for such relatively infrequent situations will be addressed later in the book).

Indirectly Uncovering Concerns About Medication Sensitivity and Medication Practices

Before wrapping up our discussion on the importance of understanding and responding to our patients' perceptions regarding their medication sensitivity, let me share one more valuable tip. It is a tip that returns us to the question of how to uncover our patients' fears or concerns in the first place. I think you will find the tip to be both a bit unexpected and novel. As it ends up, it is also quite useful. I wish I'd thought of it myself.

When providing my workshops on the MIM, one of my greatest pleasures occurs when a clinician proffers an interviewing technique that I would not have thought of using in a million years, yet I subsequently find to be quite useful. For instance, Michael Applebaum, a physician from Idaho, described a technique he likes to use when uncovering a patient's personal feelings about medication sensitivity and dosage.

You will note that our techniques thus far, such as the Medication Passport Question, are fairly direct in their wording. Applebaum suggests a technique that is indirect, yet because of its indirect nature may uncover information – with reticent or more wary patients – that may not have surfaced with a more direct approach. Not only does Applebaum's tip provide a novel way to uncover patients' perceptions of how sensitive they feel they are to medications, but an adaptation of it can also shed light on another key aspect of patients' medication passport – the patients' medication practices in the only world that really counts: What do they do at home after leaving our offices? Applebaum's technique looks like this:

TIP 6 Let's See, What Dose Should I Try?

"Mr. Jamison, when you take an aspirin or Tylenol or Motrin for a headache or pain of some sort, how much do you usually take?"

As the patient goes about nondefensively describing his or her medication practice toward an over-the-counter commonly taken medication, all sorts of little secrets can emerge. A patient with a fear of medication sensitivity will often betray that concern by his or her choice of a low dosage, or the patient may make a revealing spontaneous comment (while shaking his or her head) such as, "Oh, I don't like to take medications at all, so I only take a few tablets, if any." Such a comment provides a surprisingly good glimpse at our patient's feelings about medication use in general while offering us an indirect hint at his or her current medication practice. More than a hint about potential future medication practice will emerge when a different patient responds to the Let's See, What Dose Should I Try? inquiry with the following words, "I prefer naturopathic remedies. I can't remember the last time I took an aspirin or Tylenol. Don't like 'em. Doesn't Tylenol hurt your liver or something?"

On the other end, one may find a patient who sheepishly answers, "Probably more than I should?" With a gently phrased follow-up question (sometimes accompanied by a gently teasing tone of voice by the clinician) such as, "How do you mean 'more than you should?'" Overmedicators or self-medicators may unexpectedly reveal themselves often with a bit of an embarrassed chuckle.

As mentioned earlier, one can extrapolate on this indirect technique by asking the patient to elaborate about a commonly prescribed medication, which the patient is not currently taking (so there is no reason for defensiveness in the patient's answer) as with, "I'm just curious, if you take something like an antibiotic, say something like penicillin or ampicillin, how do you feel about taking it in the sense of do you worry about taking such medications, or are you ever concerned that you're taking too much of them or taking them for too long?" Said in a nonaccusatory tone, such questioning can bridge into an exploration of important material related to our patients' medication practices with regard to a medication that they are currently taking, as seen in the following prototypic illustration. In this illustration, an internist is picking up a new patient, who has a history of migraine headaches, diabetes, and epilepsy, who is concurrently being followed by a neurologist, Dr. Nylan (fictitious name):

Clin.: You know, I'm just curious, if you take something like an antibiotic, say something like penicillin or ampicillin, how do you feel about taking it, like, do you worry about taking such medications in general, or are you ever concerned that you're taking too much of them or taking them for too long? (variation of **Let's See, What Dose Should I Try?**)

Pt.: I don't know . . . I don't usually have any problem with them. I once had a pneumonia, and I really was grateful for whatever the hell they gave me. It worked great.

Clin.: Good to hear . . . Are you pretty careful about how much medication you take? I know you're on a few medications now, some of which I'll be following you for.

Pt.: Oh yea, my wife and I are not real keen on medications unless you really need them (pauses) like when I had that pneumonia. And I know I have to take my medications for my sugar and my seizures.

Clin.: Good to hear. Makes sense to me. You don't want to take any more medication than you need to be effective (the clinician is deftly taking advantage of a naturally arising chance to gently move with the patient on the Agreement Continuum to enhance the feeling of "going with" the patient in a nonoppositional sense, furthered by the next statements). I'm careful like that for myself. It's smart. (slight pause) Do you ever find that you don't always need the amount of medication that has been prescribed.

Pt.: You mean, like stop it early or something?

Clin.: Yea, something like that, or cut back on it, like with an antibiotic.

Pt.: (patient smiles) I suppose so . . . actually, I sort of stopped that antibiotic, the one for the pneumonia, a few days early . . . it had, sort of, you know, once I knew it had worked and stuff.

Clin.: You know what, Martellus, truth be told, you can sometimes get away with not finishing up with a medication like that (pauses) and sometimes you can't. It's usually best to stay on antibiotics till all the pills are done, just to make sure the bacteria are all dead, but it looks like you were lucky and it worked out okay for you with your antibiotic in this case (notice that the clinician effectively makes her point – it's best to stay on medications until they are done – without lecturing or scolding the patient). On the other hand, there are a few medications that you can't stop quickly. It actually can be dangerous. I'll always let you know if I'm prescribing a medication like that, if that's okay with you.

Pt.: Sure. I'd always want to know that. (pauses) Am I on a medication like that now?

Clin.: Actually, yes. Do you have any idea which one?

Pt.: Not for certain. No, is it the Tegretol, no wait, is it the, no, no, I think it's the Tegretol . . . over the years I've been on so many, I don't know for sure.

Clin.: You're right on the mark, Martellus, it's the Tegretol. If you stop it all of a sudden, you definitely could increase your risk of having a seizure.

Pt.: Whoaa . . . I think Dr. Nylan told me that once, but I sort of forgot it.

Clin.: I'm sure he did. He's a good doctor.

Pt.: It was years ago when I started . . . How many days can you miss?

Clin.: If you don't mind me asking, why are you asking? (smiles)

Pt.: (smiling) Oh, I don't know, I might miss a day or two once in a while, just once in a while.

Our clinician's indirect chit-chat about medication practice (which is far from chit-chat and is quite intentional by the prescriber) has not only uncovered, in a very conversational fashion, some important factual information about the medication attitudes and practices of Martellus, but also actually strengthened the medication alliance in a subjective fashion. Factually, Martellus might have a proclivity to "play around with his medications," which as we shall see in future chapters is a normal human proclivity. I might add that physicians and nurses (including myself) are notorious patients for doing such things when we are on the other end of the stethoscope.

In addition, Martellus, as is the case with just about all patients, will need to have intermittent reenforcement about how to use medications. *Whether one is a prescriber, a clinic nurse, or a case manager, when picking up a patient from another provider, never assume the patient has adequate knowledge about his or her current medications.* Even if the provider gave excellent education about the medication usage, it is all too easy, as was the case with Martellus, to forget information or confuse it.

With regard to subjective material, the informality of this exchange may prove to be quite useful in the future. It has created a unique exchange of shared experience for the newly evolving clinician-patient dyad. Martellus has shared some potentially sensitive or embarrassing details (about not always taking medications as prescribed) while he has learned that his new prescriber is not one to pass judgments, and, indeed, seems to have a sense of humor housed in a genuine concern about his safety regarding medications. All good stuff!

I think you will find that this type of naturalistic engagement, initiated by indirect questioning, provides a rich substrate for future interactions. Later, perhaps months or years later, if this clinician prescribes a medication that is dangerous to abruptly stop, it will be meaningfully *personalized* for the patient when he hears the clinician say, "Martellus, you remember when I told you about your Tegretol being important to never stop abruptly, this new medication for your irregular heartbeat is just like it. You should never just stop it, without first checking with me, let me explain what could . . ." The shared past experience will tend to make this new information stick better. It's more vivid, and it has a shared foundation to build on. Put simply, it will be easier for Martellus to remember.

Eliciting the Patients' Views on Their Interactions with Previous Prescribers

As intimated above, during the patient's treatment journey the patient has often encountered many prescribing clinicians. Patients may have experienced not only "problematic drugs" but also, unfortunately, "problematic prescribers." Thus, patients come to our offices carrying a passport regarding their interactions with previous prescribers in the same sense that they have a passport regarding their experiences with previous medications. If a patient has a history of bad encounters with prescribers, it is very easy for the patient to anticipate that we will fit the same mold. Such a projection can be devastating to the patient's future interest in our medication recommendations. Our next interviewing principle mirrors our previous one, *Before prescribing a first medication, try to review the patient's passport regarding previous prescribers*. The following interviewing technique, which can be worded with some degree of variations, puts the principle to use:

TIP 7 Exploring the Patient's Passport on Previous Prescribers

"How have you felt about your previous doctors, nurse clinicians, physician assistants or anyone else who has prescribed medications for you? Did any of them seem particularly good at helping you to understand your medications and any concerns you had about side effects or were any of them particularly bad at doing that?"

or if the patient is a direct transfer

"What are your feelings about your last doctor (use name of appropriate professional discipline as fits the situation)?"

Note that if you are nurse or social worker functioning as a case manager following the patients use of medications and integrated care, the Patient's Passport on Previous prescribers is easily modified as, "What are your feelings about your last case manager."

Introducing Your Personal Approach to Using Medications to the Patient

In the initial appointment, there exists no single correct way for a clinician to introduce his or her approach to prescribing medications. Each of us will vary what we say depending on our own beliefs and the differing needs of each of our patients. The following approach is not presented as the "right way" to do it, but it emphasizes that we must all give considerable thought to how we do it.

Even more important, if the student (as well as the more experienced prescriber) is to take one thing away from this section, it is the recognition that discussing one's personal approach to medication use is of vital importance. It is not some secondary task that "I'll do if I have time."

From the very first courses on clinical interviewing and the development of the therapeutic alliance, the *pivotal importance* in treatment outcome of securing and enhancing the medication alliance *in the initial appointment* should be "front-and-center-stage." Unfortunately, in the harsh time demands so common to this age of mixed-payer care, it can be easy to omit the few minutes it takes to effectively introduce one's prescribing practices, yet these 3 or 4 minutes may prove to be the defining moments for establishing a powerful ongoing medication alliance. They may well set the stage for all future medication interest in the patient.

Although this particular chapter is addressed primarily to prescribing clinicians, bear with me as I diverge for a moment from prescribing clinicians in order to emphasize a point often not emphasized enough: learning how to effectively talk with patients about their medications – so as to enhance medication interest and ongoing use – is a concern for *all* health care providers, *not* just prescribers. In this light, the many nonprescribing readers of this book mentioned earlier, such as nursing students who do not ultimately choose to pursue advanced degrees and all case managers (both degreed and nondegreed), will find some of the MIM principles and techniques from this chapter to be generalizable for use in ongoing medication monitoring and case management.

Moreover, I can assure my nonprescribing readers, that most of the principles and interviewing techniques of the remaining chapters will prove to be of great importance to you when providing ongoing medication monitoring and management whether in an inpatient unit or in an outpatient clinic. The reader may recall from Chapter 2 that the MIM was born from observing and obtaining input from the case managers and other clinicians on my original outreach team. Indeed, case managers, and other nonprescribers, play pivotal, often determinative, roles in enhancing effective ongoing medication use, for they may see the patient much more frequently than a prescribing clinician.

Let us now return to the focus of this chapter – there is another important and practical, reason for taking the time to effectively introduce one's prescribing practices. These 3 or 4 minutes – if they successfully result in enhancing the patient's subsequent medication interest and use – may save many hours of preventable wasted time for yourself and your staff. The return on your time investment can be enormous. Patients, decompensating because they have discontinued medications, will demand progressively larger amounts of time as they place an increasing number of phone calls and e-mails requiring responses, as well as frequently necessitating an increased number of appointments (some squeezed – because of their urgent nature – into an already tight schedule). It is exactly the type of time consumption that can lead to burn-out in your administrative staff, clinical staff, and yourself. Moreover, patients, who have discontinued their meds, may require hospitalization requiring large amounts of time on the part of the treating clinician whether it be a hospitalist or yourself.

The interviewing principle at hand is a simple one: *Before recommending your first new medication, take the time to introduce your personal approach to prescribing medications in general*. The following three interviewing techniques provide prototypes for putting this principle into practice. Clinicians tend to use them near the end of the first appointment usually directly before discussing their recommendations. The bridging statement might sound like this: "You know, before I discuss any of my thoughts on a particular medication, I thought it might be of value, since we have never worked together before, to share with you how I like to approach the use of medications just in general. Does that sound okay with you?"

TIP 8 The Medication Interest Opening

"My goal as a physician (substitute appropriate prescriber discipline) is to always give you my best advice, whether that advice is to start a medication, stay on it, or get off it. Together we want to find a medication that you're genuinely interested in taking because it makes you feel better and/or is doing what you want it to do. You're the one who is putting the medication in your body, so it's your opinion that is most important, not mine. Obviously, as a physician (substitute appropriate prescriber discipline), I have tremendous respect for medications and I have found them to be very helpful in many patients. I also have a healthy respect for the fact that medications can cause problems too. In my own life, I only take medications when I feel that I really need them and I feel that the benefits will outweigh the costs. I take the same approach with my patients. So, I don't suggest a medication unless I really have a feeling it will help you. I would never recommend a medication that I myself would not take or give to one of my family. And I always try to fill my patients in on possible side effects and the pros and cons of using the medication. How's that sound to you?"

With a single elegantly effective statement – "Together we want to find a medication that you are genuinely interested in taking because it makes you feel better and/or is doing what you want it to do" – the clinician fosters both a sense of collaboration and spotlights the goal that such a shared decision making can achieve – relief from suffering.

While forging the initial medication alliance, it is useful to further highlight the importance of the patient's input. I am once again reminded of the wise words of Robert Schuman in the opening epigram of Chapter 2, "People want to know that their opinions and concerns are worthy of interest and response." The following technique reassures the patient that such shall be the case by stamping it into the initial bond between the prescriber and the patient:

TIP 9 Introducing Shared Expertise

"I look at it that you and I are both experts. Hopefully, I know a lot about medications and how different medications can help in different ways, and I can call on years of experience, as well as other colleagues, to help. You are the expert on your own body. The medication goes in you, not me, and so I'm totally dependent on you to tell me if it's helping or not and also if it's causing any side effects. I'm counting on your input. You know your body better than I do. And I think we can be a great team in finding a medication that works well for you – that really makes you feel better. How does that sound to you?"

As with all of our tips, you can both modify them to fit your own style of interaction and have variations of the same tip that may, in your opinion, fit a bit better with a particular patient. While providing a MIM workshop in Saskatchewan, Canada, Norm Grayston described an elegant adaptation of Introducing Shared Experience that he found to be quite effective with his patients, an adaptation that I like to call the "Shared Journey Analogy":

TIP 10 Shared Journey Analogy

"When we try a medication, I always like to remind myself that, although we have lots of research on each of these medications, all people are unique and each person will handle medications slightly differently. I have lots of confidence in this medication. Our goal is to make sure the benefits definitely outweigh any potential side effects for you. So we are on a joint journey or trial of sorts to find the best possible medication for you. You are the most important partner in our journey, for I am dependent on you to tell me what is working or not working. So, please be very open about all the benefits of the medication and any concerns you may have about side effects. As a team, I feel confident we will get you some help. How does that sound to you?"

Both Introducing Shared Experience and its variation (the Shared Journey Analogy) acknowledge the fact that almost all patients have legitimate concerns about side effects. In Chapter 9, we will delineate interviewing techniques and strategies that will help patients to effectively sort out whether the pros of a medication are worth the side effects caused by it. Sometimes they are, and sometimes they're not, as amply highlighted by serious adverse reactions.

Despite an almost universal concern about side effects, patients vary greatly on how comfortable they feel about sharing those concerns with physicians and other prescribers. Some of this hesitancy has been inculcated by long-standing, but outdated cultural norms, such as the paternalistic concept that "one should do whatever the Doctor says." Note the capital "D."

Peter Weiden, whose outstanding insights regarding improving medication interest resonate wonderfully with the spirit and principles of the MIM, emphasizes that interviewers must sometimes actively help patients to move away from this "obedience mode" as he describes it in his insightful article, "The Adherence Interview: Better Information, Better Alliance."[4]

This process of deactivating the obedience mode is an ongoing endeavor that must be addressed again long after the first meeting, as we shall see Weiden demonstrate with several specific techniques in later chapters. In any case, it is often expedient to start this deactivation from the very first encounter when it comes to reporting side effects. In short, the phrase from the technique of Introducing Shared Expertise, "The medication goes in you, not me and so I'm totally dependent on you to tell me if it's helping or not and also if it's causing any side effects," may not be enough. At times, I have found it useful to be even more specific:

TIP 11 The Call-Me-First Invitation

"By the way, I really do mean that I want to hear about any side effects you may be having. For different reasons, people sometimes are hesitant to let their physicians and nurses (insert whatever professions seem appropriate) know about side effects, but I really want to know. Sometimes we can reduce them or even get rid of them, and sometimes we may need to stop the medication. And if for some reason you start getting a side effect, please call our office before you do anything. I'll let you know what I think is happening and you can decide what to do. Even if I'm not available, one of our staff will talk with you and provide advice. But try not to stop any medication without talking with me or one of my staff first. Sometimes it isn't a side effect. And some types of side effects even go away shortly after appearing as your body adjusts. In any case, I really am your consultant. In the end, you've got to call the shots, but be sure to use me."

Sometimes at the end of the Call-Me-First Invitation, I'll utilize an interviewing technique called "Feel Free to Discontinue." I learned about the technique during a workshop I was giving on the MIM in Waterloo, Iowa from a nurse practitioner, Cyd Q. Grafft. I add it to the Call-Me-First Invitation with a patient who, in my gut, I sense is particularly frightened or hesitant about a medication but genuinely wants to try it. The following tip can help to relieve some of this fear:

TIP 12 Feel Free to Discontinue

"We have really covered the side effects carefully, and hopefully you won't get many or any. But if for some reason, before our next appointment, you feel concerned about a side effect and you can't reach me or one of my staff by phone or e-mail, feel free to stop the medication immediately. You can give me a call afterward and we can see if we can come up with a better fit at our next appointment."

My only caveat here is that one can only use this technique if, indeed, it is safe for the patient to discontinue the newly prescribed medication abruptly.

We began this section with an interviewing principle, "Before prescribing your first medication take the time in the first appointment to introduce your medication-prescribing approach." We have now looked at five interviewing techniques of use when introducing one's approach to using medications (the Medication Interest Opening, Introducing Shared Expertise, the Shared Journey Analogy, the Call-Me-First Invitation, and Feel Free to Discontinue). These techniques show us how to implement the above abstract principle in the real world of a hectic clinic. If the reader, whether a student or more experienced clinician, finds that it is useful with certain patients to pair two of these techniques sequentially (or perhaps three or more), the reader will have created a personalized interviewing strategy that can be easily remembered for practical use (or taught to other students, residents, or staff).

I frequently weave together three of the above techniques into an interviewing strategy I like to call *Forging the Medication Alliance*. This interviewing strategy consists of the following three interviewing techniques sequentially employed: 1) the Medication Interest Opening, 2) Introducing Shared Experience, and 3) the Call-Me-First Invitation. Let's see how a clinician can effectively and naturalistically use it by imagining a bit of prototypic dialogue.

Illustration of Forging the Medication Alliance

We will imagine that the patient, a mid-level manager from a large retail chain, has just moved to Sacramento, California from Los Angeles secondary to a job relocation. In this instance, the patient, whom we shall call Juan, is being transferred from one clinician to another. He presents as a 55-year-old, who could afford to lose a good 20 lb, but is otherwise in reasonably good shape. He has been coping with type 2 diabetes, high blood pressure, and dysthymia for more than 15 years, all of which his primary care doctor has been successfully managing with medications. He really liked his previous doctor, and, as one might expect, he is worried about finding a new one. In particular, he has fears that the new prescriber will "monkey around with my meds."

We are picking up the conversation in the closing phase of the initial appointment in which, following the H&P, the clinician and patient are collaboratively sharing opinions on what is going on and how to proceed with treatment planning. You will also notice that our interviewer, before employing the three techniques of the strategy of Forging the Medication Alliance, will use the technique of Exploring the Patient's Passport on Previous Prescribers. In addition, she will opt to use the technique of

Exploring the Patient's Medication Passport after she finishes forging the medication alliance:

Clin.: Juan, this is your first appointment here, and before we talk a little about our possibly working together long term, I'd like to talk a little bit about how I approach using medications. First let me just reassure you that unless there is an important reason to do so, or unless you really want me to, I generally don't make any suggestions about changing medications in a first appointment when picking up a patient transferred from another doctor. Before doing so, I would like to get to know you better and what you thought about your work with your previous treatment team before I make any suggestions for changes, if indeed I have any. I also know it can be a little unnerving to switch doctors. Especially if you've . . . I see that you've been seeing Dr. Travis for almost 15 years. That's a . . .

Pt.: Long time?

Clin.: Right.

Pt.: Yea, I really liked her.

Clin.: I can see why. From her notes, it looks like she took great care of you. What did you like about her? **(Exploring the Patient's Passport on Previous Prescribers)**

Pt.: I don't know exactly, hmmm, she was just, I don't know, low key, sort of an average kind of person, but really bright. I just liked her. I felt comfortable with her. I don't know.

Clin.: Well, I'm hoping you'll like me too. In fact, it's very important to me that you feel comfortable with me and how I use medications, so that's why I thought I should share with you a little bit about how I approach medications in general, because each doctor may be a little different. Is that okay?

Pt.: Yea, sure.

Clin.: My goal is to always give you my best advice, whether that advice is to start a medication, stay on it, or get off it. Together, if we decide to try another medication, we want to find a medication that you are genuinely interested in taking because it makes you feel better and is doing what you want it to do, like lowering your blood pressure. You're the one who is putting the medication in your body, so it's your opinion that is most important, not mine. Obviously, as a physician (use appropriate discipline), I have tremendous respect for medications and I have found them to be very helpful in many patients. I also have a healthy respect for the fact that medications can cause problems too. In my own life, I only take medications when I feel that I really need them and I feel that the benefits will outweigh the costs. I take the same approach with my patients. So, I don't suggest a medication unless I really have a feeling it will help you. I would never recommend a medication that I myself would not take or give to one of my family. And I always try to fill my patients in on possible side effects and the pros and cons of using the med. How's that sound to you? **(Medication Interest Opening)**

Pt.: Sounds good.

Clin.: I look at it that you and I are both experts. Hopefully, I know a lot about medications and how different medications can help in different ways and I can call on years of experience, as well as other colleagues, to help. You are the expert on your own body. The medication goes in you, not me. And outside of some diseases like your diabetes and high blood pressure where lab work and blood pressure readings can help guide us, I'm basically dependent on you to tell me if it's helping or not and also if it's causing any side effects. Make sense? **(Introducing Shared Expertise)**

Pt.: Sounds good to me (pauses) I hope you know what you're talking about (smiles with a joking tone of voice).

Clin.: (smiles, pleasantly reflecting the patient's use of humor) Yeah, let's hope so. (smiles, pauses) I'm curious, how comfortable do you feel talking with your doctor about side effects and things like that because people vary on that point (interesting variation on the **Call-Me-First Invitation**, for the interviewer has decided to start the technique with a question).

Pt.: Oh, I'll tell you, you can count on that. I want to know what's going on. I'm not a big one for surprises (smiles).

Clin.: Neither am I (smiles). Which brings up another point. If for some reason you start getting a side effect, please give me a call before you do anything. I'll let you know what I think is happening and you can decide what to do. But try not to stop any medication without talking with me first, or if I'm not available one of my staff will be sure to talk with you, and they're great. Sometimes it isn't a side effect. And some side effects even go away shortly after appearing as your body adjusts to the medication. In any case, I really am your consultant. You get to call the final shots, but be sure to use me. (pause) I got some good ideas. (smiles) Deal?

Pt.: Deal. (**Call-Me-First Invitation** completed. Also note that the clinician has effectively used all three techniques comprising the strategy of **Forging the Medication Alliance**. And she is about to use this gateway to further her collaborative exploration and shared decision making.)

Clin.: By the way, if we run into major problems with side effects, I'll be the first one to tell you to get off the medication. Our goal is to help you to find a medication that you genuinely are interested in taking because it makes you feel better, not because I tell you to take it. I'm always interested in your input (clinician continues with the spirit of the MIM emphasizing moving with the patient along the Agreement Continuum by indicating that she too will be a watchdog for problematic side effects; the interviewer's goal is not to keep the patient on a medication but to find a medication that the patient is interested in keeping). In fact, I'm curious, how are you feeling about your current medications. **(Medication Passport Question)**

Pt.: Pretty good. Dr. Travis felt things were going pretty good, but she'd said something about being worried that my A1C – I think it's called – was creeping back up. I had the feeling that Dr. Travis was thinking of maybe making a change. I don't know. But she didn't get a chance to say so at the end. I transferred so quickly. (pauses) I don't want to change any medications unless it's really necessary. Although if she felt it was, I'd be fine with that. (Notice that the patient is subtly indicating that he is still very interested in the opinions of Dr. Travis. At some level, his words are an invitation of sorts, an invitation that the new clinician wisely accepts.)

Clin.: She doesn't mention that in her note, but maybe I should give her a call before we meet next time. I'd like to tap her opinion more directly. (The clinician could not give a more convincing message that she will listen carefully to the patient's input and act on it).

Pt.: That's a great idea! (patient looks animated and pleased)

In the above dialogue, the clinician has nicely set the stage for a true partnership. She has deftly, yet quickly, debunked any misconceptions that she may be a "pill pusher" while establishing her role as a consultant who feels comfortable with her expertise in using medications effectively. Importantly, she sought out the patient's ideas on his role and clearly stated that she values his input. But, as powerful as her statements of interest in Juan's input might be, it is the questions that she asks – and the actions that she takes – that truly prove her interest to him.

It is striking that even on topics unrelated to symptoms or diagnosis, she is clearly interested in what Juan thinks. When he comments that he really liked his previous physician of 15 years, our interviewer inquires,

"I can see why. From her notes, it looks like she took great care of you. What did you like about her?"

Concerning shared decision making, right from the first mention of medications, this physician talks the talk and, more importantly, walks the walk. She has also managed to match her style to the needs, educational background, and cultural feel of her patient. She is talking with frankness to him, "manager to manager," a style well suited to his own. *She will adapt her style of introducing her personal approach to using medications depending on the unique needs of each patient.*

The three techniques used in the strategy of Forging the Medication Alliance (the Medication Interest Opening, Introducing Shared Expertise, and the Call-Me-First Invitation) provide her with a flexible toolbox from which she can adapt her approach to the unique needs of each patient. By previously practicing the techniques and by observing the fashion in which different people respond to them, she has gained a sophisticated, rapid, and sensitive fashion of forging the medication alliance.

Concluding Thoughts

At the beginning of this chapter, we had observed that there exist three primary tasks during a first appointment regarding medication interest: (1) uncovering the patient's views on his or her current medications (as well as the concept of taking medications at all), (2) introducing the clinician's personal approach as a prescriber to the use of medications, and (3) if one feels that a new medication may be indicated, providing ample introduction to its pros and cons, collaboratively arriving at a decision as to its use, and delineating directions for its use while checking to make sure the patient understands these directions.

In this chapter, we have addressed the first two tasks. In the next three chapters, we will fully explore the Choice Triad. In doing so, we will address elements of the third medication-oriented goal listed above. Patient-centered, shared decision making will serve as the foundation for our ongoing medication alliance.

It only seems fitting to end this chapter with the wise words of Howard Brody with which we began it: "It may be argued that the ongoing personal relationship with each patient is the . . . tool of the trade for the primary care physician. The primary care physician's approach to the patient's problem is grounded in the way the patient defines the problem." In the next three chapters, we will discover exactly how our patients go about this defining business.

REFERENCES

1. Brody H. *The Healer's Power.* New Haven, CT: Yale University Press; 1992:38–39.
2. Wilson IR, Schoen C, Neuman P, et al. Physician-patient communication about prescription medication nonadherence: a 50-state study of American seniors. *J Gen Intern Med* 2007;22(1):6–12.
3. Farell B, Szeto W, Shamji S. Drug-related problems in the frail elderly. *Can Fam Physician* 2011;57(2):168–169. Accessed https://www.ncbi.nlm.nih.gov/pmc/articles/PMC3038805/
4. Weiden P. The adherence interview: better information, better alliance. *Psychiatr Ann* 2011;41(5):279–285.

CHAPTER 7

First Step of the Choice Triad: Is There Something Really Wrong?

"One of the essential qualities of the clinician is interest in humanity, for the secret of the care of the patient is in caring for the patient."[1]

Francis Peabody, MD
JOURNAL OF THE AMERICAN MEDICAL ASSOCIATION (88TH VOLUME, 1927)

INTRODUCTION: OUR FIRST PRINCIPLE

Peabody's quotation has always been one of my favorites. It seems to embody the very essence of our work, and it is as fresh today as it was many decades ago. Having examined interviewing principles and techniques designed for use in the first appointment, we are now ready to further explore several nuanced techniques that can be of further use in the initial interview or any time we are about to prescribe a new medication in ongoing therapy. In addition, they are equally useful, or perhaps even of greater use, whenever one of our patients is wrestling with whether he or she wants to continue with a medication during ongoing treatment. It is here – at the critical junction of introducing the potential use of a new medication or of helping a patient to decide whether an old medication is worth continuing – that we can pull on the framework of the Choice Triad from Chapter 5 for on-the-spot, real-time guidance and intervention.

It is during these moments of delicate, shared decision making – ripe with the potential for disagreement – that patients often determine just how much we genuinely care about them, a judgment often determined by the words we choose. It is why the creation of the medication alliance is often the forge from which the overall therapeutic alliance will emerge. But before this collaboration can begin, its success will hinge on a simple fact – the very essence of Step 1 of the Choice Triad – does the patient truly believe he or she has something wrong? With the above considerations in mind, our first principle for navigating Step 1 of the Choice Triad emerges: *When one has picked-up a new patient, at some time in the first several appointments, and optimally in the first appointment, it is of value to directly ascertain where the patient sits on Step 1 of the Choice Triad.* Once again, clinician assumptions here can be quite misleading.

Does the Patient Truly Believe?

Exploring the Diagnostic Passport: A Simple Yet Useful Interviewing Strategy

In their therapeutic journey, our patients experience a multitude of both medications and those who prescribe them. Understanding the impact of these experiences (both good and bad) can be accomplished by exploring their so-called psychological passports regarding these issues (e.g., the medication passport and the patient's passport regarding previous prescribers) addressed in the preceding chapter. There remains one more passport of potentially great significance – the diagnostic passport.

Diagnoses carry powerful connotations that can have major ramifications for ongoing medication interest and motivation. One only needs to think of the effective motivating power of the diagnosis of cancer for enhancing medication interest to immediately see the truth of this statement.

In this regard, patients are given many diagnoses. Some of them are correct; others wrong. Moreover, even when they are correct – and can potentially help with treatment planning – patients may have misunderstandings regarding their meaning and significance. Such misunderstandings can have a significant damaging effect on medication interest and follow-through.

I find that the following three interviewing techniques (although simple in nature and obvious in name) can be helpful in exploring the patient's views regarding his or her current and past diagnoses. These intimate, and sometimes highly charged, personal views can greatly affect medication interest, for who would want to take a medication for a disorder that one does not believe he or she has? As we saw in Chapter 5 when introducing the Choice Triad, it would not be logical to do so. The trio of techniques is as follows:

TIP 13 Inquiry into Current Diagnoses

"Have you been given a diagnosis?"

TIP 14 Inquiry into Diagnostic Understanding

"What is your understanding of what that diagnosis means?"

TIP 15 Inquiry into Diagnostic Agreement

"Do you agree with that diagnosis?"

These three interviewing techniques and the collaborative exploration that follows each of them are usually done in sequence, an interviewing strategy simply called **Exploring the Diagnostic Passport**. As straightforward and simplistic as these three techniques may seem, I am consistently fascinated by how often clinicians do not ask them.

The answers are sometimes quite surprising and almost always important. Do not be surprised to find a patient who does not know the diagnoses that appear in his or her electronic health record (EHR). Clinicians are not always clear in what they tell patients, and, even when they are, patients do not always clearly hear what is said.

Clinicians often employ this very effective three-question strategy in their initial appointment, often during the history of the present illness. It is not unusual, during history taking, for a patient to spontaneously provide his or her current diagnosis without the first interviewing technique – the Inquiry into Current Diagnosis – of the three-question strategy even being asked. When this occurs, it is quite natural to follow-up with the next two questions of the strategy.

I have found that if my patient reports doubts about his or her diagnosis in an early part of our first meeting, there is no reason for me to challenge his or her doubt at that precise moment, even if I agree with the patient's current diagnosis as documented in the EHR. First, such a premature challenge may seriously hurt the therapeutic alliance. Second, it is always wise to arrive at one's own diagnosis, for previous diagnoses can be inaccurate.

Instead, *if* the patient voices serious doubts about his or her diagnoses, it is an opportune time to say something along the lines of, "One of the things we can look at today is whether or not we feel comfortable that these diagnoses are accurate – they may not be. It would be a great thing for us to explore together. And at the end of the appointment I'll share with you my own ideas about your diagnosis. How does that sound?"

Going Deeper: Helping Patients to See the Danger Behind the Diagnosis

At first glance, one would think that patients would – by the very nature of the fact that they have a disease – view themselves as having a serious problem with which they want help. Alas, we are not such simple animals. Many psychological, and even cultural, biases affect a patient's perception of wellness and illness. You will encounter many situations in which a patient – despite his or her recognition of having a disease – may not feel that he or she is particularly ill, in which case it is quite logical that the patient will question whether he or she needs a medication.

Some of these situations will be unique, but a large number will fall into one of the following four categories: (1) a patient has a serious disease, but it presents with minimal or no symptoms at first (hypertension, hyperlipidemia, diabetes); (2) healthy denial – or not so healthy denial – may make a patient hesitant to accept the diagnosis of a disabling or potentially lethal disease (multiple sclerosis, cancer, AIDS); (3) the patient is dealing with a highly stigmatized behavioral disorder (dementia, bipolar disorder, schizophrenia); or (4) the patient is hesitant to accept a disorder with which the culture assigns blame (obesity, alcohol dependence, substance abuse).

No matter which situation is operant, a patient who does not believe that there is something wrong will not be interested in taking a medication. Once again, it would not be logical to do so. Thus, when addressing the first step of the Choice Triad, clinicians are often faced with the task of helping a patient to understand the truth regarding what the ramifications are for having a particular diagnosis and, subsequently, generating motivation to do something about the problem (which may, or may not, be the use of a medication).

Moreover, just because a patient, newly referred to you, has been carrying a diagnosis for years does not guarantee that he or she understood its ramifications while under the care of previous providers. It is not so much that a patient intellectually understands that he or she is, indeed, dealing with a given disease that is important; it is whether the patient believes, in his or her gut, that this disease is truly dangerous if untreated. A Princeton-educated corporate executive may intellectually recognize that she has high blood pressure, but not really understand – in her gut – how much she is at risk of a debilitating stroke or a lethal myocardial infarction.

Curiously, even with a well-known patient under your care for years, who, earlier in your care, was fully aware that he or she had a serious disease, you may need to intermittently return to addressing Step 1 of the Choice Triad. With the passing of time, as well as with success (patient's symptoms abating) it becomes all too easy for patients to lose a compelling, gut-level understanding of the dangerousness of their disease. With the dissipation of this understanding, there can be a corresponding dissipation of medication interest and commitment to use.

Whatever the case, before one can begin to transform a patient's inaccurate belief system regarding the presence of a disease and its severity, one must ascertain what the patient believes in the first place. One must ask directly for surprises are not uncommon. Too often clinicians begin trying to convince their patients that the pros of a medication will outweigh its cons (third step of the Choice Triad) before the patient even agrees that there is something seriously wrong enough to warrant such a medication (first step of the Choice Triad).

I have found the following two questions to be of value in this task. The first question addresses, in an open-ended fashion, the patient's general understanding of the disease as it might appear, for the sake of discussion, on Wikipedia, hence its name. Indeed, many patients will have actually looked up their disease in Wikipedia! The second question directly taps whether the patient truly has registered the potential range of symptoms, eventual severity of symptoms if unchecked, and prognosis including potential for death if indeed present.

TIP 16 The Wikipedia Question

"Mrs. Jenkins, what is your understanding of what diabetes is [substitute the disease in question] and what it is doing to your body?"

TIP 17 Gut-Check Question

"What's your understanding of how dangerous diabetes can be?"

Because of their open-ended nature, these two questions frequently open a doorway into important patient beliefs that may impact directly, or indirectly, on the patient's medication interest and follow-through. When answering the Wikipedia Question, the patient may share a surprisingly sophisticated knowledge base regarding his or her disease process or perhaps almost no understanding at all (a situation certainly not conducive to high medication interest and follow-through).

Patients may also spontaneously hint at their personal understandings of the etiology of their diseases when responding to the Wikipedia Question. We will see in Chapter 13, on the cultural aspects of talking with patients about medications, that both cultural and psychological beliefs regarding etiology may play a major role in determining medication interest. If a person feels that diabetes is caused by spiritual weakness or a demon, it is unlikely that medications will be viewed as relevant. If a person is in the throes of a guilt-laden major depressive episode, he or she may believe that he or she deserves to develop serious complications or even death, "Everyone would be better off without me."

When using the Gut-Check Question, it is important to observe how the patient describes possible sequelae to the disease as it unfolds. I have found that I can frequently intuit from nonverbal cues, such as the patient's tone of voice and general affect, whether he or she is truly worried about symptom progression and prognosis or just intellectually cognizant of it. The former state bodes well for high medication interest, the latter bodes poorly. It is hard to take a medication, frequently expensive in nature with potentially serious adverse reactions (or to undertake difficult behavioral interventions such as losing weight or dieting for that matter), unless one deeply feels that there is something seriously wrong.

Initial Foray into the Art of Patient Education

With the above ideas in mind, we have arrived at the topic of the art of patient education. How does one transform patient belief by the process of sensitive education? It is a good question. Patient education is indeed an art, to which much attention and thousands of pages have been dedicated – many of them were penned from the discipline of nursing, which has long recognized the importance of training clinicians how to teach. A full discussion would take us well beyond the intended domain of this book, but I believe it is important for us to examine a few core principles as related to Step 1 of the Choice Triad.

I am sometimes asked, "Should we scare patients?" The question can be rephrased as, "To what degree does fear play a role in providing motivation to take a medication (exercise regularly, change diet, etc.)?" It is a legitimate question, and the answer is a bit complicated. It is complicated because the words "scare" and "fear" are loaded with negative baggage in most cultures. Put bluntly, they sound bad. Truth be told, the words make more sense when provided with qualifiers.

Obviously, with regard to Step 1, fear plays a role, in the sense that one may be motivated by a legitimate and *well-informed* fear of the consequences of an unchecked disease as would occur when an indicated medication is not used or used improperly. The operative term here is "well-informed." Our goal is not to terrify our patients but to provide them with a well-informed understanding of what is at stake for each of them individually so that they can make a well-informed decision regarding their own level of concern and motivation.

If one creates too much fear, the result can backfire. Humans generally cannot tolerate constant or overwhelming fear for too long. Unconscious defense mechanisms will kick in and mute the message so that the intense fear goes away. With it, so goes motivation. Thus, terrifying patients is not the path to medication interest, but creating appropriate and well-informed fear is. To do so requires the clinician to approach this creation in a flexible manner with each unique patient, for patients may vary in how much fear is required in order to be well informed.

Each person will process potential difficulties in a different fashion. For some patients, a low-keyed and matter of fact description of possible symptoms and problematic outcomes (including death if it is part of the potential picture as with hyperlipidemia or hypertension) will be enough to motivate them to an effective level of medication interest and subsequent action. Others may need some time to process what is often difficult information to process. They may require subsequent, and more intense, discussion of the consequences of a stroke or heart attack on both themselves and those who love them. A few may need frequent, and fairly intense, illustrations of their dangers. Each person handles potentially frightening news in varying fashions. Like coaching, the art lies in matching the approach to the needs of the player. In this regard, I always suggest starting gently. See how your patient responds. Increase the intensity of your depictions and illustrations of potential bad outcomes as needed.

There are many more interviewing principles and techniques for enhancing patient education. We have just touched on one set of patient education principles utilized when addressing Step 1 of the Choice Triad. We will return to the topic of patient education in future pages because it pertains to specific educational challenges addressed by the Medication Interest Model (MIM).

The Hunt for Target Symptoms

From What Does the Patient Most Want Relief?

Once a patient realizes that he or she has a serious disorder such as congestive heart failure (CHF) or systemic lupus, the clinician's exploration of Step 1 often becomes more nuanced in nature. It is no longer an issue of whether the patient feels that there is something seriously wrong; he or she does. Instead, the emphasis now shifts to the equally important task of finding out which symptoms the patient most wants relief from at this moment. Medications that provide relief of this symptom or set of symptoms will frequently stimulate the most interest and subsequent motivation for use. Curiously, the symptoms with which the patient has the most concerns and from which he or she wants the fastest relief may not be as obvious as one might think at first glance, unless one asks the patient directly. The reason for this subtly hidden roadblock lays in the fact that we are on one side of the stethoscope and the patient is on the other. We think clinically. Patients think experientially. We hear about symptoms from our patients. Patients live with them.

To some degree, medical, nursing, physician assistant, and clinical pharmacy programs teach clinicians to treat diseases, but people generally take medications not so much because they have a disease but to get relief from the symptoms and the suffering their disease is causing. The difference in perspective is subtle, but it is real, with potentially telling ramifications for the building and maintaining of the medication alliance.

Obviously, in the long term, a potent driver for medication interest and use is a patient's belief that a medication can reverse or ameliorate a potentially lethal or disabling disease. But one should never underestimate the fact that in the short term, the trust that a patient has in his or her health care provider – from prescribing clinicians to case managers – is often largely determined by how hard he or she feels that the provider is working to bring relief from that individual's *self-identified* most pressing symptoms.

Wisdom from a Past Century

The great physician, Sir William Osler (pronounced with a long "O"), might be able to provide some practical insight here. Osler was knighted for his pioneering work in advancing Victorian and Edwardian medicine. He was born in 1849. By the time he died 70 years later in 1919, he had left quite a legacy, having been one of the greatest physicians to have practiced at McGill University in Canada. He was also a founding father of Johns Hopkins

University in Baltimore, Maryland, and later retired as Regius Professor at Oxford, England. In his spare time, he managed to write one of the greatest general textbooks of internal medicine in the history of medicine and nursing. Busy guy. But what I liked best about Osler was the fact that he was a bit of a renegade.

Osler was a renegade in the sense that, in a time when the "science" of medicine was all the rage, he always held compassion as the foremost principle of medicine. It is said that he had a remarkable way with his patients. He was known as much for his kind bedside manner as he was for his splendid diagnostic innovations. In a sense, one could argue that he was a forerunner of "person-centered medicine" about 100 years before it was formally delineated. To illustrate my point, we only need to look at the following oft-quoted axiom by Osler:

> "It is much more important to know what sort of patient has a disease than to know what sort of disease a patient has."[2]

According to Osler's perspective, each patient will uniquely view the impact and importance of his or her symptoms. A symptom (or a side-effect for that matter) that bothers one patient immensely may be perceived by a different patient as a mere nuisance. Patients' perceptions of their symptoms depend on who they are as people (psychologically, spiritually, and culturally).

Patients will be motivated to stick with a medication to the degree that they personally feel the medication is relieving them of their most problematic symptoms. We need to find out what symptoms these are for each unique patient. To do so, we must understand who the person is beneath the diagnosis, a theme we have repeatedly emphasized in this book. To punctuate the point, let us look at an example commonly encountered in any primary care setting – CHF.

First, let us picture a 76-year-old woman, whom we shall call Mrs. Hayes. Mrs. Hayes presents with severe dyspnea on exertion (DOE) to the point that she literally can barely get up the stairs to the second floor of her house. It would be easy enough for a clinician hearing about such a disabling symptom to feel that offering relief from it would be a powerful motivator for medication interest and use. The prescribing clinician might say, "Mrs. Hayes I think I may have a medication that might really help you to get up those stairs" thinking that the patient would find such an offer powerfully motivating. One problem. The second floor of her house only contains bedrooms for her children who are long gone. She seldom has a desire to go up those stairs.

Now picture a 32-year-old patient, Barry Mack, who suffers from equally disabling CHF after having contracted a viral myocarditis. His new family practitioner, as the history of the present illness unfolds, takes the time to uncover that Barry is a professional artist, at present, struggling mightily. We will soon see why he struggles so. Like Mrs. Hayes, Barry also has debilitating DOE. It makes reaching his second floor nearly impossible. And here is the catch.

It is on the second floor that Barry has built his studio. He has had huge ceiling windows installed that allow natural light to flow into the room. He comments to his physician, "It's the only place I can work, I have to have natural light to do my painting. My career is essentially over." Now imagine a physician who says, "Barry, I think I may have a medication that might really help you to get up those stairs."

The difference in medication interest between these two patients is staggering, even though the physicians each pinpointed the same symptom (severe in nature with both patients) for relief. The second physician has taken the time to find out what sort of patient has the disease and the first one has not. The second physician, who understands the needs of his artist patient, will have treatment success. The former physician, who does not understand the needs of Mrs. Hayes, probably will not.

Both Mrs. Hayes and Barry are presenting with advanced disease states. But attention to the patient's perspectives on what symptoms need attention *right now* is also important even with patients in the early stages of a disease process. To make the point, let us picture our Mrs. Hayes several years earlier. Mrs. Hayes is presenting with milder DOE, yet still bothersome in nature according to her own self-report, as well as other early symptoms of CHF. Also imagine that Mrs. Hayes is medication shy for she has had a series of nasty side-effects and adverse reactions over the years for a myriad of other diseases. Her DOE is bad enough that it makes going up to the second floor quite unpleasant. Once again, it would be easy for a prescribing clinician to assume that her DOE would be an excellent target symptom.

Fortunately, our prescriber, using an interviewing technique we are about to delineate, comes upon an unexpected discovery. Mrs. Hayes does not view her DOE as her most problematic symptom. Upon gentle questioning, she belatedly describes her intense embarrassment at the appearance of her ankles, as well as having problems getting into some of her shoes, because of the edema in her ankles and feet caused by her CHF. Her shame has prevented her from going to shoe stores for months, a shopping ritual she sorely misses, for she had always prided herself on having "nice, nothing fancy mind you, but nice shoes."

This tiny snapshot of "humanness" may seem, at first glance, mundane and unimportant, but it is not. It is exactly what Sir William Osler was looking for – what kind of person has a disease. It may, in its own unassuming way, hold the key to creating a powerful and lasting alliance with this elderly patient, for if a medication can be used, such as a diuretic that rapidly takes away her edema, the clinician may have found a medication that the patient is probably going to want to stay on. More importantly, the patient has found a clinician that she is probably going to want to keep. As we mentioned in Chapter 2, when one forges a sound medication alliance (the microcosm), one is often simultaneously forging a sound overall therapeutic alliance (the macrocosm).

Techniques for Uncovering the Patient's Priorities for Symptom Relief

We can now translate Osler's axiom into the following interviewing principle: *Before recommending a medication, directly ask patients from which of their symptoms they most want relief. Assume nothing.* Let us examine two interviewing techniques that can allow us to more effectively apply this principle. Both techniques were relayed to me by primary care clinicians in one of my MIM workshops. Let us continue with our elderly CHF patient as an example:

TIP 18 Target Symptoms Question

"Mrs. Hayes, of all of your different heart symptoms, which are the ones that you most want me to help you with today?"

TIP 19 Magic Pill Question

"Mrs. Hayes, if I had a magic pill – and I don't – but if I did, and it could completely take away just one of your heart symptoms which one would you want me to get rid of today?"

When through the use of such questions a prescriber can uncover which symptoms are most discouraging from the patient's standpoint and then agree to do something about those specific symptoms, patients truly feel that they are being heard, and, in fact, they are. Each of the techniques provides a succinct and effective way to employ Osler's axiom. Both ends of the stethoscope can start liking each other a good deal more. A team is being forged within minutes of the initial meeting.

Also note that both the Target Symptoms Question and the Magic Pill Question are nice examples of interviewing techniques (easily learned and taught questions or statements that are behaviorally specific and tagged with a name) that were derived from a single interviewing principle – *Before recommending a medication, directly ask patients to tell you from which of their symptoms they most want relief. Assume nothing.* The behavioral specificity of the two techniques allows us to employ this interviewing principle in differing ways depending on the needs of the patient. Note that these two questions are not identical in phrasing, request, and tone. Consequently, their subsequent influence on patients is not necessarily the same. The Target Symptoms Question asks the patient for multiple symptoms, whereas the Magic Pill Question requires the patient to choose a single symptom.

Picture an elderly patient who is constantly second-guessing everything and everyone by his very nature. Throughout his long life, he has second-guessed every decision he has made. He hates being asked to make decisions for he always feels he has made the wrong one, spending hours of time ruminating about his decision. If I wanted to uncover from which symptoms of his CHF he himself most wants relief, the Magic Pill Question (which forces him to make a specific *single* decision) might be quite disturbing. He might spend the next two days worrying, "Oh my God, I told the doctor the wrong thing to help me with!" This patient may find the Target Symptoms Question much less unsettling for it allows him the freedom to share a variety of symptoms related to his CHF.

In contrast, picture a 10-year-old girl who is developing heart failure related to congenital heart defects that have not been completely alleviated by surgical intervention. She walks into your office wearing a "magic cape" and carrying three Harry Potter books. This 10-year-old is practically begging the interviewer to use the Magic Pill Question, "Now if I had a magic pill, like Harry Potter might have – and I don't – but if I did and I could help you with just one of your symptoms from your heart problems, which one would you like me to try to help you with first?"

In both of the above instances, the clinician has matched the interviewing technique to the unique desires and psychological functioning of the patient. Using such information to intentionally utilize a specific interviewing technique may lead to the discovery of a more powerful personal motivator for enhancing medication interest, a more effective use of the medication, and a significantly improved outcome for each of the patients.

A slightly different technique – the List Maker's Question – is a variation of the Target Symptoms Question and seems to be of use with patients with a leaning toward, as one would guess, the making and utilizing of lists. The technique, a superb example of shared decision making, was provided by a child psychiatrist Amit Gupta during one of my workshops. I think you will find it to be of use with selective patients:

TIP 20 List Maker's Question

"If you can give me an idea of which of your symptoms are the most bothersome for you, you know, cause you the most problems, I think it might help us to choose the best medications for you. Let's see if we can list them in order of most bothersome to least bothersome. And we'll try to figure out which medication or medications might help with what is bothering you the most."

In our discussion on patient-identified target symptoms, we have inadvertently come upon an important realization. It is not only the presence of a disease and its accompanying symptoms that drives medication interest and follow-through. The suffering *(unique to each patient)* caused by the disease and its symptoms functions as a major motivating factor. Both Mrs. Hayes and Barry had the same disease, CHF (and a similar severity of symptoms), yet the suffering caused by each of their symptoms varied greatly between the two of them.

This immensely important principle is often made more concrete and user-friendly by making a distinction between the words "disease" and "illness." A **disease** is the disruption of the patient's biologic structure and physiology (objective in nature). An **illness** is the amount of experiential suffering (subjective in nature) caused by this disease to this particular patient. The intensity of the **illness** – a major driver toward medication interest and use – is determined by a complex matrix including the patient's health beliefs, psychological perspectives and defenses, cultural influences, familial supports and pressures, spiritual beliefs, and the direct impact of the disease on the patient's means of livelihood, housing, and safety.[3]

The distinction between disease and illness is at the root of innovative movements such as patient-centered medicine/nursing and person-centered medicine/nursing. It is eloquently captured by Juan Mezzich, one of the founders of person-centered medicine, and his colleagues:

> ".... asking patients how they feel about their illness, how it affects their lives, rather than focusing only on the disease, results in substantially increased trust and treatment adherence. This often allows the patient and clinician to find a common ground on treatment, prevention and health promotion. Thus, person-centeredness offers a 'clinical method of participatory democracy', a factor in success of treatment and improvement of the patient's quality of life; better understanding of the psychological aspects of a patient's problems; and improved patient confidence regarding sensitive problems."[4]

This distinction between disease and illness – and the principles of patient-centered and person-centered medicine which follow from this distinction – will serve us well throughout the remaining chapters of this book as we move ever deeper into the practical application of the MIM.

Conclusion

From the above discussion, we can see the power of the interviewing principles and techniques of the MIM emerging. Techniques such as the Wikipedia Question and the Target Symptoms Question allow us to more effectively demonstrate the caring that Francis Peabody highlighted in our opening epigram. It is one thing to care. It is another thing to effectively demonstrate that care. Both are critical for healing to be maximized and medication interest to be generated.

In this chapter, we have developed a toolbox that contains a variety of specific interviewing techniques that will allow us to better gauge a patient's position regarding the question, "Am I really sick?" But even if a person feels that there is something seriously wrong, he or she may still lack interest in using a medication, for the patient must also believe in the power of the medication, itself, to fix what is wrong.

This search for motivation to use a specific medication for a specific patient-identified reason is the topic of our next chapter. It will prove to be a nice example of shared decision making. Curiously, we will find that the promise of symptom relief, powerful as it might be, is not always the most powerful motivator for medication use. It is our patients who hold the secrets to these motivators. We need only ask the right questions to unlock them.

REFERENCES

1. Peabody F. A medical classic: the care of the patient by Francis W. Peabody. *JAMA* 1927;88:877.
2. Osler W. *The New Medicine website*. http://www.thenewmedicine.org/timeline/doctor_patient_book.html. Accessed June 11, 2016.
3. Jakovljevic M, Ostojic L. Person-centered medicine and good clinical practice: disease has to be cured, but the patient has to be healed. *Medicina Mostariensa* 2015;3(1-2):2–5.
4. Mezzich J, Appleyard J, Botbol M, Ghebrehiwet T, Groves J, Salloum I.M., and van Dulmen S. Editorial Introduction: Primary health care and person centered medicine. *Inter J Person Centered Med* 2015;5(2):45–50.

CHAPTER 8

Second Step of the Choice Triad: Can a Medication Help Me?

"People are the undisputed experts on themselves. No one has been with them longer or knows them better than they do."[1]

William R. Miller

From MOTIVATIONAL INTERVIEWING: HELPING PEOPLE TO CHANGE

The Challenge

Having developed an effective toolbox for navigating Step 1 of the Choice Triad, we are now ready to move on to Step 2. Before proceeding, it may be useful to review the Choice Triad itself. If you will recall, the motivational model provided by the Choice Triad suggests that, for a patient to show a genuine interest in taking a medication as well as following through with its effective use, the patient must embrace the following three beliefs:

1. The patient must feel that there is something wrong from which he or she personally wants relief.
2. He or she must believe that the medication has the potential to bring relief from the perceived problem (or perhaps prevent a serious future problem as with a vaccine).
3. The patient must believe that the pros of taking the medication outweigh the cons.

If any one of these three beliefs is absent, or deteriorates, it is unlikely that the patient will continue with the medication, for it would be illogical to do so. With regard to Step 2, this belief will either be accepted or rejected by the patient by asking a no-nonsense question of themselves: "Can this medication help me?" Despite its simple structure, it is a deceptively complex question. The answer will depend on a multitude of factors, some of which are knowledge based – the patient understands the theory behind the use of the medication and agrees with it – and others of an interpersonal nature – the patient likes, respects, and trusts the clinician.

In point of fact, it is even more nuanced, for it has more than one step. It is not just that the patient must answer the question "Can this medication help me?" In addition, the patient must answer yet another question, for even if the answer is "yes" to the above question, patients will also need to ask themselves, "Is this medication the *best* way for me to get help?" Either the patient or the clinician (or both) may feel that an intervention such as diet, exercise, or an approach from complementary and alternative medicine (CAM) may be a better first choice.

If such is the case, and it is safe to do so, we can proceed to help the patient to effectively utilize whatever alternative approach he or she has chosen with the hope that it will indeed be successful. The less medications needed by a patient for effective healing, the better. In this regard, it is also of note that the Choice Triad (as well as many of the specific interviewing techniques of the MIM) is directly transferable to enhancing motivation and follow-through with nonmedication approaches such as diet and exercise or with CAM approaches.

Once a patient has decided that a medication is his or her preferred choice – either having chosen it immediately as the preferred choice of action when first suggested by the clinician or having had little success with an alternative approach, the patient subsequently has arrived at his or her own decision that a medication could be beneficial – the clinician will then be ready to focus on the critical process of enhancing the patient's belief in Step 2. It is the intensity of this belief that will prove to be one of the most potent drivers of the patient's motivation to stick with the prescribed medication despite the many difficulties that can arise from its use, not the least of which can be significant side effects or even more serious adverse reactions as well as financial burdens. In short, Step 2 is all about enhancing motivation.

From the clinician's perspective, the task of Step 2 becomes one of actively helping the patient to solidify his or her own personal motivational goals while tying the promise of achieving these goals (relief of symptoms, resolution or curing of his or her disease, prevention of a potential future disease, etc.) directly to the use of the medication being prescribed. *The more concretely the patient understands why he or she is taking the medication and the more deeply convinced that he or she becomes that the medication holds the most likely way to get the desired symptomatic relief or cure, the more likely that effective medication follow-through will occur.* In keeping with the spirit of the MIM, for the patient to have a robust motivation to initially use and to subsequently continue to use the medication, these beliefs must be arrived at by the patient on his or her own terms.

The Delicate Art of Enhancing Motivation

Common Sense Bridges

With some of our patients, the securing and enhancing of Step 2 of the Choice Triad is a relatively easy matter. From our joint exploration of Step 1, we will have discovered one or more powerful motivators (appearing as specific symptoms or disease states) that the patient has highlighted as problematic and with which the patient wants help. All we have to do is to make a bridge from Step 1 to Step 2 by indicating that we have a medication or medications that can help the patient to obtain relief from whatever symptoms or diseases he or she has identified as problematic. As one would expect, one of the primary factors that motivates a patient toward the use of a medication is the belief that the medication may remove a disturbing symptom. The specific symptom or symptoms will naturally vary from disease to disease.

On the simplest level, a patient with strep throat will seek relief from the distressing sore throat that is so common to strep. A patient with benign prostatic hypertrophy may want relief from urinary hesitancy or frequency. On more serious levels, a patient with congestive heart failure (CHF) may seek relief from a disabling dyspnea on exertion (DOE) or paroxysms of nocturnal dyspnea (PND). From Chapter 7, we have seen that questions such as the Target Symptoms Question and the Magic Pill Question can further secure motivation by collaboratively uncovering the patient's most desired areas for symptom relief.

For other patients, or as a second motivator for the patients already focusing on symptom relief, the Diagnostic Passport, as uncovered in Step 1, may secure yet another motivational pool. In this sense, the hope of getting rid of an identified disease, by name, can be an equally potent motivator as seeking symptom relief, or in some instances an even more potent motivator.

This situation is particularly true if a patient has a serious, or life-threatening, disease. In such instances, simple phrases emphasizing the effectiveness of the proposed medication in addressing the specific disease at hand can be particularly useful; for example, "Mrs. Anderson, this set of medications is specifically designed to hit exactly this type of cancer" or "We're going to do everything we can to bring your rheumatoid arthritis into remission, Mrs. Anderson, and I have several medications that I've found to be particularly good at doing so."

Although somewhat obvious in nature, it is surprising how easy it is, in a hectic clinic or hospital setting, to miss the opportunity for effectively using such phrases. In addition, saying the words is not enough. It is how we say them that determines their ultimate power. To maximize their power, the clinician must gracefully embed them into the ongoing conversation, do so in an unhurried fashion, and make sure that eye contact is excellent. Moreover, the conversational moment chosen for making the empowering statement must be both well timed and memorable.

Needless to say, during such conversations, the clinician's laptop or clipboard should be out of the way, either out of reach on a desk, a shelf, or on the floor. It is also often useful to repeat the connection between the use of the medication and its impact on the disease later in the conversation to further secure its impact. In short, the clinician wants to make the statement stick. Besides increasing medication interest, such statements also can generate hope and mobilize those placebo effects that seem to impact on pathophysiology.

Thus far, we have been talking about enhancing motivation by focusing on the specific symptoms and/or diseases that were uncovered during our explorations of Step 1 of the Choice Triad. But some patients are motivated to use their medications effectively by factors that are unrelated to symptom relief directly. These personalized *situational* motivators are unique to the patient's worldview and interpersonal situation. They are sometimes surprisingly powerful, indeed sometimes more effective at enhancing medication interest and follow-through than symptom relief or the targeting of the patient's disease per se.

Put succinctly, these personalized motivators arise more from the patient's illness than his or her disease. I am reminded of yet another quotation from William Osler: "The good physician will treat the disease, but the great physician will treat the illness."[2] Indeed, we have already discussed the fashion in which motivation for medication use can be mined from an exploration of the patient's illness perspectives back in Chapter 2 with our very first prototypic interviewing tip – the Inquiry into Lost Dreams.

"Inquiry into Lost Dreams" Revisited

If you will recall, the Inquiry into Lost Dreams was the technique shared by a pediatrician during one of my MIM workshops. He described how he utilized it with adolescents presenting with asthma. I want to revisit it here for two reasons. First, although introduced earlier, as a teaser of sorts, demonstrating the effectiveness of a specific interviewing technique drawn from a specific interviewing principle, the Inquiry into Lost Dreams is, in reality, a tool from the toolbox utilized for navigating Step 2 of the Choice Triad. And it is here that we can better illustrate its effectiveness contextually and via clinical dialogue. Second, it is one of my favorite techniques. I have found it to be both simple to use and remarkably effective.

As noted in Chapter 2, the Inquiry into Lost Dreams evolved from the following interviewing principle: *The most powerful motivators patients may have for using a medication may be directly related to regaining a lost life activity as opposed to mere symptom relief*. Let's repeat some of the material from Chapter 2 to refresh our memories.

In the workshop, our pediatrician commented that one of the most powerful motivators for some of his adolescent patients was the obvious one: They wanted relief from their acute asthmatic attacks. But he found this to be true only if the adolescent was experiencing severe and frightening asthmatic attacks, which many of his patients were not (see pages 28–29). He discovered that with patients whose attacks were disruptive but not necessarily frightening in nature, there often existed a more powerful motivator for using medications. Curiously, it was not directly related to relief from the asthmatic symptoms themselves. Moreover, it was a motivating factor that he found he could repeatedly tap whenever his adolescents were having tough side effects even to the extent of wanting to discontinue their meds.

What was the secret to generating such tenacious medication interest? What was the personalized motivator so common with kids suffering from asthma? He went on to describe that, more often than not, his patients were not seeking relief from something that the asthma had given them – shortness of breath. They wanted back something that the asthma had taken from them – to be normal again. They wanted to play a sport again that they loved. They wanted to be able to function again just like the other kids. They wanted to be free of the stigma of "being an asthmatic."

It is no different with our adult patients. In many instances, patients with diseases from rheumatoid arthritis to chronic obstructive pulmonary disease (COPD) and CHF want back their dreams, their livelihoods, their peace of mind, their self-esteem, and the confidence to pursue goals without becoming beset with self-doubts. The desire to recover these lost dreams can often provide powerful motivators that may help patients to tolerate surprisingly unpleasant side effects.

Let's review the wording of the technique:

TIP 21 Inquiry into Lost Dreams

"Is there anything that your asthma is keeping you from doing that you really wish you could do again?"

If you will recall, if the student responds by giving the name of a specific sport or other activity, the clinician can finish the Inquiry into Lost Dreams as follows:

"Now I can't promise this, but I have had some very good luck with helping other students, with asthma like yours, to get back into their sports. We have some great medications that can help with that goal. Once again, no promises, but I would like to work with you to see if we might be able to get you back out on that soccer field. How does that sound to you?"

We now have an opportunity to bring the Inquiry into Lost Dreams to life with some clinical dialogue. Let's imagine a 62-year-old grandmother suffering from CHF and osteoarthritis (In her youth, she was a runner who ran just a little too far too often.) She is also battling about 40 pounds of uninvited weight, although she has lost about 10 pounds in the past year – not bad. In short, she would be a fairly typical patient in any primary care clinic or private practice.

In any case, our patient, whom we shall call Mrs. Moss, has been around the block with doctors, nurse clinicians, and physician assistants for many years. We shall picture that she is meeting this physician for the very first time. We are going to pick up this interview early in their initial appointment, long before we see the clinician using the Inquiry into Lost Dreams, for this early snippet of dialogue demonstrates an important aspect of the MIM: The MIM techniques are not used in a vacuum.

As discussed above, they are woven into the conversation in a naturalistic fashion that is interdependent with the interviewer's ongoing engagement with the patient. Their effectiveness is enhanced by the clinician's abilities to quickly "get a read" on his or her patient's personality style and, from this knowledge, more effectively choose and apply the MIM techniques. In this instance, the opening vignette shows us something important about

Mrs. Moss that allows the clinician to more effectively employ the Inquiry into Lost Dreams later in the appointment: Specifically, despite her anxiety, she has a sense of humor:

Clin.: I'm glad to see you could make it today. I've been looking forward to meeting you. Your previous doctor, Dr. Jamison, sent a very nice referral letter and explained some of your problems with your heart. Hopefully I can help.

Pt.: Well, the first thing you need to do, Doc, is do something about those steps of yours.

Clin.: I'm not sure I follow you Mrs. Moss.

Pt.: Your steps up from the lower parking lot. You know, the ones that look like the steps from the movie *The Exorcist* (patient gives a wry smile).

Clin.: (physician finally gets where this is going and smiles) Oh, *those* steps.

Pt.: Yea, *those* steps . . . a little rough for someone with a bad heart and bum knees to climb up.

Clin.: Oh yea (pause), we probably should have told you about the upper parking lot.

Pt.: Really? There's an upper parking lot? (patient gives a foxlike smile)

Clin.: Well, the good news is that I see that you're not out of breath now, so that says something good about your heart function, because those are pretty nasty steps.

Pt.: I hate to burst your bubble, Doc. But the reason I'm not out of breath now is that I had to wait 45 minutes in your waiting room (accented with a pointed, yet still friendly, "umph").

Clin.: Hmmm. (chuckling) You're a bit feisty for someone with a bad heart. I see I'm going to have to stay on my toes here.

Pt.: Oh, you're going to need to do better than that. You're gonna need an extra set of toes, Doc.

Well, I think it is safe to say that our Mrs. Moss is a bit of a pip, in a delightful fashion of course. But the good news is that there is a playfulness here that betrays both a sharp intellect, a pretty good sense of self-esteem, and the opening for the clinician to be able to also use humor as an engagement tool that can subsequently be utilized to provide some personalized nuances to some of the MIM techniques, such as the Inquiry into Lost Dreams.

Let's pick up our dialogue with Mrs. Moss, much deeper into her initial appointment, after the clinician's initial history and physical examination

(H&P) has been completed. Let us assume that the provider, while exploring her Diagnostic Passport, has uncovered that Mrs. Moss has a pretty good knowledge about both her CHF and her osteoarthritis.

On the other hand, while exploring her Medication Passport, the clinician has adeptly uncovered that she has considerable hesitancies about being on medications, which she has seldom taken in the fashion that her previous physician Dr. Jamison had prescribed. But she also has hesitancies about being on a diet and exercising too! In short, she is where many of our patients find themselves, between the proverbial rock and the hard place. She is obviously motivated to get symptom relief, but it's not enough to keep her on her meds.

Can our provider help Mrs. Moss to mobilize a personalized, situational motivator in the same fashion as our pediatrician so adeptly does with his adolescents with asthma? The Inquiry into Lost Dreams is designed explicitly to do just that:

Pt.: You know it's frustrating at times, the shortness of breath, I mean.

Clin.: Oh, I'm sure it is. I would imagine it is very frustrating. It sounds like it's even tough for you to get upstairs sometimes.

Pt.: Oh, I don't even go up to the third floor anymore . . . not worth the trouble, if you know what I mean. I've not only got the functional heart of a mouse, I've got the knees of a dead horse.

Clin.: Not good.

Pt.: No, not good.

Clin.: You know, Mrs. Moss, after listening to your history, I'm starting to get some ideas about how I might be able to help, but I'd like to get an even better idea of how much your heart condition limits what you can do. Think carefully about this one. Is there anything that you really want to do, that you just can't do, you know something that it really pains you that you can't do because of your heart condition? **(Inquiry into Lost Dreams)**

Pt.: (pauses, then sits up with a little more emotional charge) Why, yes there is. You know what really hurts me . . . I have the most lovely granddaughter, with the lovely name of Kamala, out in California, and when she was 3 years old I promised her that Gran "will someday take you to Disneyland." And you know what, I don't think it's ever going to happen. And what really bugs me is that she's ten now, and pretty soon, she's not going to want to go to Disneyland with Gran anyway.

Clin.: Well, that's sad. I can see why it hurts you so much. (pause) You know, what is it exactly that frightens you or makes you hesitant to go?

Pt.: Part of it is the airports and the plane. The last time I flew out there was over 2 years ago, I made it alright, but it was a real pain. It's just too much walking, and I hate being wheeled around in a stupid wheelchair, it's like I'm an old fogey or something. (pause) And I have to bring the oxygen sometimes and that's a pain in the butt. And I'm afraid that even when I get there, which I think I could manage, I wouldn't be any fun at Disneyland I'm afraid to say (almost tears up).

Clin.: Well, you know what?

Pt.: What?

Clin.: I really think I might have a medication that might help. It might actually help enough to get you out to Disneyland. I can't make a promise that it will, but I certainly can promise that I can try. And even if it can't get you out to Disneyland, I do think it might help your breathing considerably. If it's okay with you Mrs. Moss, I would like to see if you would be comfortable working with me to at least see if that is possible. What do you think? (**Inquiry into Lost Dreams** completed)

Pt.: Well . . . (sitting up, with a brighter affect, and a bit of a twinkle in her eye).

Clin.: Now don't get overexcited, (said smiling) I can't promise you a date with Mickey Mouse or anything!

Pt.: Doc. I decided a long time ago that I'm done with mice and men, ain't worth the trouble. But I'd sure like to get a picture of Kamala getting a big hug from that mouse. Now *that's* something I'd like to see.

Clin.: That's a wonderful image. Let's keep it in mind. It's a great reason to try the medication that I have in mind, and to see if it can help. Let me tell you a little bit about it, both the pros and cons, and you can see what you think about giving it a try. It's called . . .

This is an impressive demonstration of the Inquiry into Lost Dreams being seamlessly woven into an initial appointment following the H&P. Note also that, from the initial dialogue, the prescriber recognized that one could capitalize on Mrs. Moss's sense of humor to personalize the Inquiry into Lost Dreams. The clinician did so with the quip about Mickey Mouse. The resulting image that Mrs. Moss spontaneously generated – of Mickey Mouse hugging Kamala – is a potentially powerful motivator for her interest in trying a medication. It is also a motivating image she can return to over and over if her motivation might be challenged by side effects.

At such moments, it is also an image that the clinician can *intentionally* pull on, perhaps in a situation when the clinician might believe that the side effects could be reduced, if only the patient would not unilaterally discontinue the med between appointments, as with, "I know you're having some tough side effects – and they are tough – but fortunately, I have some ideas on how we might be able to make them much better, and I don't think we have seen the full power of this medication to help with your breathing just yet. Remember, we are still trying to get that picture of Kamala with Mickey, so if you can hang in there just a little bit longer, Mrs. Moss, it will give me a chance to see if I can get rid of some of these side effects for you. If we can't do that, well, then we will need to come up with something different. Here is what I suggest we try . . ."

A Variation on a Theme

In the above example, a transformative moment is occurring before our very eyes thanks to the skilled interviewing of the clinician. The Inquiry into Lost Dreams represents an easy-to-use, single interviewing technique for tapping highly personalized and, hence, meaningful motivators for patients. I have found it to be very fruitful for many patients, indeed most patients, but some patients may have difficulty identifying concrete losses or positive changes they want to make in their life.

It's my belief that such patients may cognitively handle stresses differently than others, perhaps with a little less concrete organization and directed problem solving than those patients who respond quickly and easily to the Inquiry into Lost Dreams. These patients have curiously not kept tabs on their specific losses, per se, so much as feeling a more overwhelming sense that all is lost or "everything is different." For such patients, I find that it is sometimes easier to approach the topic slightly differently by generically asking them to reflect on how their life might be different if a specific symptom or disease was gone.

This approach, which gently posits a "What if . . .?" kind of question, can often help them to discover powerful motivators that lie deep within their souls and that they had never fully consciously grasped as possibilities for achievement. I think you will find that if a patient does not offer much response to the Inquiry into Lost Dreams, you can pull the following closely allied variation of the Inquiry into Lost Dreams out of your toolbox. It is known as the Alternative History Question, and, depending on the disease in question, it sounds something along the following lines:

TIP 22 Alternative History Question

a. "If you didn't have your knee pain, what would you be doing, how would things be different?"
b. "If your prostate symptoms were gone, how would your life be different?"
c. "If your migraines were in better control, how would your future be changed?"
d. "If we could get your schizophrenia under better control, how would your life change?"

Depending on their specific disease state, the patients' answers can greatly vary but, not infrequently, they will carry a deeply personalized and emotional charge. Patients often respond to the Alternative History Question with answers like "I'd be able to play tennis again and be able to mow my own lawn instead of depending on others" (osteoarthritis); "I'd date again, I feel so embarrassed going to the bathroom constantly, and I have had so many embarrassing situations. I feel so old" (prostate enlargement); "I could work again. I wouldn't have to feel like I'm a misfit who everyone thinks is faking it" (migraines); "I'd have my own apartment," "My family would want me around, and they would want me home for Christmas again," "Maybe I could go to college, I'd really like to do that" (schizophrenia).

With regard to the latter – patients coping with schizophrenia – the answers of my own patients are sometimes so laden with pain, for the illness has decimated their sense of self-respect, that tears may follow the use of the Alternative History Question. And, indeed, if during my subsequent discussion with my patient, he or she arrives at an understanding that a medication might represent a viable pathway to regaining one of these lost dreams, we will have collaboratively found a powerful motivator for sparking medication interest.

As we did with the Inquiry into Lost Dreams above, I'd like to contextually illustrate the Alternative History Question as it is being gracefully employed in a clinical setting. To do so, I'm going to illustrate its use not with a medication per se, but with an example from surgery. I believe we will find this useful for two reasons: (1) Surgery is often one of the most difficult therapeutic interventions to convince patients to undertake, for, frankly, it *is* scary. If we can show the effectiveness of the employment of the Alternative History Question with something as imposing as surgery, we will have created a fairly convincing argument for its use with medications. (2) I had mentioned earlier in this chapter that I thought you would find many of the techniques of the MIM directly transferable to increasing interest and motivation with a variety of nonmedication interventions, such as diet, exercise, physical rehab, meditation, diagnostic procedures, and surgery. Such recommendations for interventions are part and parcel of everyday practice in primary care settings such as family medicine and internal medicine as well as in specialties ranging from cardiology, pulmonology, and endocrinology to physical medicine, psychiatry, and surgery. This example will highlight this potential.

Let us imagine an orthopedic surgeon talking with a patient in his late 60s, who has been suffering from severe osteoarthritis for over 15 years. Mr. Blount, who prefers to be called by his first name, Desmond, has been highly opposed to the idea of bilateral knee replacements. A retired lawyer, he has tried a variety of alternative treatments, such as acupuncture, which years ago had provided moderate relief but is no longer effective. He has also been tried on a variety of nonsteroidal anti-inflammatory drugs but there are concerns about creating a potential gastritis considering his advancing age. He has chosen to avoid the use of opioids for fear of addiction. Steroid injections are becoming problematic, appearing to be causing further joint damage as an adverse reaction.

The picture is further complicated by a unique factor that hangs like a shadow over Mr. Blount's contemplation of surgery. He had a nephew who developed a severe infection following a knee replacement. Within a week, his nephew threw a pulmonary embolism and died.

Mr. Blount clearly has ample reason to be hesitant about surgery. We are picking up the conversation late in a scheduled follow-up appointment in which his potential surgeon and he had once again been discussing the pros and cons of surgery, of which Mr. Blount remains leery:

Pt.: Truth be told, I'm in pretty bad pain all the time, but you know, I'd rather be in pain than dead. (pauses, looks up at the surgeon with a bit of a defeated look) I just don't know what to do.

Clin.: Desmond, you have every right to be hesitant about surgery. It's always sort of scary. I'm hesitant about surgery for myself, and I wouldn't have it done unless I felt it to be necessary. (Notice how this surgeon is deftly applying the spirit and principles of the MIM by creating a nonoppositional alliance with Mr. Blount by moving with him on the Agreement Continuum. If this has been his interviewing practice over his previous appointments with Mr. Blount, he has probably already secured some of the key interpersonal factors, such as respect and trust, that, as we mentioned earlier in the chapter, are prerequisites for a patient to answer "yes" to the question "Can this medication – in this case surgery – help me?") But I wouldn't suggest the replacements unless I really felt that they would go well for you. And we'd do them one at a time, so you'd get a chance after the first one to see if the pros outweighed the cons or not.

Pt.: Yea, yea, I know. (pauses) Don't get me wrong, I really trust you. (bingo) That's not it. I just don't know. (pauses) The pain is really bad, I, I . . . I just don't know.

Clin.: Well, it's a tough decision, and you don't have to make up your mind right now. (still no pressure from the surgeon) I think I've got a pretty good idea what your worries are, and they are legitimate, especially after what happened with your nephew. In helping you to weigh things here, I think it would help me if I had a better idea of what some of the benefits might be. (Notice that the surgeon is not going to tell Mr. Blount – or "lecture him" about – the benefits of surgery; he is going to let Mr. Blount discover the benefits for himself.) You know, what if we did the knee replacements, and you had essentially no pain when you walked, and I don't think you will, what would you be able to do differently in your life that you can't do now? **(Alternative History Question)**

Pt.: Hmmmm (pauses, then smiles) I'd get a dog. I adore dogs. I had two Springer Spaniels, Maddie and Wendy. I loved them to death. We'd go out for long walks out in a field behind my house, sometimes with a light snow falling. Really magical. (pauses) But after they both passed I realized I just couldn't keep up with a new dog. As my knees got worse, I couldn't even take them out for walks. It wouldn't be fair to a dog if I can't take them out for walks for god's sake (sighs). I sure miss having a dog, especially a Springer.

Clin.: They're sort of wild things aren't they (smiles), Springers, I mean. I'm not sure anyone can keep up with two Springers. They're not called Springers for nothing!

Pt.: Oh, they're nutballs alright! (chuckles) I love them. Really affectionate too!

Clin.: Well that sounds like a good change. I bet it would be great fun to walk with a pair of Springers again, out in a snowy field. (pauses) What else might you be able to do? (**Alternative History Question** repeated).

Pt.: Hmmm. I never really thought about this, but I'd start to travel again. My wife and I used to travel a lot, Italy, Spain, even China (looks animated), but the airports were just too much. They make them so you have to walk so damn far. It was just too much. And I hate, I mean I hate, driving in a damn scooter or being wheeled about in some cart for old people. But if my knees were okay, wow, if they were really okay, I'd be on a plane in no time.

Clin.: Sounds good to me, just get me a ticket if you're going back to Italy (both laugh). What else would be different? (Third employment of the **Alternative History Question**)

Pt.: Oh, I don't know. I, I, well, there's a brook down deep in the woods behind Laurie's and my house. We used to go down to that brook almost every week, except in the winter, and I spent a lot of time down there alone. (pauses) It's sort of place where I'd find my soul. Yea, I miss that, I miss that a lot. (pauses) Dr. Miller, are you really telling me that you think I could do these things, really? Without much pain?

Clin.: (smiles) Really. (pauses) Perhaps, no guarantee, but perhaps with no pain, but certainly with a lot less pain. Just like old times. You know, Desmond, I can never guarantee anything with surgery, but from my experience, and I've had a lot of it, I think your chances for a very good outcome are excellent.

Pt.: (sighs and sits up with a bit more spunk). I don't know, maybe I might want to try one knee. Which would you do first?

Truly skillful interviewing, and it looks like it is paying off. One would be hard-pressed to see a better example of shared decision making. In it, we have seen our surgeon intentionally use a single interviewing technique – the Alternative History Question – three times. Notice that it was the patient that produced the motivators, not the surgeon.

In a similar fashion, whether talking about surgery or using medications, I truly believe that many patients hold the keys for motivation locked inside them. They are often deeply personal motivators of which we might have no knowledge. The goal of the clinician becomes one not of telling patients why they should take a medication but learning from patients why it would be wise to do so. Skillfully, and intentionally using interviewing techniques such as the Inquiry into Lost Dreams and the Alternative History Question clinicians can optimize the chance that patients will discover for themselves why they would want to take a medication. I am reminded of the wise words of Richard Miller from our opening epigram of this chapter: "People are the undisputed experts on themselves. No one has been with them longer or knows them better than they do."

Our surgeon could have spoken in generalities to Mr. Blount, telling him that he would be much more mobile if he underwent knee replacements and, "You could do a lot of things that you can't do now." Such generalities pale in intensity compared with Mr. Blount's self-generated image of himself walking through a snowy field with two Springer Spaniels bounding about. The former is a light tug toward surgical interest, and the latter is an almost irresistible pull.

The above illustration demonstrated the use of the Alternative History Question with regard to a surgical procedure, but one can imagine its almost daily utility in a busy primary care or specialty clinic when addressing smoking cessation with a patient suffering from COPD, while recommending diet with a patient coping with obesity, or an exercise regimen for a man with progressively worsening erectile dysfunction and vision problems from diabetes. Both the Inquiry into Lost Dreams and its close sister, the Alternate History Question, are not magic, but they sometimes seem to be so. Simple. Powerful. Easily taught. Easily learned. Easily utilized.

What if the Disorder Has No Symptoms?

The power of the twin techniques of the Inquiry into Lost Dreams and the Alternative History Question lies in the fact that the symptoms caused by our patient's diseases are causing considerable pain and loss of functioning. But in everyday primary care and specialty care clinics, such is frequently not the case. Many of the diseases that clinicians encounter do not demonstrate many, if any, symptoms in the early stages of the disease (e.g., hypertension, hyperlipidemia, the metabolic syndrome/early diabetes).

One trick of the trade with such symptomless diseases stems directly from our understanding of the Inquiry into Lost Dreams. Perhaps we can adapt it for use with hidden diseases by communicating that a dream may be lost in the future if medications are not effectively utilized:

TIP 23 Protecting Future Dreams

"Mr. Tenney, you've told me a lot of things that you really love to do, from playing tennis and going skiing to playing with your new grandson, who I must say from his picture is really cute. And I don't want to be overly dramatic, but the chance of you having a stroke or a heart attack, especially with your Dad having had a stroke, is truly very real. By keeping your high blood pressure down, we might be able to prevent a stroke or heart attack so that we can keep your dreams alive for you. And keeping your blood pressure down is exactly what this medication helps to do. It's a dream protector, if you know what I mean."

If we reflect back on Mrs. Moss from earlier in the chapter (the grandmother who wanted to take her granddaughter to Disneyland), yet another avenue comes to mind for uncovering motivators for patients with symptomless diseases. Patients can have powerful reasons for taking medications that are based primarily on the idea of helping others. In many instances, these interpersonal motivators can be a great deal more compelling than simply taking a grandchild to Disneyland (important in its own right). Sometimes a patient feels that if he or she does not take a medication, catastrophic events may befall loved ones. It is this avenue that provides some keys for helping patients to find previously untapped motivators for using medications effectively.

In this regard, a primary care physician from Los Angeles shared the following technique at one of my MIM workshops. I have found it to be very effective. It introduces a theme that is of immense importance: understanding the critical need – when helping patients to find motivators unique to themselves – for interviewers to be facile at effectively navigating cross-cultural issues and divides.

The clinician was White, but much of his work was with the Latina/o population. He found that Latino males often didn't want to take medications for their symptomless diseases, such as hypertension, for "taking care of oneself" is viewed as being self-centered. On the other hand, the Latina/o culture places a profound emphasis on family ties and responsibilities, which displays itself as an intense belief in taking care of one's spouse and children (as well as extended family) no matter what the cost. Family needs first. Individual needs second.

Spending precious money on medications, when "there is nothing wrong with me – symptomless disease such as hypertension – when I need that money for clothes and food for my kids" simply flies in the face of the patient's cultural ethics. Indeed, all of the risks and dangers of undocumented immigration are often undertaken because of profound and pressing needs to help one's family survive.

The family practitioner commented that convincing young Latino fathers to take medications for asymptomatic diseases was often an insurmountable barrier to medication interest and follow-through. He related that one day he inadvertently stumbled on the solution when he was eliciting the routine family history during an initial H&P. We will call the patient Miguel. When he asked Miguel whether anyone in his family had had a heart attack or stroke, the patient commented, "Yeah, my father. He died of a heart attack (pauses), . . . it was the worst day of my life. He was the greatest man I've ever known." When asked how old he was when his father died, he commented, "Way too young, I was 12." The patient welled up with tears.

At this point, the proverbial "light bulb" went off in the clinician's mind. The light bulb in question can be summarized by the following interviewing principle: *Actively explore with each patient the potential interpersonal motivators that might ensue, regarding loved ones, if the disease should worsen or death result*. During the closing phase of the interview when the clinician was recommending the use of an antihypertensive, he put this principle into practice with the following interviewing technique:

TIP 24 Tapping Family Motivators

"Miguel, I know you don't feel much like taking these medications for your high blood pressure, and I understand that. There might be another reason, in addition to taking care of yourself, why it may be very important for you to try to take them. I think they can help you to take care of your family. You see, I don't know if your father had high blood pressure like you have, but it commonly runs in families from generation to generation. I think he very possibly did. And high blood pressure is one of the number one causes of heart attacks. I think there is a very good chance it is what caused your father to have his. This medication is designed to help prevent heart attacks, something that you know from your own experience would be horrible for your wife and kids. I can't guarantee you that it will prevent you from having a heart attack, but I think there is a good chance it will. We need to keep you healthy, not just for you, but for your two children. Our goal is to try to lower your blood pressure so that we can protect your heart. And if we do this right, we might be able to prevent your two children from going through what you went through when you were 12. (pauses) . . . You know, this warning might just be the last great gift your father gave to you. What do you think?"

To me, this interviewing exchange was brilliant. The family practitioner focused on his patient's cultural matrix both in a general sense (Hispanic pride in familial responsibility) and in a personal sense (Miguel's loss of his father at an early age).

The physician commented that he had found this tip to be useful from that day forward, with rather startling increases in medication interest in this specific population. He uses it with asymptomatic diseases, such as hypertension, hypercholesterolemia, and diabetes.

It is also useful for patients whose symptomatic diseases have been in remission for long periods of time to help them to keep in mind why they are taking the medication, for such diseases have paradoxically become symptomless because of the impact of the medications. From a personal standpoint, I have found that Tapping Family Motivators can be very useful with many psychiatric conditions, for some of which – in a primary care setting – you will be providing direct care (mild to moderate depressions) or indirect supportive care (bipolar disorder and schizophrenia). For instance, when some patients suffering from bipolar disorder move into a strong remission, they still have regrets about what the bipolar disorder "put my family through." Tapping Family Motivators can be a particularly powerful technique for keeping this motivational awareness vibrant for such patients.

This technique can also be expanded beyond family members. For some patients, such as teachers, ministers, physicians, nurses, and social workers, it is their commitment to their communities and to helping others that stands as a powerful motivator for them to stay healthy and capable of helping. As one would expect, this tip is of great use not only among the Latina/o population, but across all cultures when we find individuals possessing a high sense of responsibility to family or mission.

Ed Hamaty, a pulmonologist and hospitalist, added that such family or community motivators, as described above, can be enhanced significantly by helping patients to create individualized affirmations such as "This one is for my grandchild." Simply repeating this affirmation every time the patient reaches for his or her medication bottle can go a long way toward inspiring motivation. To optimize its power to enhance medication interest, it is important to reenforce it over time.

Another primary care clinician had an excellent interviewing technique to accomplish that exact task. A nurse from Kansas, Janet Brack, suggested a clever extension of the above interviewing technique. She asks patients whether they might have a photograph of their children with them. If they do, she asks to see it. Naturally, no matter what the appearance of the child or children might be, she enthusiastically comments how cute the kids are. She then employs the following technique:

TIP 25 Visual Reminder for Tapping Family Motivators

"Mr. James, you've already decided that one of your reasons, besides taking care of yourself, that you want to stay on your medications for your diabetes is to keep healthy for your family. That's a great goal, and I think you can do it.

Some of my patients with diabetes have found a neat trick that helps them to remember how taking their medications can help them to help their families. They get a picture like you have here of their kids, and sometimes they even make it bigger; if you happen to have it on your phone or computer, you can just print it out larger. They then place their medications on top of the picture. Every time they reach for their bottles, the picture reminds them of why they are taking the medications, and they say something to themselves like, 'I'm doing this for me, and I'm doing this for my wife and two kids. I need to be there for them, and these medications are going to help me to do that.' Many of my patients tell me this really helps them to stay motivated to use their medications wisely. How does that sound to you?"

If safety is an issue, as it would be with digoxin and two kids in the house, the photograph can be taped or placed inside a medicine cabinet that is locked or out of reach of children.

Speaking of kids, I am reminded of a very clever tip for prompting an adult patient to take medications in an ongoing fashion, once again based on the patient's concern for his or her children. This tip was provided by one of my MIM workshop participants. I never would have thought of it in a million years, yet it is not only clever, it is effective.

Having done a social history, during the initial H&P, the provider can make a concerted effort to find out whether the patient has a child or adolescent with a chronic disease that requires medications. If the child dislikes taking his or her medication or the adolescent has trouble reliably taking his or her medication, the provider can use the following tip:

TIP 26 Modeling Medication Interest for One's Child

"In a strange but useful way, Mrs. Peters, your taking your blood pressure medication may indirectly help Timmy. You can be a good role model for him on the importance of taking a medication. You can let him know that you need a medication and that you now understand how easy it is to forget to do so. And you can show him by example the importance of taking your medication on time. This sharing of the disorders you are each coping with and the problems associated with taking medications for them can actually be very bonding for the two of you. I have even had patients tell me that they decide with their children to take their medications together so that they can 'remind each other.' It could really help Timmy to feel more comfortable both about having a disorder and about taking his medications. I think he might feel less stigmatized about having a seizure disorder if he knows that you have a disorder too."

The above tip can be useful with both symptom-laden diseases and symptomless diseases – the topic of this section. But I think it is particularly useful for symptomless diseases for it reminds the patient that taking his or her medications, which might not seem so pressing a matter to the patient (for he or she is not experiencing symptoms), is important for helping his or her child who does have painful or disturbing symptoms.

With the deployment of this interviewing technique, the clinician has helped the patient – with a symptomless disease – to associate the taking of his or her medication with the relief of an actual symptom of great importance to the patient. Paradoxically, it happens to be a symptom plaguing his or her child.

With regard to helping patients with symptomless diseases not only to be aware of their diseases but also to actively consider that the control of their disease is directly dependent on effective medication follow-through, it is useful to return to the topic of patient education. The following tip can help your patients to better understand the importance of their "numbers" (whether the numbers are blood pressure readings, blood sugar values, or their A1C value), for such numbers may be the only "target signs" of their asymptomatic diseases. It can be very hard to be motivated by abstract numbers to persistently take a medication, especially if there are bad side effects. It is also difficult for patients to associate these numbers with the use or lack of use of their medications.

In any case, I think you will find the following strategy to be valuable in both highlighting the presence of the disease (reenforcing Step 1 of the Choice Triad) and tying the use of the medication directly into the numbers being used as gauges of success in treating the disease (addressing Step 2 of the Choice Triad). In short, the Back-Burner Strategy makes the "numbers" real.

TIP 27 Back-Burner Strategy

"My role is not to scare you, Rohan, but to help you to understand why it is so important to take care of your atherosclerosis, so that you have some real choice in how to keep yourself healthy. The problem with atherosclerosis is that it is the type of problem that is a delayed problem, that sort of sneaks up on us. For myself, I always find such problems to be tough ones because it's easy for me to put them on the 'back burner,' when they really need to be on the front burner.

"It's like we're cooking up a big Thanksgiving dinner, and we have some of the side dishes on the back burners of the stove hidden away behind the pots on the front burners. It's so easy, when we get busy making the potatoes and tending to the turkey, to lose sight of what is cooking on those back burners, but what's cooking is getting hotter and hotter. Suddenly, without any warning, the gravy is boiling and spilling over all over the place, and we got a real mess on our hands.

"Atherosclerosis is just like this. It may slowly, over the years, get worse and worse, so that our arteries, as I showed you before, may get more and more clogged, and then boom, like the pots on the back burner boiling over, our arteries may shut down suddenly even if they are not entirely clogged. And just like it's too late with the burned gravy or the scorched vegetables, we have a real mess on our hands. Only this time, the mess isn't a ruined meal; it could be something like a heart attack or a stroke.

"We need to bring the problem of treating your atherosclerosis onto the front burners, where you can take care of it, to help prevent it from 'boiling over.' And it's keeping track of those numbers we talked about that can help keep it on the front burner for you, that will let us both know how 'hot the food in your pot is getting,' if you know what I mean. By following your blood pressure numbers, we may have a much better idea of what is going on with your arteries. Then we can use your medication to lower your blood pressure, to make things safer for you."

Depending on the patient's cultural context, I have found it to be useful to flexibly change the metaphor used in the Back-Burner Strategy. For instance, if the patient is a trucker or mechanic, one can talk about the need to routinely check the oil in the engine, and that it's easy to forget to do so, but it's very important to do so for the engine can be destroyed if one does not "keep up with the numbers." Techies can be reminded of the importance of keeping up with recommended virus updates or their computers can become hostages to ransom-ware. Whatever metaphor fits the patient best becomes the metaphor of choice for a skilled clinician.

In addition to interviewing techniques such as the Back-Burner Strategy, well-organized educational approaches such as the use of illustrations, models, and web-based animations can help patients understand the potential consequences of unchecked symptomless disease states. In addition, the entire process can become more personalized and reality based for some patients by having the patient chart his or her own numbers or perhaps by downloading an app that does the charting for the patient and subsequently shows the patient's progress graphically.

Generalized Techniques for Bolstering Belief and Excitement About Medications

We are not going to have the same confidence in all of our medications, and we should never feign confidence when we do not have it. But if you feel a medication has a good chance of helping, it is often useful to share that optimism with the patient. Keep in mind that all medications carry within them a potential placebo effect. This placebo effect is not something to be ignored; it is something to be enhanced. Placebo effects sometimes bolster the pharmacologic efficacy of medications or independently change pathophysiology by themselves, as has been seen in several antidepressant studies.[3,4]

If the prospective medication has demonstrated good results in well-controlled clinical trials, I go out of my way to let the patient know of this fact. I also find it useful to be specific about instances in which the medication has personally been valuable with my own patients. Such personal endorsements by me are often much more persuasive to patients than a horde of research studies. Fortunately, we can take advantage of both approaches as follows. Imagine for a minute that we are talking with a patient about one of the newer medications for psoriasis:

TIP 28 Instilling Positive Expectations by Highlighting Previous Success Stories

"This medication has really proven itself in recent research, and I, personally, have had some great luck with it. I would say that in the last 3 months alone, I've had at least a dozen patients, sitting in that exact chair, who have had very significant improvements in their skin since we started them on it. There are no guarantees, but it can be really pretty striking how much this medication has decreased their skin lesions, occasionally even completely."

Another rich yet often overlooked opportunity for enhancing patient belief revolves around the process of writing out prescriptions. Our written prescriptions are not only sterile communications to pharmacists about medications, but also, for some of our patients, they are tangible symbols of hope. Curiously, from the perspective of cultural anthropology, prescriptions share some striking similarities to talismans, even to the point of being partially written in a secret language (Latin) that is understood only by the healers of the culture but not by those people seeking the help of those healers. I'm not suggesting that prescriptions are talismans, but I am suggesting that symbolically, like talismans, they may be powerful enhancers of the placebo effect in their own right.

As such, it may be useful, from a psychological perspective, "to charge them" with the power of our own belief. A patient with intractable pain, debilitating depression, or AIDS is looking for hope, even if the hope is for just a small relief in suffering. This is a hope that talented physicians sometimes enhance, not only by their choice of medications, but by how they handle the pieces of paper that procure those medications.

TIP 29 The Talisman Effect: Optimizing the Power of the Prescription to Symbolize Hope

If I have a good feeling that a particular medication is going to help a patient, I have found it useful to do the following. As I hand the prescription to the patient, *while we are both holding it,* I explain the directions. After I'm done, I look the patient directly in the eye and say the following: "Well, good luck with this. I've got a really good feeling it is going to help you." It is a simple gesture. It takes no time. But it is the type of gesture from which hope is sometimes kindled.

Obviously, a handwritten prescription lends itself admirably for use in the Talisman Effect, for it represents something the patient can tangibly hold and take home. It may also be bolstered by the presence of "magical" Latin script. But as many of us are moving toward electronic scripts, the savvy clinician can still employ the Talisman Effect. Even though the formal prescription may be sent electronically, one can still write down the directions for the medication on a separate "official" piece of paper with the letterhead of the clinic or hospital certifying its importance.

One can then undertake the exact same protocol with regard to "charging the talisman." In addition, as research has shown, carefully reviewing how one should take one's medications enhances the likelihood of effective medication follow-through. With a single technique – the employment of the Talisman Effect – the clinician can simultaneously enhance the likelihood of a placebo effect while increasing the likelihood of effective medication follow-through. Not bad for a single interviewing technique.

A very simple variation of the Talisman Effect was given to me by a physician, Grant Chernick, during one of our MIM workshops. When handing a patient his or her prescription, he looks the patient right in the eye while confidently commenting, "Well, here's your prescription, I trust it will help!" It can be surprising how something as simple as this variation of the Talisman Effect can provide a potent jolt of hope in a patient, especially if the clinician in the previous ongoing therapeutic alliance has secured the patient's trust and respect. Patients do care what we think, especially if they like us.

As I end this section, I am reminded of one of my favorite tips. It was provided by a pediatrician, Dipankar Mukhopadhyay, and it delightfully captures the magic and unique solutions sometimes required when working with small children. If you have built up a good ongoing relationship with a child and his or her parents, the following approach can be both great fun and highly effective for improving medication interest in a small child.

The tip addresses a common problem in pediatrics: toddlers fussing about taking medications. Sometimes, it is hard for small children to truly understand why they are taking medications, and once they decide they don't want to be bothered, tantrums and tightly clamped lips are not far behind.

The tip is based on the fact that little kids sometimes get a kick out of the idea that they have to "keep tabs" on Mom or Dad rather than vice versa. This phenomenon can be put to good use in helping kids to get interested in taking their medications. After writing out the script, the clinician turns and hands the script to the young patient, saying as in the following tip:

TIP 30 Mommy's Little Helper

"Now this piece of paper will allow you to get your medicine from the pharmacist. This medicine will really help your sore throat to feel much better. But the only way it will work is if your Mom remembers to give it to you once in the morning and once at bedtime. Do you think you can make sure your Mom remembers to do this?"

Engaging these young patients in the "monitoring" of their parents' behavior usually gets a chuckle from the parent and an enthusiastic nod from the child. This technique is a wonderful example of "externalizing the problematic behavior," a technique often useful with children and adolescents. For instance, a child who has been teasing another child may be told that there are problems with teasing at school (and why it is a problem) and then may be asked to help make sure it is not happening anymore in the hallways, perhaps being used as a hallway monitor. Having been "hired" as a monitor, such a child may suddenly cease all teasing behaviors. When you see it work, it is really quite remarkable. In any case, you may be able to find other uses for "externalizing problematic behaviors" when attempting to increase medication interest even with adults.

Having created a practical toolbox filled with interviewing techniques for helping patients to find personalized motivators for medication use, one more step in the Choice Triad must be navigated before medication interest is solidified and medication follow-through is secured. Patients can believe that there is something wrong with which they want help (Step 1), and they can believe that a medication may be the answer for achieving specific personalized goals and symptom relief (Step 2), but unless they believe that the pros of the medication truly outweigh its cons, they would be foolish to take it. I would never take a medication that I felt would hurt me more than help me. Would you?

REFERENCES

1. Miller WR. *Motivational Interviewing: Helping People Change.* http://goodreads.com/author/quotes/128663.William_R_Miller. Accessed December 02, 2016.
2. Jakovljevic M, Ostojic L. Person-centered medicine and good clinical practice: disease has to be cured, but the patient has to be healed. *Medicina Mostariensia* 2015;3(1–2):2–5.
3. Leuchter AF, Cook IA, Witte EA, et al. Changes in brain function of depressed subjects during treatment with placebo. *Am J Psychiatry* January 2002;159:122–129.
4. Mayberg HS, Silva JA, Brannan SK, et al. The functional neuroanatomy of the placebo effect. *Am J Psychiatry* May 2002;159:728–737.

CHAPTER 9

Third Step of the Choice Triad: Do the Pros Outweigh the Cons?

"If you are trying to make a difficult decision and you're weighing up the pros and cons, you have frank conversations. Everybody knows this in their walk of life . . ."[1]

Tony Blair
FORMER BRITISH PRIME MINISTER

QUESTIONS, CONCERNS, AND "COMMITTEES"

Hidden World of Patient Concerns

In our walk of life – functioning as healers in our cultures – there is arguably no greater truth than Tony Blair's comment, for we will find ourselves having many frank conversations with our patients about the pros and cons of our medications. These conversations can range from a fairly low-key discussion concerning the pros and cons of taking an antibiotic for sinusitis to the far-from-low-key discussion revolving around the use of a chemotherapeutic agent for cancer that could, itself, be lethal. Conversations don't get much more frank than the latter.

In our last two chapters, we explored Steps 1 and 2 of the Choice Triad. From our explorations, we gained a clearer understanding of how patients decide to try a medication. But one last hurdle remains before a patient will try a medication and subsequently choose to continue it. As we noted at the end of our last chapter, even when a patient feels that there is something wrong and is motivated to do something about it via the use of a medication, if that patient is not convinced that the pros outweigh the cons, the medication bottle will remain on the shelf. Period.

We are about to discover that there are remarkable differences in how individual patients go about this business of weighing the pros and cons. The differences arise because the patient's biologic disease is often not the sole – or even primary – determining factor of the patient's weighing of the pros and cons. It is the patient's illness, the fashion in which the patient's biologically rooted symptoms metastasize throughout all the elements of the patient's life that creates many of the patient's pros and cons.

What is unique to each patient is how the patient perceives his or her symptoms (as well as the side effects created by the agents offered to treat those very same symptoms) and their impact on the patient's intimate relationships, livelihoods, daily activities, and spiritual/cultural beliefs. Understanding this uniqueness is at the heart of understanding how we can increase medication interest and follow-through. Our goal by the end of this chapter is to have developed a toolbox (in fact, three toolboxes) that are rich with interviewing techniques for more effectively, and sensitively, engaging in the frank conversations of which Tony Blair hints in our opening epigram.

We must begin our exploration of the third step of the Choice Triad – the ultimate deal-maker or deal-breaker with regard to medication interest – by asking ourselves the most basic of all questions. What is it that our patients are weighing in the third step of the Choice Triad? The answer is not as simple as one might expect, for our patients are weighing a surprisingly large number of quite specific concerns about taking medications. These concerns might vary in nature from concrete cognitions that could be written down to more evasive "gut feelings" that elude capture by words.

Near the turn of the last century, Robert Horne and John Weinman, in an innovative article, attempted to categorize the numerous factors facing our patients as they weigh the pros and cons of putting a medication into their mouths. At its simplest level, they found that patients "weigh their beliefs about the *necessity* of the prescribed medication for maintaining health now and in the future" with their "*concerns* about the potential adverse effects of taking it."[2] Makes sense. The question now becomes how is this abstract process translated into everyday clinical experience.

In this regard, I have found that most of our patients' concerns cluster around three factors: Cluster A – Efficacy, Cluster B – Cost, and Cluster C – Symbolic Meaning of Taking the Medication. Better understanding of these three factors, and how to effectively ask questions that allow patients to openly and honestly share their concerns about these three factors, is, in many respects, the key to securing the third step of the Choice Triad.

As you will recall from Chapter 5 (see page 61), Colleen McHorney had found that two of the most powerfully predictive factors for "adherence" lay within the three clusters our patients use when weighing the pros and cons of taking a medication.[3] Specifically, the cost of the medications and the fears that the medication will do more harm than good were, according to McHorney's data, determining drivers during the patient's decision making.

But as important as this quantitative data are regarding ultimate patient choice, one must delve more deeply into its qualitative implications if one wants to have the frank conversations our patients need. Our patients' concerns about cost and their fears of potential harm are determined by a complex variety of factors unique to each particular patient and each particular patient's culture.

The factor of cost is not limited to financial burden. There exist a variety of other "costs" to the patient from stigmatization to familial discord related to differing family opinions regarding the medication in question. Moreover, the patient's fears are driven by a remarkable number of factors in addition to side effects or adverse reactions.

Let us now return to our clusters in more detail. We will find that exploring these clusters will allow us to address just about any concern a patient may be weighing during the final, and crucial, step of the Choice Triad:

Cluster A: Concerns about the efficacy of the medication

Cluster B: Concerns about the cost of the medication

Cluster C: Concerns about what it symbolically means to take the medication

Each of these three clusters forms its own continuum or axis. Each of our patients, as he or she is sitting in our exam rooms or hospital units, has a position along these three axes concerning the pros and cons of the medication – toward one end or the other. For instance, concerning the efficacy of the medication, each patient has a personal belief about the extent to which a medication is "working." Some patients are convinced that the medication is helping a lot, whereas others are convinced that it is not helping at all. Of course, many are in between. But the closer the patient is to believing that the medication is not helping, the less his or her interest will be in staying on it.

The point at which the above three axes (efficacy, cost, and meaning) intersect can provide us with a remarkably clear idea about which way the patient is leaning: "Should I take this medication or not?" or "Should I continue to take this medication or not?" By weighing the concerns on each of these three axes, our patients decide whether the *necessity* of the medication outweighs their *concerns* about the medication exactly in the fashion outlined by Horne and Weinman.

Consequently, learning to have a frank discussion with our patients regarding all three of these axes is a critical skill set for any sophisticated clinician to master. Fortunately, there exists a practical toolbox for each axis of the third step of the Choice Triad. But before we can address how to utilize these toolboxes effectively, we must examine one more intrapsychic phenomenon.

Where Does the Patient Weigh the Pros and Cons?

There exists a "catch" to addressing and transforming any concerns our patients may have in Step 3 of the Choice Triad. A metaphor will help us understand this catch. It is important to realize that few, if any, patients are sitting around, with a pencil in hand, making lists of the pros and cons. Patient beliefs are often a somewhat chaotic potpourri of opinions on numerous aspects of the medication, from side effects to convenience, from financial cost to what the patient's partner and family think about the medication. These beliefs, some conscious, others preconscious, are all simmering in a stew from which a decision will emerge.

When people (whether it is ourselves considering medications for ourselves or our families or patients considering medications for themselves) are weighing the pros and cons of taking a medication, there exist a multitude of beliefs to be weighed. Each of the pros and cons is considered in the decision-making process. For a person facing the formidable decision as whether to place a foreign substance in his or her body, it is as if – *metaphorically* speaking – the person has a committee inside his or her head. Each member of the committee represents a differing opinion the patient holds about the medication.

For instance, if the medication in question were an antidepressant, part of the patient might be saying, "This medication makes me feel better because it helps me stop crying." But another part of the patient might chime in, "Yeah, but I can't sleep on it." A third member of the committee might add, "But I can get back to work again." This positive vote may be quickly countered by another "committee member" arguing, "But this medication is costing us an arm and a leg!" and so on and so on, until it is as if the committee chair (the patient's ego) suddenly says, "We've heard enough, let's vote!" And they do. The patient makes a decision – either to continue the medication or to stop it.

Here is the catch: I have found that roughly 90% of the time, when this metaphorical "committee" votes – that is, the patient decides to stop the medication or continue it – the committee votes outside of my office. In short, the patient has either stopped the medication or has already decided that he or she does not like it before we meet again.

If the committee votes outside of my office, I have no opportunity to sway the committee before it votes. It's a done deal. I generally find that if a patient has already stopped a medication, it is frequently hard to persuade the patient to try it again. To do so, the patient must first acknowledge in his or her own mind that he or she has made the wrong decision. Admitting that one is in error is not the most natural of human inclinations. Even when the clinician has persuaded the patient to try the medication again, the reluctant patient is now coming from a perspective of looking for the slightest evidence that he or she was right in the first place as in, "This medication is bad for me." Such a patient is preloaded to experience low medication interest.

On the bright side, clinicians are, by definition, important resources of information about medications for the patient's internal committee and, at times, strong lobbyists for their use. Patients value our opinions. Indeed, the more powerful our medication alliance, the more our opinions are valued. Perhaps the patient stopped the medication because he or she had some negative experiences with the medication that we could have helped with, as with a method of decreasing an unwanted side effect. Or perhaps the patient simply had some misinformation about the medication, perhaps discovered on the web, that we could have clarified very easily. In any case, we can do neither of these interventions if the "committee" has already voted.

Another interviewing principle now begins to emerge. It is a simple one. It is also one of the most important interviewing principles that I have found for enhancing medication interest: *Invite the patient's committee to vote inside your office not outside it by asking specific questions concerning the patient's emerging views of the pros and cons of the medication during each medication evaluation. Once again, assume nothing.* In short, the clinician wants to hear the patient's views on the three axes concerning efficacy, cost, and meaning while the patient is sitting in his or her office.

To continue with our metaphor, the answers uncovered provide a means for the clinician to see where the patient's internal committee members are sitting on the axes. The answers allow the clinician to address misinformation, allay unwarranted fears, and, in some instance, to learn from the patient that the cons of the medication do, in actuality, outweigh the pros. If possible, we want the patient to decide to stop or to continue the medication while we are there, that is, functioning as a trusted member of the committee during the appointment itself. Attending to this interviewing principle has become one of my major *conscious* goals during medication checks over the years.

Uncovering the Patient's Pros and Cons Regarding Cluster A – Efficacy

> The most common rationales for altering medication practice are drug related: the medication is perceived as ineffective or the so-called side effects become too troublesome.[4]
>
> Peter Conrad, PhD

Efficacy from a Patient's Perspective

As we continue to explore what makes patients interested in taking medications, we inevitably must examine the issue of efficacy because efficacy is at the very heart of how patients weigh the pros and cons. Despite this fact, in over 20 years of clinical experience I have yet to have a patient plop into a chair in my office and comment, "I'm having some concerns about the efficacy of my Haldol."

For prescribing clinicians, the word "efficacy" has various technical connotations. Research literature makes distinctions between efficacy (the ability of a medication to achieve its goals in more idealized settings such as research projects and academic centers) versus medication effectiveness (how well the medication is able to achieve its goals on the clinical frontlines of community practice and outpatient clinics, where various psychological, cultural, and sociological factors impact on the use of the medication).

From the patient's perspective, it is a good deal simpler. As Iqbal Ahmed cogently points out, clinicians often prescribe according to the "proven clinical efficacy" of the medication as opposed to its "effectiveness."[5] For patients, there is no distinction between efficacy and effectiveness. Instead, the patient decides on the usage of a medication on the basis of *the patient's perception of its efficacy in layperson's terms (e.g. "Does it work or not work for me?")*. Put into even simpler terms, patients tend to perceive efficacy by asking themselves the following question: "Does this drug make me feel better?" or "Is this drug doing what I want it to do?" The patient's answer to this question of "efficacy" will frequently tip the scales in one direction or the other regarding medication interest.

As Peter Conrad suggested in the opening quote from his article, *The Meaning of Medications: Another Look at Compliance*, the answer to the patient's question, ultimately, comes down to whether the patient's perception of symptom relief outweighs his or her perception of side effect damage. From the view of understanding medication interest, the key word in the last sentence is *perception*.

We often hear, in both research and clinical parlance, that a patient discontinued a medication because of a side effect. No patient has ever stopped a medication *solely* because of a side effect, unless the side effect killed him. Patients stop a medication because of their *perception* that the costs of the side effect are not worth the benefits of the medication, not because of the mere presence of the side effect itself. *Side effects don't lead to discontinuation; perceptions do.*

By way of illustration, we all know patients experiencing severe side effects who, nevertheless, stay on a medication because they believe that the pros of the medication outweigh the costs of its side effects. To make our point, we need only look at instances when patients tolerate the severe side effects of chemotherapeutic agents for treating cancer because they believe that the agents can save their lives.

Returning to our committee metaphor, the perceptions of these cancer patients represent determinative positive votes in the patient's internal poll on medication interest. As stated earlier, our goal is to get the committee to vote in front of us. The art of securing this "in-house" vote lies in skillfully questioning our patients about their core beliefs regarding efficacy from a person-centered perspective.

Opening the Door to a Frank Conversation About Efficacy

Initiating the Discussion of the Pros and Cons Before Writing an Initial Script

With many patients, raising the concept of their weighing the pros and cons is a pretty easy task for the prescriber, for the patient was already doing so in his or her own head. In such cases, patients generally respond readily to a simple question from the prescriber such as, "Let's take a look at some of the pros and cons of starting up a medication for your hyperlipidemia."

On the other hand, via earlier conversation, as when reviewing the patient's medication passport, you may sense that a given patient is particularly leery about medications (or it may be the case that the medication in question carries the potential for serious adverse reactions warranting genuine patient concern such as bone marrow suppression with Tegretol or chloramphenicol, loss of hearing with an aminoglycoside, severe immunosuppression with chemotherapeutic medications or AIDS medications). In either case, such fears may make it difficult for the patient to objectively weigh the pros and cons.

In one of my MIM workshops, Sharon Laval, an obstetrician/gynecologist from Canada, passed on an effective approach for helping patients to develop the ability to more realistically weigh the pros and cons of a medication in such a situation. She accomplishes this task by gently reminding the patient that – throughout his or her life – the patient has often decided to try something, or to undertake a task, despite the presence of a certain degree of risk. This reminder serves to foster a more comfortable acceptance of relative risk. See what you think:

TIP 31 Remembering Reasonable Risk

"Taking medications is sometimes a bit like driving a car. We all know that there are risks to driving a car – some quite serious. Some of these risks might also be out of our own hands. But we all choose to drive a car because we believe that the relative risks to driving the car are outweighed by the convenience, fun, and benefits of driving. In short, the risks are outweighed by the simple fact that we need to get from point A to point B, and we think the benefits are worth the risks. What we will do concerning potential medications is to look carefully at the pros and cons. I can't tell you that you will not have any side effects. But you may decide that it looks like there is a good chance that the side effects will be outweighed by the benefits. If you think that will be the case, it may be worth giving the medication a chance. I'll give you my best advice of the pros and cons and you can figure out what would be best for you. How's that sound?"

Helping the Patient Weigh the Pros and Cons During Follow-Up Med Checks

Generally speaking, one of the best ways to begin the discussion regarding the patient's experiences on a medication prescribed during the last appointment, telephone call, or e-mail exchange is to simply ask directly:

TIP 32 "Since Last Time" Question

"How's that medication working out that we started up last time?"

or

"Since the last time we met, what have you thought about that medication we started?"

The value of the "Since Last Time" Question lies in its open-ended nature. It allows the patient to bring up any kinds of concerns, which, at times, may reveal concerns not related to efficacy in which case you can flexibly address those issues as described later in this chapter. But, generally speaking, I find that in response to the "Since Last Time" Question, patients frequently bring up either concerns about the medication not working or concerns about its side effects.

Pay attention to how rapidly the patient answers, as well as the enthusiasm voiced, for hesitancy or lack of enthusiasm may reflect significant concerns hidden behind the content of a response such as, "I guess it's okay." The truth often lies less with the patient's words and more with how the patient voices them. Any nonverbal indication of concern can easily be tapped with a follow-up question such as, "Heather, you seem a little hesitant, is there anything, even a small thing that concerns you about the medication?"

The "Since Last Time" Question also appeals to patients because the clinician's unprompted inquiry about the new medication metacommunicates two things to the patient: (1) the clinician is well aware that a medication was started up during the last visit and (2) the clinician is genuinely interested in the potential impact – both good and bad – of the medication. The clinician's interest is not limited to a generic interest in how the patient feels about the medication; the clinician is also interested in specifics – such as the patient's feelings about the dosage of the medication.

Addressing the Patient's Concerns About Dosage: Trapdoor Question Redux

We can now return to an interviewing technique introduced, to wet our appetites, as another prototypic interviewing technique back in Chapter 5, the Trapdoor Question. As mentioned then, it is a technique of use in helping patients weigh the pros and cons related to efficacy in Step 3 of the Choice Triad. I want to readdress it here, not only because it is one of the foundation stones of uncovering our patient's views on the delicate balancing of benefits versus side effects, but also because we can now see it put into action via clinical dialogue.

If you will recall, one of the most likely periods for medication interest to plummet is when a prescribing provider – focusing on inadequate relief of target symptoms – suggests increasing a medication to a patient *who already feels that he or she is on too high of a dose* but does not spontaneously voice that concern to the provider. I believe that a large portion of such patients – who do not immediately voice concerns about the suggested increase in dosage – will be inclined to lower or stop the medication before the next appointment. Patients may be hesitant to voice concerns at this junction for a variety of reasons including: fears of displeasing the clinician, ambivalence about the suggestion, feeling that their family wants them "to do whatever the doctor says," and so on.

In Chapter 5, we called this phenomenon – patients not informing clinicians that they are displeased with a dosage increase and subsequently stopping the medication in the weeks after such an increase has been made – the "trapdoor effect." The name, which was subsequently applied to the resulting interviewing technique designed for its resolution, came from the fact that when this situation arises, the medication interest of the patient seems to disappear as if a trapdoor had opened beneath it resulting in medication discontinuation.

Before proceeding, let us review the exact wording of the Trapdoor Question:

TIP 33 Trapdoor Question

"At this point in time, in your own opinion, do you feel that you are on too little, too much, or just the right amount of this medication?"

As you might recall, one of the strong points of the Trapdoor Question is that it inquires along a continuum and thus does not bias the patient in any specific direction. The important point is to directly ask for the patient's opinion about the current dosage before suggesting an increase. Once again, assuming nothing.

In this chapter, we now have the opportunity to see the Trapdoor Question put to the test, doing what it does best, helping patients to share the truth about their feelings concerning their medications and their current dosages. We will see how we can gracefully weave the Trapdoor Question into an unfolding conversation with our patients in a naturalistic fashion. We will also see how this style of questioning can not only provide information regarding our patient's views on dosage, but also open the conversation into a wealth of patient concerns, some idiosyncratic in nature, that may be critical to enhancing our patient's medication interest and follow-through.

Let us imagine a woman in her late 50s with chronic hypertension. She has been about 25 lbs overweight for years, coming on and off diets rather regularly. When younger she had been a fairly keen athlete, including running marathons, but has lost her exercise bug over the years. She is both intelligent and motivated for help. On the other hand, she is a bit shy and is consistently hesitant to share her opinions whether it is with her husband, her friends, her employer, or her health care providers.

About a year ago, she moved her residence and switched to a new provider, who happens to be a nurse practitioner. Her relationship with her nurse practitioner is a good one, but they have had trouble getting her hypertension under control. At last, by adding and then gently increasing Lopressor (a beta-blocker), her blood pressure readings have, for the very first time, been within normal limits (although barely). Her nurse practitioner is pleased with finally getting close to the results she wanted to achieve, but feels that a little better control is warranted and is planning on recommending another mild increase in dose.

We will pick up their dialogue, during a routine scheduled appointment, on the day of first success, moments after the clinician has taken her blood pressure. In their conversation, we will see the clinician use the Trapdoor Question to tap into the concerns of her patient (whom we shall call Beth).

In the ensuing dialogue, we will also see the clinician use two additional interviewing techniques, not yet discussed, which are designed to uncover a patient's true feelings as he or she weighs the pros and cons of the medications (the interviewing techniques will be noted in the dialogue). The effective use and timing of these techniques will be explored in an appropriate later chapter. At present, it is valuable to see the fashion in which a clinician can utilize several interviewing techniques of the MIM in tandem to create a naturalistically flowing conversation when exploring the third step of the Choice Triad:

Clin.: Beth, I'm really excited. When you came in today, our medical aid noted that your blood pressure readings were within normal limits. I just did them again to make sure. You're not gonna believe it.

Pt.: What?

Clin.: Normal . . . Both your systolic pressure, you know, the upper number and your diastolic, the lower one, were normal (clinician smiles).

Pt.: Good (pauses) good.

Clin.: (smiling, genuinely pleased) Don't get me wrong, they're both just barely within normal limits. But this is the first time we've ever gotten them within normal limits.

Pt.: That's really good to hear (said with little enthusiasm). Is it the Lopressor?

Clin.: Probably. We've had you on your diuretic for a long time without a lot of luck and added the Lopressor about 5 months ago. Every time we've raised it, your pressures have gone down a bit. (pauses) So I think it's most likely the beta-blocker. They're really good medications. (pauses) Your pressures are not quite where we want them, and we've some decisions about what to do next. I'm just curious, from your own perspective, at this point in time, do you feel that you're on too little, too much, or just the right amount of the Lopressor? **(Trapdoor Question)**

Pt.: I don't know. I think it's okay where it's at, I guess (not looking overjoyed).

Clin.: You look a little hesitant there. If I was going to buy a car from you, I wouldn't be overly convinced I should, you know what I mean?

Pt.: (Beth smiles) I don't know. I'm glad my pressures are better, that's for sure. I just don't know.

Clin.: Is there something you're experiencing that you're concerned whether it might be a side effect of the Lopressor? **(Direct Side-Effect Inquiry)**

Pt.: I don't know. Maybe it's nothing, but it's bothering me a fair amount.

Clin.: Go ahead. All side effects are important. What are you worried about?

Pt.: Well, we've talked about it before, feeling weary all the time, you know, no energy to do stuff. It's not getting any better. I think it's getting worse.

Clin.: How do you mean?

Pt.: I've got two rescue dogs and I have to take them both out about three or four times a day to do their business. And I need to take them down to the edge of the woods behind my house, but it's a really steep hill to get down there, and they're jumping all over the place dragging me by their leashes. It's crazy. And when I climb back up that hill, I'm really winded and really exhausted. It's really strange. And it makes me worried I'm having a heart attack or something. I've never had anything like that. I know I'm in bad shape, but this just seems weird.

Clin.: Hmmm. (pauses) Actually, like we've discussed before that's sometimes seen with beta-blockers like the one you're on. They lower pulse rates, which can make it harder to exercise. When people exercise, their pulses tend to go up naturally to make sure their muscles are getting enough oxygen. That's normal. But if you're not in good shape – and you're not exactly the well-toned marathoner that you were in your 20s (Beth smiles) – you're gonna get pooped real fast if your pulse doesn't go up, and the Lopressor can, with some people, tend to stop it from doing so. If you recall the technical name for that is "exercise intolerance" . . . (this side-effect had been discussed before, but the clinician realizes it's useful to reexplain both the side effect and its cause in the context of Beth's current concerns to help lessen her fears about the medication. It is time well spent. But, as we are about to see, there's more to the story opened by the clinician's judicious use of the **Trapdoor Question**).

Pt.: Yeah, I remember, but I didn't think it could be this bad. It's just a hill in my backyard for God's sake.

Clin.: I know. It can be pretty bad, but it's a side effect, an unpleasant one for sure, but the good news is that it is unlikely you're having a heart attack, it's probably all an example of the exercise intolerance . . . And we can have you run a tread-mill test if you want just to be certain . . . In the long run, I think you'll need to weigh how much that fatigue bothers you compared to what we're trying to prevent, you know, a true heart attack, a stroke, or even death. I'm not downplaying how uncomfortable exercise fatigue is . . . you'll just have to make a decision for yourself after weighing the pros and cons.

Right now, I'm sort of leaning toward staying on the med, if you can tolerate the fatigue. We'll check your heart out too, just to be sure.

Pt.: Yeah, that's good to know, about the exercise fatigue I mean, but . . .

Clin.: And? . . . You still look like you've got a concern of some sort.

Pt.: Well, I've gained a lot of weight . . . I'm not certain you realize how much.

Clin.: Yeah, I noticed that too, let me just make sure I do know how much. Let me just check here (checks on her laptop) . . . Wow, more than I realized.

Pt.: Yeah, according to your scales, I've gained close to 20 lbs.

Clin.: Yeah. No, you have.

Pt.: Is that caused by the Lopressor?

Clin.: Could be. (pauses) It's not a real common side effect on the Lopressor, but it does happen with some people. Usually it's a small amount of weight, but there are some people who gain a lot of weight. Those patients also tend to find it's hard to lose weight. It just depends on the individual.

Pt.: Yeah, I thought so (said sort of forlornly). I went out on the web, and a lot of people are complaining about gaining weight on these drugs. (pauses) That really really bothers me. And I'm eating much less than I usually do, and I'm one of those people who can't seem to lose the weight. Not only that, but despite feeling tired all the time, I've been walking a mile or more every day like you suggested last time. It's exhausting and I'm still not losing weight.

Clin.: Well, that's a bit of a more serious problem. To be honest, if we raise the dose, and I was considering suggesting doing so, just to get a little better control, I think there's a good chance the weight problem is gonna stick around if it is caused by the Lopressor, which it might or might not be.

Pt.: I really don't want to raise this.

Clin.: I can see why. The extra 20 lbs added to the 25 you already had is really making your weight a more major problem. It's sort of undercutting what we're trying to do by lowering your blood pressure. (pauses) How are you feeling about your weight?

Pt.: What do you think!?

Clin.: Probably not too good . . . I'm sure you're unhappy with how it makes you feel and look. Who wouldn't be. Has your husband said anything to you? (**Intimate Relationship Inquiry** – family members often have strong opinions about side-effects) I know you two communicate pretty well.

Pt.: (sheepishly smiles) No. He's too nice a guy. But we haven't had sex in 2 months. And that's really unusual for us. I know it bothers him. It bothers me. It's just a mess.

Clin.: I get you . . . And to think I was so excited too, about the good pressures I mean. (smiles)

Pt.: Me too. But I can't do this.

Clin.: Let's regroup. I want to make sure I'm following how you're seeing all this. The exercise intolerance is bothersome, truly bothersome, but you could probably tolerate it if that was the only side effect.

Pt.: Yeah.

Clin.: But the weight gain is a different story. It bothers you a lot personally. For the record it would bother me too, I know that. And you're really worried about how this is impacting on your marriage. Is that about right?

Pt.: You got it.

Clin.: You know what?

Pt.: What?

Clin.: I think we need to change direction here. We've still got some other medications we can try . . .

Pt.: Thank god!

Clin.: (smiles) You know, Beth, I'm just curious about something.

Pt.: What's that?

Clin.: What would you have done if I had suggested raising the Lopressor? You wouldn't have taken it would you?

Pt.: (smiles sheepishly) Nope . . . In fact, I almost stopped it last week after reading about it on the web.

Clin.: You wouldn't have told me, would you? (smiles)

Pt.: (smiles sheepishly again) Probably not. At least not for a while . . .

I have included this extended dialogue, for it is ripe with information that demonstrates the immense importance of exploring a patient's process of weighing his or her pros and cons. *Note that both anecdotal and research evidence has shown that many patients often do not tell prescribers or other health care providers when they have unilaterally decreased or discontinued a medication.* This lack of communication is, at best, misleading for clinicians when treatment planning and, at worst, frankly dangerous.

If Beth had abruptly discontinued her Lopressor, she could have been headed for some real problems, probably not fatal but definitely not good. In patients with fragile diseases – where the prescribed use of their medications is critical – such unilateral and abrupt changes can be life threatening. A patient with AIDS or a poststent procedure on his or her coronary arteries who abruptly stops an indicated medication risks severe repercussions including death.

Beth also illustrates that even though a medication achieves symptom relief (or in her case, the achievement of a desired physical sign or lab value), it may not be the medication of choice. As former Surgeon General Koop had admonished earlier in our book, no medication works inside a bottle. Despite its apparent efficacy from a clinician's standpoint (effectively lowering the patient's blood pressure), I don't believe Beth would have continued her use of the Lopressor. From a patient's definition of efficacy (Is this drug making me feel better?), it was definitely not efficacious. As we have noted earlier, an ideal treatment plan that the patient is not going to follow is not ideal, it is foolish.

If her nurse practitioner had continued to push on the use of the Lopressor, something even worse potentially could have unfolded – Beth might have lost trust in her clinician. Moreover, Beth would have begun to withhold information from her clinician as well. The therapeutic alliance would have begun to deteriorate, never a good sign for therapeutic success.

By contrast, because the clinician deftly, *intentionally*, and with an open mind chose to explore the third step of the Choice Triad, the clinician uncovered material that changed her own mind about the use of the Lopressor. First, on a purely physiologic level, her discovery of Beth's significant weight gain on top of her already problematic weight suggested that the deleterious effects on her lipids and triglycerides – potentially caused by her increasing obesity – could outweigh the benefits of the lowered blood pressure regarding atherosclerotic plaque. Although it is far from certain that the weight gain was being caused by the Lopressor, it is possible. It is certainly worthy of consideration. Second, as she uncovered the psychological, and legitimate, concerns of Beth about the side effects of her Lopressor, including fears of marital damage (a major con), it became apparent to the clinician that Beth would not stay on this medication. This treatment plan was doomed to failure.

It is also worth noting that when people weigh long-term benefits (preventing a stroke, a myocardial infarction, etc.) against immediately problematic side effects that are causing marked problems right now, it is all too easy, for the patient, to lose sight of the importance of the medication's long-term benefits. *In short, it is human nature, when weighing the pros and cons of just about anything, to give more weight to immediate problems than potential future benefits.*

Another positive effect of the clinician's careful exploration of Beth's weighing of her pros and cons is worth noting. Returning once again to Robert Schuman's comment that "People want to know that their opinions and concerns are worthy of interest and response," nothing convinces a patient that we have listened to their opinions and concerns as convincingly as having their opinions change our own. Nothing.

Beth's relationship with this talented nurse practitioner has been powerfully solidified by seeing the clinician change her recommendation for continuing on the Lopressor. Indeed, if at a future point, this clinician feels that Beth should continue with a different medication despite some very difficult side effects caused by that medication – or perhaps even return to the Lopressor if deemed necessary – it is much more likely that Beth will value her clinician's advice and be more willing to do so. Once again, we are reminded of two compelling truths: (1) discontinuing medications – or not using them as prescribed – is the number one cause of treatment failure and (2) by improving medication interest and follow-through, we can decrease our patients' suffering and, in some instances, prolong or even save their lives.

A Frank Discussion Among Ourselves

Finally, we cannot leave this illustration without acknowledging an important element – time. This exchange took about 5 minutes. That doesn't sound like much time, but in a busy clinic where one is seeing around 20 patients a day, it is. Anyone who claims that it does not take time to ask questions about patients' interests and concerns with medications (and to subsequently take the time to sensitively listen to their answers) is not telling you the truth. The trick is to do so in the most efficient fashion possible, exactly what the MIM was designed to do.

And here we come upon a paradox. Using interviewing techniques such as the those illustrated in the above dialogue, and those techniques described in the remaining pages of this book, can save time – a lot of it. Apparently, what is true in business, "one must spend money to make money," holds true in clinical work with regard to time management: "one must spend time to save time."

Picture patients with serious illnesses such as congestive heart failure (CHF), rheumatoid arthritis, multiple sclerosis, diabetes, chronic obstructive pulmonary disease (COPD), cancer, and AIDS. By way of example, let's look at a patient with CHF who, because the clinician took the 5-10 minutes to discuss and collaboratively decide on the patient's CHF medications, is in strong agreement with the use of his or her medications. This patient religiously uses the medications exactly as directed. The result is a patient whose CHF is in good control. Such a patient may be scheduled for relatively infrequent appointments and may remain an outpatient for years.

By contrast, picture that a different clinician does not take the time to carefully uncover our imagined patient's concerns and hesitancies about his CHF medications. Such clinicians may have saved 5 or 10 minutes of time, or did they?

In the weeks that follow, this patient fails to take his medications as recommended. Soon enough his CHF is acting up. Like clockwork, the calls start coming into the clinician's office at the most hectic of times. The patient is calling because of increased symptoms. Appropriately, frightened family members may also start calling concerned by their father's striking shortness of breath and fluid retention. Staff is starting to get frustrated by the number of disruptive calls, including the prescribing physician, who must handle some of the calls personally, in an already overloaded day, and is also dealing with e-mails from the patient and his family! Soon enough the patient must be seen monthly or even weekly in an effort to control the CHF. Vastly more time is being eaten up by this patient's care than the 5 to 10 minutes that would have been used applying the principles of the MIM. But we're not even close to being done clocking the time that is lost by *not* taking the time to collaboratively agree on a medication regimen with the patient.

This "noncompliant" patient's CHF is going to worsen. The result is a hospitalization or many hospitalizations. Now the clinician (or perhaps a hospitalist to whom the patient's care has been transferred) is going to be doing an initial H&P, rounding daily, and dictating or typing up a lengthy discharge summary while intermittently dealing with unpleasant insurance hassles. It is not an exaggeration to say that the 5 to 10 minutes it would have taken to explore the steps of the Choice Triad – to use the MIM to share decision making – could have saved hours and hours of time. If this patient ends up in an ICU, the number of lost hours is staggering.

And here we have stumbled on yet one more advantage – a financial one – to implementing shared decision making with strategies such as the MIM. With the advent of the Affordable Care Act (ACA) and other foreseeable systems that may supersede it, it is likely that the government intends to financially reward clinicians and health care systems that can concretely demonstrate improved rates of "medication adherence," which demonstrably drive down health care costs.

The Subtle Art of Exploring Side Effects

In Chapter 6, where we discussed MIM approaches for use during the initial appointment and the writing of the "first script," we saw two techniques – Introducing Shared Expertise and the "Call Me First" Invitation – that are effective ways to directly invite the patient to share future side effects. Let us now see how we can follow-through with this invitation during subsequent med checks as the patient wrestles with his or her concerns about efficacy. The patient's potential conundrum will be triggered by the all too common appearance of unwanted side effects that must be weighed against wanted benefits (some of which might not have shown up yet!).

Peter Weiden points out that our initial invitation to share side effects is not always easy to accept in subsequent sessions. Part of the problem lies in the very nature of the more traditional models of "medication adherence" that sometimes, inadvertently, create an oppositional dynamic. As Weiden cogently states, such oppositional dynamics can result in a relationship "encumbered by obedience issues" as described in Chapter 6.

These obedience issue dynamics must be dismantled quickly if the medication alliance is to be a healthy one, in which both parties truly share expertise and decision making. If the patient does not share his or her concerns about side effects, there is nothing the clinician can do to alleviate them. Weiden proposes two techniques for dismantling the obedience rut, which can be adapted to address side effects, as well as further reenforce the "shared-expert" spirit of the MIM.[6] Here is a slight adaptation of one of Weiden's techniques that I have found to be useful:

TIP 34 Hurt Feelings Observation

"Sometimes patients are nervous about telling me what is really going on about their side effects because they are afraid of hurting my feelings or making me angry. Please always let me know if you are having any side effects. Our goal as a team is to limit them and, if we have to, change medications. I promise you I won't take it personally if you decide you need to stop the medication because its side effects outweigh its benefits for you."

Weiden's original technique was designed to help a patient *who has already stopped a medication* to relay "the secret" with a minimum of shame and/or guilt. When used for this purpose, it reads exactly as Weiden delineates:

"Sometimes patients are nervous about telling me what is really going on about their side effects because they are afraid of hurting my feelings or making me angry. Although I certainly think it is a good idea for you to stay on medication, I promise you I won't take it personally if you've stopped."

Below, another one of Weiden's techniques for uncovering completed discontinuance can be adapted to spotting impending discontinuance related to the patient's side effects perceptions.

TIP 35 The "Let's Get Off the Medication Together" Invitation

"If you are like many patients, at some point you might decide that you want to stop a medication, perhaps because of its side effects. Although there might be a part of you that doesn't want to tell me, please do. It's okay. I want you to tell me about any side effect concerns, and if you feel we need to stop the medication, let's do it together. If I know that's what you want to do I can help you to get off the medication in the safest possible way. Even if we decide we have to agree to disagree about whether or not stopping the medication is wise, it doesn't matter, you have to make the final decision and my goal is to make sure that whatever decision you make, we do it safely. Hearing your concerns will also help me to make better recommendations for you down the road. We are a team here."

Recognizing the inherent hesitancies that patients may have about reporting side effects, we come to our next interviewing principle: *Always directly ask patients in each encounter about the presence of side effects*. Without asking directly about side effects, clinicians and case managers invite misunderstanding. This misunderstanding can be a harbinger of discontinuance. The following technique in its differing variations is an antidote to the problem, and we already saw it illustrated in the above conversation with Beth:

TIP 36 Direct Side Effect Inquiry

"Are you getting any of the side effects that we talked about last time?"

or

"Are you having any problems that you are wondering whether or not they might be a side effect?"

Weiden adds the following variation:

"Are there any side effects that cause distress or discomfort?"[7]

Once a patient has shared a concern about a side effect, the goal is to ascertain how the patient experiences the side effect and how the patient feels the problematic side effect stacks up against the benefits of the medication. The clinician should guard about preconceived ideas that the benefits outweigh the cons. Once again, the ultimate decision maker (unless a medication is being court-ordered) is always the patient. I believe this collaborative exploration of how the patient views the personal impact of the side effect on his or her functioning is enhanced by the number and specificity of the interviewer's questions about the side effect being reported.

For instance, let us look at some questions that can be useful in ascertaining the impact, from the patient's perspective, of a commonly encountered side effect – nausea. We will use nausea as our prototype for exploring a side effect, for I think you will find the type of questions that follow to be of use with almost all side effects. Common triggers for nausea include NSAIDs, antibiotics, antidepressants, chemotherapeutic agents, and narcotics, but a myriad of other agents can cause nausea including cardiac glycosides, certain antihypertensives such as potassium sparing diuretics, and oral hypoglycemic agents such as metformin. In short, whether one is a physician, nurse clinician, physician assistant, or clinical pharmacist, one will be involved in many a frank discussion with patients about nausea.

Even mild nausea can be a surprisingly potent con to the use of any of the above medications. And it can be easy to underestimate the impact of nausea on any given patient, for each person responds to nausea differently. For some patients nausea is reasonably tolerable if mild, for other patients it is simply intolerable even when mild in nature. And for most patients moderate to severe nausea of a persistent nature is often intolerable. No matter who the patient or how mild the nausea, it is important that he or she feels the clinician is taking his or her concerns seriously. The following types of questions can be useful in metacommunicating the genuine concern and interest these patients are seeking:

TIP 37 Techniques for Conveying Concern About Side Effects

a. "Tell me about a specific time you felt nauseated and walk me through what happened."
b. "Just how bad does the nausea get?"
c. "How often are you feeling it?"

d. "How many days this week did you get it?"
e. "Is it making it harder for you to do anything?"
f. "On a scale from 1 to 10, with 1 meaning 'it hardly bothers me' and 10 meaning 'I can't stand this side effect,' where would you put your nausea this past week?"
g. "I have some ideas about what to do to get rid of the nausea, but if we can't, do you think the nausea is bad enough that it outweighs the good things your medication is doing. Sometimes it's a tough call, but only you can make it. The bottom line is: do you think the benefits (name them) are outweighing the problems with the nausea at this point?"

Such questions cut to the core of the matter so that there is no miscommunication possible here between the patient and the prescriber. By understanding how problematic a side effect is, we can help the patient weigh the pros and cons more effectively. Moreover, it allows us to brainstorm with the patient on various options for attenuating the nausea caused by the medication in question, if possible, or switching medications, if necessary. Now that we have examined the issue of common side effects, let's take a look at a significantly less common side effect, but one that presents our patients with an extraordinarily difficult decision. Indeed, we have entered the arena of the most frightening of all potential adverse reactions.

How to Present a Medication When One of the Potential "Side Effects" Is Death

When clinicians propose a treatment that carries risks of dangerous adverse reactions, they must inform the patient of those risks.[8] For instance, some medications in internal medicine carry a distinctly increased risk of death, as is seen with chemotherapeutic agents in oncology. Medications used to treat illnesses such as rheumatoid arthritis, psoriasis, or AIDS may so compromise the patient's immune system as to allow the emergence of potentially life threatening opportunistic infectious agents or cancers. Some of our antiepileptic medications carry an increased risk of potential lethality such as carbamazepine (agranulocytosis), divalproex sodium (chemical hepatitis), and lamotrigine (Stevens-Johnson syndrome). In psychiatry, clozapine may lead to agranulocytosis, cardiac myopathy with sudden death, or the metabolic syndrome and diabetes. These potentially lethal adverse reactions must be discussed openly with patients. The question becomes, "How does one raise these issues in such a way that one is effectively describing risk without generating inappropriate fear?"

One solution lies in an interviewing technique called Personalizing the Risk. I'll use an example – clozapine – from my own discipline (psychiatry), for I am familiar with presenting this medication and its potentially serious adverse reactions to patients. Clozapine also provides a particularly convincing prototype of the power of Personalizing the Risk as a method for sensitively introducing lethality as an adverse reaction, for it is not only scary in its lethality, it also requires the patient to undergo frequent blood drawing (an accompanying con that many patients are not eager to embrace) to monitor for the emergent signs of impending agranulocytosis. In short, the use of clozapine can be a bit of a hard sell. Nevertheless, I have found Personalizing the Risk to be effective at helping patients feel more comfortable with giving clozapine a chance and the results have often been life transforming, for clozapine has proven to be a frequently effective antipsychotic when other antipsychotics have failed.

Imagine a clinician who has been working for years with a patient, whom we shall call Roberto, whose schizophrenia has responded poorly to antipsychotics. They have established a robust therapeutic alliance, having navigated some rough roads together. Roberto has been doing somewhat better but is still hounded by disabling voices and intermittent delusions. Psychologically, Roberto has successfully embraced both Step 1 and Step 2 of the Choice Triad – he believes he has schizophrenia and he believes that medications may help, although he has been sorely disappointed by their lack of effectiveness to date.

The clinician is personally convinced that clozapine could be potentially lifesaving (preventing suicide) and/or life transforming for Roberto. After explaining the pros and cons of clozapine effectively, including the potential for death, the clinician might proceed as follows:

TIP 38 Personalizing the Risk

"You know, Roberto, when thinking about using clozapine, one has to give a lot of thought to it, because of the dangerous side effects that I mentioned. You and I have a pretty good relationship and have known each other for a long time now, and I think we trust each other. Considering the fact that every medication we've tried has failed, and this medication has a definite tendency to help when other medications have not helped with schizophrenia, if I was in your spot, I would absolutely take it myself. Not only that, but the risk of the bone marrow problems and the possible problems with your heart and diabetes is relatively low, if we carefully keep our eyes out for them and take protective steps if any changes are seen. When a team carefully monitors for these side effects and, trust me, we will, I feel very confident that this is a generally safe medication to use – so much so that I would give it to a member of my own family if he or she were in your spot. I wouldn't say that to you unless I meant it."

By utilizing Personalizing the Risk, based on a genuine belief in the relative safety in using clozapine when monitored properly, the clinician has helped the patient to address one, if not *the*, most difficult decisions that a person can make in Step 3 of the Choice Triad – weighing the pros of a medication against the possible con of death. No doubt, it is of value to hear from a trusted clinician an honest and spontaneous sharing of the clinician's personal opinion when suggesting the use of potentially dangerous medications from chemotherapeutic agents to agents for the treatment of autoimmune disorders, seizures, and AIDS. This interviewing technique can also be of use when introducing other agents, where the clinician needs to discuss potentially significant or unpleasant, but nonlethal, side effects or serious adverse reactions. *One should never use Personalizing Risk unless one has a genuine belief in one's recommendation and would, indeed, be comfortable taking the medication if one were in the patient's circumstances.*

As we wrap up our discussion of Personalizing the Risk, it is worth returning to a peripheral, yet important, point made earlier in the book. The principles and techniques of the MIM are obviously focused on issues surrounding the use of medications. Yet the Choice Triad construct of the MIM is, in actuality, a generalized motivational theory that can be applied to almost any health-related patient choice including patient decisions about agreeing to undertake specific forms of case management, wellness programs, and exercise protocols.

In addition, almost all of the specific interviewing techniques of the MIM as they stand – or in some cases if modified only slightly – are prototypic examples of shared decision making. One can use them when helping patients to review the pros and cons of all of the above health options. After a patient has made the choice to try a specific intervention – whether it be a smoking cessation program or a physical therapy program status post a hip replacement – many of the specific interviewing techniques of the MIM can subsequently be utilized to enhance patient motivation for follow-through. No place is this useful generalizability better illustrated than with surgery and the use of Personalizing the Risk.

As we saw illustrated in Chapter 8 with our patient, Mr. Blount, who was contemplating knee surgery, the three steps of the Choice Triad are as reliable a construct for understanding how a patient chooses surgery as they are for understanding how a patient chooses a medication. A patient contemplating surgery will have to navigate all three steps of the Choice Triad: (1) feel something serious is wrong, (2) feel that surgery may be the best choice for relief, and (3) believe that the pros of surgery outweigh the cons. In this regard, if the reader is considering surgery as a career (or perhaps is already a surgical resident or surgeon), I believe you will find Personalizing the Risk, in particular, to be a surprisingly useful technique when collaboratively helping a patient to weigh the pros and cons of surgery where the "side effect" of potential death is not infrequently present.

Questions for Uncovering Positive Effects of Medications

As important as the task of eliciting, and subsequently helping to relieve side effects is, it is equally important to help the patient obtain a clear picture of the medication's benefits, for side effects can quickly become preoccupations that hide benefits from the patient's awareness. Once again, the simplest approach is to ask directly:

TIP 39 Symptom Relief Inquiry

"Is the medication helping with any of your symptoms?"

If the patient answers yes, add, regarding the symptom in question, "Give me a rough estimate, has it barely helped, helped a little, helped a lot, or totally gotten rid of the symptom?" With sophisticated patients, one can ask them for a percentage of relief provided by the medication from 0% to 100% relief. As time permits, you can repeat such questioning with other symptoms that the medication appears to be relieving.

Depending on the disease for which the medication is being prescribed, as we have seen earlier, it is often less the patient's direct symptom relief and more the indirect alleviation of the detrimental complications of the patient's illness that convinces a patient that a medication's pros outweigh its cons. Such benefits can include an improvement in functioning, an increase in mobility, an increase in a sense of self-worth, an enhanced ability to enjoy life, and, not least of all, hope. In this regard, the following questions can be useful for uncovering those reductions in the costs of the illness that can be tapped as powerful enhancers of motivation for continued medication use:

TIP 40 The "Life Is Better" Inquiries

"Is your medication helping you to get around better?"
"Is your medication making you feel more hopeful about the future?"
"Is your medication making it easier to be at work?"
"Is your medication helping you to enjoy your family/friends more?"

If you know specifically what activities and pleasures have been disrupted or discontinued for the patient by his or her illness, one can be more personalized as with:

> "Tyra, I know how much you've missed going on social media since your illness, because you just feel so wiped, have you been able to get back on Facebook and your Twitter feed again since beginning your (name of medication)?"

> "Julio, have you been able to get back to your online gaming since we started you up on (name of medication)? I know you've missed your gaming friends a lot."

Curiously, despite being positively experienced by the patient, such major indirect "pros" of a medication are not always immediately ascribed by the patient to the use of the medication. Medication interest and motivation for follow-through can be enhanced, sometimes to a significant degree, merely by helping the patient more concretely associate such indirect benefits with the use of the medication itself. You might recall that the Inquiry into Lost Dreams technique from Chapter 8 was designed to proscriptively create such associations in the mind of the patient.

In a similar light, regarding psychological benefits more directly, many readers, especially those readers that enter fields related to primary care will be prescribing many antidepressants and antianxiety agents. Indeed, more antidepressants are prescribed in the field of primary care and associated subspecialties, than in the field of psychiatry itself. Whenever, and by whomever, they are prescribed, Weiden describes several variations on the Life Is Better Inquiry that can help patients recognize the benefits of their psychotropic medications including[9]:

"Is your medication helping you to feel better in any way?"
"Is the medication helping you deal with stresses or day-to-day problems?"
"Does the medication make life easier for you in any way?"
"Is the medication helping with any of your relationships?"

Before leaving the area of discussing the pros of a medication, it is useful to remember another important interviewing principle from Peter Weiden: *Don't oversell the benefits of a medication.*[10] It is important to communicate both confidence and hope regarding any medication that one is prescribing, but it is important that the clinician be aware of the limitations of the medication as well. As Weiden points out, some medications may not be curative or may not even be able to restore "normal functioning."

It is important that the patient be aware of the legitimate benefits of the medication so that he or she is not disappointed by inappropriate expectations for relief. Such disappointments can also deleteriously impact on the medication alliance, for the disappointed patient may feel that the clinician is not a credible source of information or, even worse, is willing to purposely mislead the patient.

Uncovering the Patient's Pros and Cons Regarding Cluster B – Cost

> You tell them – you tell them there's a cost . . . Every decision we make in life, there's always a cost.[11]
>
> Brad Meltzer
> *The Inner Circle*

Cost is the second major cluster of beliefs that patients weigh while deciding whether to continue or to stop a medication. Cost is translated by most patients into a question such as, "Is it worth it to me to take this drug?" As clinical experience suggests – and McHorney's research verifies – money is a major issue regarding medication interest and follow-through. Returning to our "internal committee" metaphor, on the pro side, the patient may have many internal committee members singing the praises of a medication, but all one needs is one member of the committee to say, "That's all well and good, but we simply don't have the money and that's that."

Moreover, money is not the only issue. There can be other costs to taking medications. These costs include concerns such as inconvenience, workplace disruption related to medication use, and interpersonal challenges. We will examine how to address all these costs in this section.

Interviewing Techniques for Addressing Financial Costs

The Art of Sensitively Exploring Cost: More Taboo than One Might Think

We want to be aware of cost issues as a potential serious problem, not only because they can lead to medication discontinuance but also because we may be able to do something constructive to prevent such discontinuance. Financial cost is a major impediment to medication interest, but it does have a surprising number of potentially helpful solutions, including use of generics, use of medication samples, formal use of pharmaceutical programs for indigent patients, and supplemental governmental and insurance programs related to the ACA (or whatever future governmental programs may be in effect).

As we discussed in Chapter 6, Howard Brody makes the point that not only is the personal relationship *the* tool of the trade for clinicians, to use this tool effectively the clinician's "approach to the patient's problems must be grounded in the way the patient defines the problem."[12] In this regard, we need to see how each patient is defining the problem of cost, because patients may be embarrassed by their financial situations. In such instances, instead of viewing money as the problem, patients may view themselves as the problem for not having enough money. This type of negative self-impression can make the topic of cost a taboo.

If we don't know of the problem, then there is nothing we can do about it. While sitting in a café, busy at work with the first edition of my book introducing the MIM,[13] a nurse, who happened by, provided me with the following interviewing principle: *Develop the habit of routinely asking every patient about the cost of his or her medications, because if you don't ask, you often will not be told.*

As prescribing clinicians and as case managers, it is sometimes a sobering realization to see the financial burdens of our prescriptions. Despite its best intentions, it is not clear yet the extent to which the ACA will help with these costs especially if it is ultimately repealed and replaced or modified. In any case, the importance of applying this interviewing principle will probably only increase in time. Let us look at a variety of variations on a single interviewing technique that effectively allows the employment of the above interviewing principle:

TIP 41 Gently Exploring Cost Issues

1. "Mrs. Phillips, I'm always curious about how much my patient's medications cost. How much did you end up having to pay for the (insert medication in question) this past month?"
2. "Were you surprised by the cost?"
3. "How much of that did you have to pay for yourself?"
4. "It can be tough for anyone to pay for his or her medications; how much of a burden do you think this will be for you and your family?"

Routinely asking such questions assures insight into the financial cost issues potentially impacting on our patients' medication interest. Using these interviewing techniques, the clinician can gently open the door into this critical topic. Naturally, the next question is, "Having uncovered prohibitive cost issues is there anything we can do about it in an immediate sense?"

Generic medications of a certified bioequivalence are certainly a reasonable first answer. Another thing to keep in mind is that, regarding a specific medication, a pill that is twice the dosage of another one may be only fractionally more expensive. In such a case, if the pill is scored, you can write the script for pills of the double dosage and then instruct your patient to cut the pill in half, being sure that the patient is able to do so effectively. *I sometimes have patients demonstrate in front of me how they halve the dosage to make sure that they can do so appropriately, keeping in mind that patients with rheumatoid arthritis or failing eyesight may have trouble with such a task.*

On a more systems-wide perspective, with the hectic pace of our clinics, anything that slows up a prescriber is going to have a tendency to not get done. Sometimes a lot of chart culling and paper processing is needed to get a patient enrolled in one of the pharmaceutical plans for the indigent.

If there are particular medications that a clinician often uses in his or her clinic – that are available on such plans – it may be useful to have the office manager type up a list of those medications, including whom to call, the telephone number, and what information will be needed from the chart for that particular pharmaceutical company plan. Such a list posted on the wall of the examining office serves both as a prompt to consider such programs and as a much appreciated way of getting the job done quickly, with the least amount of hassle. The bottom line of such a posting is that more patients may get the advantage of some of these generous pharmaceutical programs.

A Paradox: When High Prices Are Good

In our ongoing efforts to help patients maintain an interest in staying on medications, a nurse from Oklahoma, Rosemarie Borjon, shared a counter-intuitive, yet very sound insight in one of my MIM workshops. We humans "like a good deal," and it can be very appealing to patients to understand fully the magnitude of the deal that they are receiving when pharmaceutical companies provide medications free of cost or at reduced prices (or insurance benefits are kicking in from plans made available from the ACA). Before I had heard Rosemarie's tip, I would normally just say something like, "Boy, it's great that we are going to be able to get these meds for free, they cost a fair amount." But Rosemarie shows how it is wise to be a bit more specific:

TIP 42 Making the Most of a Good Bargain

"Mrs. Timkins, I just checked on the regular price of [name of medication in question] for a 30-day supply, and it would normally cost you [give unadjusted cost]. You'll be getting it at the price of only [give adjusted price after insurance discount, pharmaceutical house discount, or free as with a 'sample']. You're getting an extraordinary bargain on a very expensive and effective medication. I'm very excited about it."

According to Rosemarie, informing the patient of the actual dollar cost of a medication (provided free from a pharmaceutical or at a lowered cost from a governmental agency/insurance program) can help enhance both medication interest and follow-through in several ways:

1. The patient may attach a higher degree of efficacy to the medication as in, "a medication that costs $380 per month must be better than one that only costs $12 per month."

2. Patients may be more hesitant to miss doses because they are thinking about how much money they wasted when they just tossed $15 (three pills) down the toilet because they weren't used as prescribed.
3. They don't feel so bad about their co-pay. For instance, a patient may not feel so intimidated by a $30 co-pay, if they are aware that without their insurance, they would be paying $450 per month.
4. Truly understanding the excellent value that they are receiving makes it significantly easier for patients to feel that it is worth doing the extra paperwork for verification documents.

Interviewing Techniques for Addressing Costs Unrelated to Money

The Hidden Cost: Inconvenience

James Ellison makes the following point that is often not given enough attention: "In general, patients should be discouraged from beginning a treatment that is likely to become burdensome as a result of inconvenience."[14] At first glance, the point seems painfully obvious, but I have been surprised at how often I seem to ignore it.

I ignore it, not because I do not believe it, but because I am unaware just how inconvenient this particular regimen for this particular patient has become, because I have not asked about it directly. Once again, our interviewing principle is simple: *Ask patients directly about inconvenience, paying particular heed to the patient's perception of its degree of burdensomeness*. As with financial cost, subtle taboos push patients toward silence on this topic.

Inconvenience can manifest in many ways, and it often occurs as a daily problem. On a mild side, with a patient who is easily forgetful, multiple dosing schedules frequently result in missed doses. The hassles inherent in trying to remember when to take one's medications can create an ongoing and unpleasant inconvenience. On a more moderate side, a disabled or elderly patient may find it difficult to drive to the pharmacy. Sometimes the waits at the pharmacy are surprisingly punishing for a patient with COPD, who is uncomfortably short of breath, or a patient, with a social anxiety disorder, who is acutely intimidated by a crowded pharmacy waiting room.

These practical concerns – which can create daily moments of inconvenience and worry – actually move us into the topic of how do we, as clinicians, help patients with medication follow-through *after they have decided to try a medication*. Such a shift in topic, if we chose to pursue it, would take us outside the realm of the relationship between enhancing patient choice/motivation with interviewing techniques, which is the primary focus of the MIM and our book. Fortunately, for any readers interested in this very important topic (enhancing medication follow-through) you will find it concisely addressed in Appendix B (e.g., case management, smartphone prompts, easier-to-use pillboxes, behavioral tailoring, dosage simplification, etc.).

On the other hand, such practical concerns cannot be addressed unless the clinician is aware that problems with inconvenience exist in the first place. It is to the initial unmasking of such problems in the interview that we can now turn our attention. Several problems and interviewing techniques for uncovering them come to mind:

TIP 43 Inquiry into General Inconvenience

"Are you finding that taking the medications is inconvenient for you in any way?"

TIP 44 Inquiry into Timing Inconvenience

"Sometimes it can be hard to remember when to take medications. Are you finding that it is hard to remember to take your medications at the times that I had suggested. If so, we might be able to figure out better times?"

TIP 45 Inquiry into Transportation Inconvenience

"Have there been any problems for you in getting to and from the pharmacy for your medications?"

Let us look at an example of an interviewing technique that can address one of these problems once uncovered: an elderly woman who finds driving to the pharmacy to be frightening. She has a son who can do it for her, but he lives 30 minutes away. She feels guilty (a psychological cost of her illness) that he has to drive this distance to get the prescription from her and then drive another 15 minutes to the pharmacy. Our patient is between the proverbial rock and the hard place. She needs the medications. It is daunting to go herself. She does not want to inconvenience her son. If we remember the advice of Ellison, it looks like we are setting up a situation where inconvenience is going to become burdensome.

While presenting a workshop at Riverview Physician Services in Wisconsin, a certified medical assistant provided me with a readymade tip for this problem. She commented that with the elderly or disabled (or with anyone who had transportation problems), especially when regarding the first script, she asks:

TIP 46 Calling in Prescriptions for the Patient

"Would you like me to call that prescription in for you? Once I've called it in, you won't have to wait as long at the pharmacist and, if you like, someone else could pick up the medication for you. He or she doesn't have to get the prescription from you. Your medications will be waiting for him or her at the pharmacy. You can even call ahead and make sure the prescription is ready to be picked up."

She reported that these patients often seemed visibly relieved and were appreciative of this simple act of kindness. Not only had a potentially disengaging roadblock to medication interest been dismantled, but the patient had also found a clinician who cared. With the advent of e-scripts, this tip has become even easier to employ.

The Stigmatization Cost: Problems at the Workplace

If a patient's boss has created a pervasively hostile environment toward employees who are coping with long-term illnesses, a patient may experience anxiety several times a day as he or she sneaks off to the bathroom to quickly gulp down a tablet or two. In other instances, patients with specific diseases, such as epilepsy, depression, and AIDS, may be wary of sharing this information at the workplace, secondary to stigmatization issues in the culture.

Because these concerns are universal in nature, I have found it useful to raise the issue of workplace stigmatization with my patients even when they do not raise it spontaneously. On occasion, I have been surprised by the intensity of the problem, an intensity that had clearly led to missed doses and, at times, had given the patient thoughts of stopping the medication altogether. The following simple question serves as a nice introduction to the topic:

TIP 47 The Workplace Inquiry

"Are you having any problems with taking your pills at work?"

At one of my MIM workshops, Samir Tuma, a clinical Associate Professor of Medicine at the University of Texas Medical School, offered a clever strategy for dealing with workplace stigmatization whether it results from employer or fellow employee stigmatization. He finds that the following advice is often greatly appreciated:

TIP 48 The "Vitamin Bottle" Decoy

"I have found that there is a very simple way to deal with this problem. At home keep your medication in its standard bottle. But bring a couple of your pills to work in a tiny, but well-labeled empty 'vitamin bottle.' Then you can pull the bottle out anytime at lunch or where most appropriate, and, if anybody asks, just rave about how much benefit you've been getting from vitamin C or whatever vitamin you choose to rave about. No one will give it a second thought."

The Tragic Cost: Disruptions in Relationships

A Matter of Safety and Needed Deception

A patient's choice to use medications can have unintended and marked interpersonal costs that can become surprisingly dark in nature all too quickly. Some patients may be coping with an alcoholic spouse/partner who is highly opposed to the use of medications and could erupt into physical violence if his or her spouse's "dirty little secret" is revealed. With such severe consequences – including the possibility of physical assault – the patient's internal committee may wisely answer the question, "Is it worth it to me to take this drug?" with a flat out "no." As we have seen so many times before, the healer's art is to help the patient share these concerns during the office visit itself. I have found that the easiest approach is to gently ask:

TIP 49 The Dangerous Secret Inquiry

"Have you been able to share with your partner (husband, wife, spouse) that you're taking this medication or have you decided to sort of keep it hidden for a while."

The indirect, unassuming quality of this question can gently open the door for a patient to share his or her troubling fears. I want to emphasize to the reader that domestic violence is truly ubiquitous, and it is a secret that will often be withheld without skillful interviewing as reflected by the Dangerous Secret Inquiry. As one can well imagine, a negative response (e.g., the patient has not shared the use of the medication) to the Dangerous Secret Inquiry may be the clinician's first hint of the presence of domestic violence, which the clinician can subsequently explore in a sensitive fashion.

Side Effects Are a Family Affair

At other times, a partner/spouse may disagree with the use of medications because of the impact of the patient's medication-induced side effects on him or her. These collateral side effect concerns represent potentially powerful cons to the use of our prescribed medication from a different light. The question for the patient is not, "How is this side effect making me feel?" It is, "Is the side effect causing other people problems whom I love?" In this regard, sexual dysfunction and weight gain can create powerful problems between a couple. To uncover such sensitive issues, Weiden suggests the following general technique[15]:

> **TIP 50 Inquiry into Med-Induced Relationship Problems**
>
> "Are there any side effects interfering with your relationships?"

Even if one receives a negative answer to this question, if the medication in question is known to cause sexual side effects, I have found it to be useful to directly ask about them because of the strong social taboo against admitting sexual dysfunction. Moreover, sexual dysfunction is often not raised spontaneously by patients. Instead, affected patients tend to simply stop the medication. Once the topic has been raised, it is valuable to ask how the person's spouse or partner feels about the dysfunction, for his or her voice will cast a powerful vote on the decision to continue on the medication.

This area of relationship-related discontinuance (and the opinions of family and friends on shaping the patient's final decision in the Choice Triad) is so important that we will devote an entire chapter to it (Chapter 14).

An Unexpected Cost: Thwarted Goals

As with relationships, side effects can cause problems unrelated to how they make the patient feel physically or psychologically. Instead, the problem created by the side effect involves impairment in the ability to achieve a much-desired life goal of the patient. Such examples might include cognitive impairment caused by an antipsychotic preventing a patient from attending college or participating in job training or perhaps weight gain preventing a patient from becoming a personal trainer or model. Even a supposedly minor side effect such as a dry mouth can become a major side effect for a teacher, minister, or actress, all of whom must engage in public speaking frequently. In the same fashion that – as Sir William Osler pointed out – it is critical to understand what patient has a disease, it is equally important to find out what patient has a side effect. Patients will respond differentially to the presence of their side effects.

Even cross-cultural issues can play an intriguing role in how patients view their side effects. In one study of Hong Kong Chinese patients, few of the patients complained about the polyuria (frequent urination) and polydipsia (need to frequently drink fluids) so often seen with the use of lithium. These side effects are commonly problematic with patients of all races in Western countries, for they can cause significant problems in job settings where one is expected to stay in place for hours at a time as well as disrupting sleep. By contrast, most of the Hong Kong Chinese patients viewed these side effects in a positive light. They believed that the increased water consumption and excretion was evidence that the body was ridding itself of toxins and aiding digestion.[16]

A minor side effect to one patient may present as a major side effect to another and vice versa. Peter Weiden posits a simple question for uncovering the patient beneath the side effect:

TIP 51 Dream Destroyer Question

"Are any of your side effects interfering with any of your future goals or work?"[17]

Or a subtle variation that I use:

"Is your [mention specific side effect being discussed] causing you problems at [whatever situation is appropriate, such as school, work, or recreational activities]?"

Uncovering the Patient's Pros and Cons Regarding Cluster C: The Soul of the Pill – Symbolic Meaning to the Patient

I doubt whether a doctor can answer this question in general terms. For the meaning of life differs from man to man, from day to day

> and from hour to hour. What matters, therefore, is not the meaning of life in general but rather the specific meaning of a person's life at a given moment.[18]
>
> Victor Frankl
> *Man's Search for Meaning*

A Most Curious Puzzle

It is not so much that a pill has a soul. It is that each pill has an impact on the soul of those who take it. This impact is particularly marked with patients with severe and chronic illnesses, who are destined to be on medications for many years, perhaps indefinitely. If you must reach for a pill bottle several times a day, over 700 times a year, tens of thousands of times over a lifetime, then that pill is going to assume a meaning to you, personally. The pill will become a symbol. In this sense, when weighing the pros and cons of meaning, the question for many patients becomes one of, "What does it say *about me* that I *have* to take this drug?"

Such a question moves patients inexorably toward deeper questions concerned with meaning – who they are, and why do they need to take this drug that other people do not? "Why am I so different than all of the other kids?" (asthma meds), "Have I become addicted to this drug?" (arthritis pain meds), "Was I born defective?" (seizure meds), "Shouldn't I be able to handle life's stresses without needing a crutch?" (antidepressants), "Shouldn't I rely on God to heal me instead of taking these toxic drugs?" (all medications). For many patients, these are disturbing questions with disturbing answers; for others graceful resolutions exist. The former patients stop their medications, and the latter patients stay on them.

The symbolic meaning of the medication has particular significance when working with patients suffering from severe and chronic illnesses including multiple sclerosis, rheumatoid arthritis, epilepsy, cancer, schizophrenia, bipolar disorder, lupus erythematosus, renal failure, CHF, strokes, chronic pain syndromes, AIDS, and the list goes on and on. It is a list that none of us would like to be on, yet one that all of us know may await us someday.

The truth be told, these are diseases of fear, and the medications that help control and occasionally cure them assume a larger-than-life meaning to both the patient and the clinician trying to comfort that patient. These strikingly high stakes are another reason that these medications cut directly to the substance of the patient's soul and, for that matter, the soul of the clinician.

As we have seen while we examined the issues of efficacy and cost, the patient's perceptions shape the only viable reality with regard to medication interest. As Osler said, it is critical to understand what type of patient has a disease because it is the uniqueness of the patients that will determine the uniqueness of these perceptions. Ultimately, to understand our patients, we must also understand not only what they think about their diseases but also what they think about the medications that they are now forced to take because of their diseases.

Peter Conrad's article, *The Meaning of Medications: Another Look at Compliance*, mentioned earlier in the chapter provides a wonderful introduction into this highly private world. In the concluding pages of this chapter, we will often refer to it.

Over the years, I have come to realize that it is the Cluster C concerns – originating from patients' perceptions of what their need to take medications says about them as people – which is often the major determinant of long-term medication interest. An understanding of this set of beliefs is of particular value in explaining the many instances in which patients suddenly stop an extremely important medication – such as an antiseizure medication or a medication for AIDS – for what appears to be no good reason.

In such situations of puzzling medication discontinuance, we often find, concerning the Cluster A concerns, that the patients feel that the symptom relief brought by the medication outweighs its side effects. Relating to Cluster B concerns, these patients also view the benefits as outweighing both the financial costs and the costs to convenience and psychological well-being. Yet these same patients stop the medications anyway (in which case the results are often catastrophic) – the patient with a stable bipolar disorder goes into a series of manic rages, the MS patient returns to the confines of the wheelchair, and the AIDS patient plummets into a death spiral. Everyone is puzzled.

AIDS: The Hidden Loss

The list of potential losses that a patient with AIDS may face is staggering: loss of functioning, loss of livelihood, loss of financial security, loss of friends due to stigmatization, loss of a sense of well-being secondary to symptoms, and, not least in nature, potential loss of life. These losses are so dramatic that they often overshadow another much more subtle but intensely painful loss. It is a hidden loss that most of our AIDS patients and, indeed, most of our patients with severe and chronic illnesses must deal with on a moment-by-moment basis.

The loss stems from the fact that from the moment we turn to one of our patients and say, "I'm sorry to have to say that it looks like you have AIDS (or cancer or Alzheimer's disease)," the lives of these patients will never be the same again. They immediately, in a matter of seconds, lose the ability to live life without thinking that they may soon lose that life or the ability to enjoy it. It is a haunting fear and a nagging enemy. In some respects, this hidden loss, the ability to not think about "being diseased," may be one of the greatest losses of all.

An understanding of this loss and its immense ramifications pulls us into the heart of our discussion concerning the meaning of medications and the patient's soul. At first glance, one might think that AIDS patients would have minimal problems with taking their medications because the cost of not taking their medications, that is – death – is so striking. But medication interest is sometimes quite problematic with AIDS patients. The answer to this puzzling state of affairs seems to lie in how the patient perceives his or her medication symbolically.

For some patients with AIDS, these medications come to symbolize hope. They are viewed as a godsend. These patients have high medication interest and will tolerate surprisingly severe degrees of both side effects and inconvenience. But for other patients, these medications come to be almost more like enemies.

Part of their low medication interest is logical and easily recognized by all. It has to do with legitimate concerns from Cluster B – cost – both cost of the medications and the disturbing inconvenience related to swallowing the pills themselves. Although the advent of ART (antiretroviral therapy) has decreased the number and size of many AIDS-related medications, certain pills and regimens remain challenging. Some patients experience gagging down their medications, a remarkably unpleasant activity that can be a leading cause of ineffective medication use and even discontinuance.

But the other part of the problem stems directly from the hidden symbolic concerns that we have been discussing and their impact on the meaning of the medications to the patient. These patients are coping with the constant awareness of their disease and the appalling shadow that this awareness casts on their ability to simply "enjoy life" without fear and worry. Some patients coping with AIDS would figuratively "give their right arms" to be able to live a 3-month period again, during which time they would have absolutely no idea that they had AIDS – to savor once more the immense luxury of living life without this lingering shadow.

For these patients, the pills and their pill bottles can come to symbolize not hope but despair. Several times a day, just as they were about to lose awareness of their illnesses, they must reach for these bottles to be reminded of it. Our medications, without any intention on our parts, have come to symbolize, for these patients, not that there is help for their disease but that they are "diseased."

The medications have become constant reminders that life can never be the same again. For some of these patients – and I feel it is a very human and very normal response indeed – it all just becomes too much. They think, "I can't put up with this anymore. I just don't give a damn." Such patients may skip some doses or even stop them altogether.

Described here is a prime example of how a patient's perception of a medication can help define that patient's perception of himself or herself. What, at first glance, had appeared as a puzzling discontinuance of medication, at second glance, makes sense. The discontinuance of the medication is a protective response for a person who is striving to get away from the self-perception that "I am diseased."

I want to return for a moment to an interviewing tip briefly mentioned in Chapter 8, which was provided by a pulmonologist, Ed Hamaty. His tip was mentioned when we were discussing the approach of motivating patients via their desire to "be there" for their families. If you will recall, he had suggested that helping patients to create a phrase to repeat when reaching for their medications, such as, "This is for my granddaughter," could be powerfully motivating (when taking medications for illnesses that may not have immediate symptoms such as hypertension).

Hamaty, in a personal communication, described a sophisticated and practical method of conceptualizing these affirmations that went far beyond their use as family motivators. He suggests that patients often unknowingly adapt some of the demoralizing thoughts, described previously, into psychological scripts that are automatically played with every dosage.

He first noticed this counterproductive process with his AIDS patients but soon found the problem to be ubiquitous across many chronic diseases. As taking the pills becomes more psychologically painful, patients begin to anticipate the unpleasantness of the upcoming "pill-taking ordeal." In essence, they begin to "play a tape" that sounds something like, "Oh God, not this again" or "I'm so sick of being sick."

Hamaty suggests that we can work with these patients to create positive affirmations designed to replace their naturally arising negative ones. The patient's demoralizing tape can thus be "rerecorded" into something much more comforting and inspiring for use as the patient reaches for his or her medications.

TIP 52 Changing Tapes

Picture a patient fighting AIDS, who feels a certain pride in his or her efforts against the AIDS virus, despite the fact that he or she is slowly becoming demoralized. For such a patient, the following two-word affirmation – "Take that!" – directed toward the AIDS virus itself may function almost like a personal act of releasing defiance.

To be maximally effective, Hamaty emphasizes that each aphorism must be individually generated by the patient and have unique meaning to that patient. For instance, if the patient is suffering from intractable pain as he takes his pain medication, the patient might say, directed toward the pain, "Not today you don't."

The creation of such affirmations can be effective with patients dealing with psychiatric disorders as well. For example, many of my younger patients with OCD find it reaffirming to say something like the following: "This one is for you OCD, I'm gonna kick your butt today." Such affirmations externalize the disease so that the patient does not view himself or herself as the problem while focusing the patient on his or her ability to control the OCD symptoms, frequently using cognitive behavioral therapy techniques as well.

When "Cure" Is Not an Option

We can see that there are many things we can try to do to help with the intense demoralization that our patients with chronic illnesses often encounter, from checking to see whether a major depression is on board that may respond to antidepressants, to rallying the patient's support systems, to changing the patient's demoralizing "tape." But even our best efforts do not change the fact that there is ample reason to be demoralized by the presence of a fatal or lingering illness. The acceptance of such a momentous loss is never an easy path for anyone, patient or clinician. Nor can it be.

When discussing the pros and cons of taking a medication – as much as we, or our patients, wish that one of the pros of taking the medication is "cure," we may have reached a stage of the disease process where the only pros are decreased suffering as death approaches. Thus, in addressing Cluster 3, the symbolic meaning of the medication to the patient, both the patient and the clinician may inexorably come upon the fact that the patient must face death.

This inescapable dilemma of both past and modern medicine – that our medications are not always able to stop death – reminds us of a very important point from Chapter 1, a point pertaining to the role of the therapeutic alliance that bears repeating now: "The remainder of this book is an effort to show some of the concrete techniques that can help prescribing clinicians effectively do their part to define this potentially powerful alliance, the alliance that helps us to heal when healing is possible and to comfort when it is not."

It reminds us that one of the most important functions that we serve as physicians, nurses, physician assistants, and other providers is to be there not only when we are offering hope for cure but also when we are communicating that no such hope exists. Such moments of exquisite anguish, and their aftermath, may very well be the moments in which it is most important for us to be there for our patients.

As Thomas Gordon and W. Sterling Edwards point out in their sensitive and insightful book, *Making the Patient Your Partner*,[19] one of the greatest fears that a patient with a fatal illness has is that once the physician or nurse clinician cannot offer a cure, the clinician will disappear. Gordon and Edwards go on to add that simple comments such as, "Don't worry, despite the bad news, I have no intention of abandoning you. I'll see you as often as necessary and we'll fight this thing together" can be extraordinarily reassuring to patients.

It is over the effectiveness or ultimate impotence of our medications that these moments are most apt to arise, hence the importance of their discussion in this book. It is an opportune time to remember that it is our ability to convey our caring that is often the cornerstone of our healing and our ability to comfort. It also reminds us that when our patients or their family members find themselves crying as they face the loss of hope for a cure, the greatest gift we have to offer is often simply our own tears.

The Curious Paradox of Success: Why Patients "Test"

Perhaps one of the most frustrating phenomenon for clinicians occurs when patients, devastated by illnesses such as epilepsy and bipolar disorder – who have finally achieved some freedom from their symptoms – suddenly choose to stop their medications. Many of these patients are intelligent, motivated for health, psychologically intact, well aware of the potential risks of stopping their medications, and are even vocal proponents of the usefulness of medications. Yet, they suddenly stop them. What gives?

These patients are often a puzzlement and a frustration for their prescribers, case managers, family members, colleagues, and even themselves. For me, the insight into these patients and their self-induced relapses came not from my own clinical work, but once again from the writings of Peter Conrad and his work with patients with epilepsy. Let us see what Conrad uncovered.

First, Conrad discovered that patients who had their epilepsy in excellent control would sometimes do exactly what my patients with bipolar disorder would do: abruptly stop their medications. Let us hear why this occurred from one of Conrad's patients herself:

> When I was young I would try not to take it . . . I'd take it for a while and think, "Well, I don't need it anymore," so I would not take it for, deliberately, just to see if I could do without. And then (in a few days) I'd start takin' it again, because I'd start passin' out . . . I will still try that now, when my husband is out of town . . . I just think, maybe I'm still gonna grow out of it or something.

Conrad's patient sheds a brilliant light on the curious paradox that unfolds when medications are effective in relieving symptoms. Indeed, if a medication removes all symptoms – whether in a seizure disorder, an arrhythmia, or bipolar disorder – the paradox is at its maximum. Simply stated, if a medication successfully removes all symptoms, it removes any ability for the patient to know whether the disease is still active.

When medications completely relieve symptoms, paradoxically, the problem with the meaning of the medication is that patients no longer know what it means. They no longer know what they really have and, indirectly, it can feel as if they do not know who they really are. Conrad summarizes far better than I can, what intelligent patients with epilepsy will face if their medications remove all symptoms:

> But how can one know that a period without seizures is a result of medication or spontaneous remission of the disorder? How long can one go without medication? How "bad" is this case of epilepsy? How can one know if epilepsy is "getting better" while still taking medication? Usually, after a period without or with only a few seizures, many reduced or stopped their medicine altogether to test for themselves whether or not epilepsy was "still" there.

With such patients, the discontinuance of their medications is no longer a mystery or a puzzlement. It makes good sense. It is not comfortable or natural to not know what is going on inside one's body. The urge to "test" is not the hallmark of "opposition" or "lack of insight." It is the attempt to gain insight. When I have a patient in good remission, I will periodically ask something along this order:

TIP 53 Testing the Waters

"Jim, you've been doing great on your medications now for over a year. It's wonderful that you have your seizure disorder [substitute whatever illness the patient is dealing with] in excellent control. Some of my patients tell me that after a while they get curious about whether or not they still have their seizures or even need their medications. I think that is a natural curiosity. Do you ever have thoughts like that?"

Depending on what the patient says, one can gain insight as to whether the patient's internal "committee" is getting ready to vote for a unilateral "med-free trial." Sometimes the clinician can convince the patient's committee that such a trial is not advisable. Such proactive questioning by the clinician can prevent a serious relapse.

I should add one other note. Sometimes it becomes obvious to me that a patient is absolutely determined to discontinue his or her medications. After carefully reviewing such a patient's history, *if I determine it is safe to do so*, I will proactively suggest that we taper the medication together under carefully controlled circumstances and with support systems well alerted. In contrast to the frequently deep tailspins that patients experience when they secretly and abruptly stop all their medications without informing their providers, I have found that, in some instances, such controlled tapers allow the treatment team to halt any ensuing decompensation much earlier and to restabilize the patient with much smaller doses.

I generally do this type of taper if the patient agrees to carefully look for early warning symptoms of relapse and to restart the medication, if necessary, and the patient agrees to view it as a legitimate test to see whether the disease is still present. If relapse occurs, it is not uncommon for such patients to gain insight into the need for their medication. This genuine openness on my part – to initiate a taper – often generates a significant increase in the patient's subsequent openness to restart a beneficial medication if problems arise.

For example, I had one patient, with schizoaffective disorder, who had resisted medications for years and had consistently been in and out of hospitals several times every year. He hated being in the hospital but always ended up creating long hospitalizations for himself by stopping his medications secretly and abruptly. Eventually, he agreed to a controlled taper. After three such controlled trials – and resulting brief hospitalizations – he walked into my office and said, "You know what, Dr. Shea, I guess I really need this shit!"

He has continued on his medications since that day. At a later point, he added, "I still don't think I have this schizo-whatever thing. But I am sick of landing in the hospital, and I do get wired up without my lithium."

When Medications Become Symbols of Weakness

General Considerations

We have already seen with Conrad's patients coping with seizure disorders that medications can be viewed by patients as evidence of "being diseased" or may even generate the self-perception that one is somehow weaker than other people because one *needs* to take a medication. Indeed, bearing a chronic illness requires patients to carry the weight of two crosses. They must not only bear the weight that their illnesses bring to them but also the weight that other people foster on them for having those illnesses. Stigmatization can occur across a wide range of diseases, including juvenile onset diabetes, seizure disorders, AIDS, cancer, and, of course, mental illnesses.

Weiden has delineated several questions that can be used across disease states as sensitive probes regarding the impact of the use of a medication on a person's self-perception[20]:

TIP 54 Tapping for Med-Induced Shame

a. "Do you ever feel that taking your medication is a sign of weakness?"
b. "Do you ever feel embarrassed or ashamed to take your medications?"
c. "Does taking your medication make you feel good about yourself?"

Of course, mental illnesses may very well stand as the "granddaddys of stigmatization." As such, gathering an understanding of the impact of stigmatization with these diseases may help us to better understand how to transform the stigmatization that can be found in many other nonpsychiatric diseases. But there is another reason for us to take a closer look at the impact that our prescription pads or e-scripts may have on our patient's self-image when treating their mental disorders, for many of the readers of this book will be treating many of these patients. And I'm not talking about those readers who choose to enter psychiatry as a specialty.

Prescribing Psychiatric Medications in Primary Care and in Specialties from Endocrinology to Cardiology: The Role of Stigmatization

From epidemiologic studies, we have known for several decades that clinicians working in a primary care setting will be seeing a large number of people coping with psychiatric disorders.[21–24] Just how many can be a little surprising. In fact, *roughly* ***one in every four patients*** *seen in a primary care setting is likely to have a co-morbid psychiatric disorder* with major depressive disorder and dysthymia, anxiety disorders, substance use disorders, and somatoform disorders often topping the lists.[25] Moreover, nearly half of these patients may have two or more psychiatric disorders. These findings are not surprising since nearly half of the people living in the United States will develop a mental health disorder during their lifetime.[26]

In addition, the future of much of mental health care, in my opinion, is going to focus on integrated care in psychiatry. With integrated care, mental health professionals will be housed directly in primary care clinics allowing for an immediate ability to provide sophisticated consultation to primary care providers as well as providing direct care with more complex patients.[27] The bottom line of all of this is simple – if you eventually work as a primary care physician, advanced practice nurse, physician assistant, or clinical pharmacist – you are going to be writing a lot of prescriptions for patients with psychiatric conditions.

If you eventually choose to specialize or subspecialize, whether your ultimate specialty is cardiology, pulmonology, or endocrinology, you are destined to find your clinic waiting rooms filled with patients coping with painful psychiatric disturbances. As mentioned in Chapter 1, such disorders – if untreated – may actually decrease your ability to treat the patient's non-psychiatric disorder (*patients with untreated depressions frequently find it difficult to take the medications prescribed for their nonpsychiatric disorders*). Adequate care for the nonpsychiatric diseases of these patients will require that either you or a trusted colleague will need to prescribe psychotropic medications.

The purpose of this section is not to explore all of the complex nuances related to the stigmatization of people who have mental illnesses. Rather, the purpose is to uncover the role of the stigmatization – associated with the use of the psychotropic medications prescribed for these illnesses – in creating damage to the patient's self-image. As we saw earlier, the negative views that patients have toward their medications is often insidiously transformed into a negative view of themselves. This negativity can drop the bottom out of medication interest. This damaging phenomenon is well worth our attention because we can frequently transform it through the use of sound interviewing techniques.

The stigmatization of psychiatric medications, and, consequently, of oneself for needing them, is not solely the domain of psychiatric disorders such as schizophrenia and bipolar disorder, where psychotic process is often encountered. It can also be seen with the more common psychiatric disorders mentioned above (from major depression, generalized anxiety disorder, and PTSD to panic disorder and alcohol and substance abuse disorders), which are seen in the offices of primary care physicians, nurses, and specialists on a daily basis.

For instance, a high functioning woman who was the manager of a medical office and was suffering from a moderately severe depression poignantly described her feelings of stigmatization to me as follows:

> Please don't get me wrong. I really appreciate how much this medication has helped me. But if I'm honest with both you and myself, every time I reach for it, I feel as if I am defective. I just do. I don't know why.

Experiencing such a negative feeling about oneself once, and sometimes multiple times, every day, as one uncaps his or her pill bottle, is no small matter. Returning to our metaphor of the patient having an internal committee that is voting "yea" or "nay" on the issue of staying on a medication, it is easy enough to guess this member's vote. From this point of view, considering stopping the medication, despite it working effectively, is logical; taking the medication is causing psychological damage at least once or twice every day. Such psychological damage is a very real and a very bad side effect.

Imagine the negative consequences of this stigma for patients coping with schizophrenia or bipolar disorder. When these patients are reaching for their medications, they are often experiencing profoundly disturbing thoughts, such as, "They all think I'm crazy. Maybe I am after all. Maybe I'm just worthless. The only way I can function is if they drug me." Needless to say, this type of brutal self-denigration is a significant "con" to taking any medication. It is not illogical for a patient experiencing this type of daily psychological battering to consider discontinuing his or her medication. It is common sense.

Especially with psychotropic medications, one of the major myths widely associated with their use, especially antidepressants, is one that predisposes patients toward such damaging self-denigrations. It is the myth that "I should be able to handle my depression or anxiety without the need for a medication." In this regard, patients often view that the medication in question is an unnecessary – and often expensive – crutch. After providing education on neurotransmitters and their possible role in certain depressions, I like to proactively address such a myth as follows (using an SSRI as an example):

TIP 55 Dismantling the "Crutch Myth"

"There is another common misconception that these medications are crutches that somehow you should be able to cope with depression without medications. But if your brain is not making enough serotonin, it simply isn't making enough serotonin, and you can't just 'will it' to make more, any more than a person with diabetes can will his or her pancreas to make more insulin. We would never tell a person with diabetes that his or her insulin is a crutch because it isn't. We are simply getting that person's insulin back to the normal level that everyone else has.

"It is exactly the same with your depression. Your brain is not making enough serotonin, and we are just going to get your serotonin back to the normal level that everybody else has. It isn't a crutch. It is getting your serotonin level back to normal, so that you then have a fair chance to effectively cope with your stresses. Don't let anyone tell you it is a crutch, because it is simply not true."

The small amount of time this technique requires – and although it is a relatively small amount of time it is not an insignificant amount when you only have 7 to 15 minutes with a patient – can pay off in a big way in increasing medication interest. Without such proactive comments, many patients will have stopped their antidepressants by the next visit, necessitating the time-consuming process of introducing yet another new medication. Furthermore, if, following the medication discontinuation, the patient's depression worsens it may, ultimately, require more frequent appointments or even hospitalizations.

As we have seen so many times before in this book, in such instances, these few comments, which indeed cost us a few minutes, may save many hours of clinical time as well as thousands of dollars if hospitalization results. The proactive use of Dismantling the "Crutch Myth" is a win-win-win situation (saves the patient from suffering, saves the clinician time, saves the system money).

A Surprisingly Indirect Way for Decreasing the Stigmatization of "Needing" a "Drug"

As we wrap up our survey of interviewing techniques for use in navigating the tricky waters churned by stigmatization, an underutilized technique in my opinion might be staring us in the face. Patients often have a high regard for our opinions that leads us to the topic of *selective* "self-transparency." If the clinician feels comfortable with self-transparency – *and is judicious as to when to use it* – sharing something about oneself can be a surprisingly effective tool for helping a patient feel more comfortable about "needing" a medication.

A MIM workshop participant of mine, Aida Li, has found self-transparency to be occasionally useful in destigmatizing. For instance, if the patient appears frightened about a medication, such as an asthma medication or a medication for CHF, she might comment, if true:

TIP 56 Selective Use of Clinician "Self-Transparency"

"You know, my mother is on this medication and thinks it is just great."

At times, it can be useful to share one's own experience:

"You know, Jim, I've been on this same medication for my high blood pressure for years, and it has been an awesome med for me. My blood pressure has been great and any side effects went away quickly."

When a patient hears that the prescribing clinician is using the same medication, it is hard to imagine a more credible endorsement.

Proactively Transforming Medication Stigmatization with Children and Adolescents

For most kids and teenagers, considerable stigma still exists with taking medications, from asthma medications to attention deficit medications.

Few students are comfortable pulling out an inhaler before gym class or trotting off to the school nurse to get a pill. Consequently, it is useful to ask younger patients what it is like to be taking a medication at school or on the playground.

On the other hand, a pediatrician, who treats many children with hyperactivity, told me that he has noticed a change in attitude in a growing number of adolescents over the past decade regarding their medications. Some students are now talking about them a lot. "I'm taking this." "I'm taking that." "I'm on Ritalin." "I'm selling Ritalin, best prices in the school district – locker # 67." You name it, it comes out of their mouths. For a small number of students, especially those students in middle or high school, being on a psychiatric medication has become an "in thing."

Consequently, it is possible that the teenager you are prescribing for has already heard something at school about the medication that you are about to prescribe. As with adults, that "something" might not be too good. In addition, the student may know somebody who is taking the medication and his or her associations with that student may not be positive ones. The following question can ferret out this roadblock to medication interest quite easily:

TIP 57 Teenager Bad Association Inquiry

"Do you have any friends or know of anyone at school who has taken this medication?"

The subsequent exchange may go something like this:

Pt.: Yea . . . (The student starts squirming in his or her seat.) . . . Jimmy Wilson.

Clin.: Who is Jimmy Wilson?

Pt.: (Further squirming) He's the biggest geek in the school. I'm not kidding you. Geek city, dude.

If so, at such moments the astute clinician has the choice of proceeding, "Well, if you just take this medication that I'm offering you, you too can become a geek in just under a month" or "Well, perhaps we can find a medication that works in a similar fashion but which you might be more comfortable with. How does that sound to you?" It doesn't take a rocket scientist to figure out the more effective path for increasing medication interest. But the choice of paths would not have been known, unless the clinician had asked the above question.

Concluding Comments

We have finished our exploration of the Cluster C concerns with which our patients wrestle when weighing the pros and cons of taking a medication or staying on a medication in the third step of the Choice Triad. Indeed, we have discovered that the weighing of the pros and cons – with regard to what the medication may symbolize to our patients – is a complex phenomenon that sheds a penetrating light on the distinction between illness and disease and the importance of understanding the person beneath the diagnosis. This does not surprise us, for we have emphasized the uniqueness of each of our patients throughout the pages of this book. The ability to recognize this uniqueness, and to subsequently tailor the discussion of medication use to the unique perspectives and beliefs of each patient, is at the heart of the MIM, as it is with all shared decision making and person-centered medicine approaches.

I am reminded of the epigram by Victor Frankl that opened our discussion of this section of our chapter: "I doubt whether a doctor can answer this question in general terms. For the meaning of life differs from man to man, from day to day and from hour to hour. What matters, therefore, is not the meaning of life in general but rather the specific meaning of a person's life at a given moment." And so it is with our medications.

With each patient, the meaning of the medication is of the utmost importance in the final weighing of the pros and cons, and this meaning may shift over time. Thus, the question for us is not so much, "What does it mean to this patient to be taking this medication?" Rather it is, "What does it mean to this patient to be taking this specific medication at this specific moment in his or her life?" The only way to know is to ask. And in this concluding section of our chapter, we have learned techniques for effectively doing so.

With the completion of this chapter, we have finished our review of all three steps of the Choice Triad. Regarding its navigation, a few more critical principles and useful tricks of the trade await us in the next chapter.

REFERENCES

1. Blair T. www.brainyquote.com/quotes/keywords/cons.html. Accessed December 12, 2016.
2. Horne E, Weinman J. Patient's beliefs about prescribed medicines and their role in adherence to treatment in chronic physical illness. *J Psychosom Res* 1999;47(6):555–567.
3. McHorney C. The adherence estimator: a brief, proximal screener for patient propensity to adhere to prescription medications for chronic disease. *Curr Med Res Opin* 2009;25(1):215–238.
4. Conrad P. The meaning of medications: another look at compliance. *Soc Sci Med* 1985;20(1):29–37.
5. Ahmed I. Psychological aspects of giving and receiving medications. In: Tseng W-S, Streltzer J, eds. *Culture and Psychotherapy: A Guide to Clinical Practice*. Washington, DC: American Psychiatric Publishing; 2001.

6. Weiden PJ. The adherence interview: better information, better alliance. *Psychiatr Ann* 2011;41(5):279–285.
7. Weiden PJ. The adherence interview: better information, better alliance. *Psychiatr Ann* 2011;41(5):280.
8. Grant JE. What to tell patients about side-effects: when well-intentioned treatment goes wrong. *Curr Psychiatr* 2006;5(2):67–74.
9. Weiden PJ. The adherence interview: better information, better alliance. *Psychiatr Ann* 2011;41(5):280.
10. Weiden PJ. The adherence interview: better information, better alliance. *Psychiatr Ann* 2011;41(5):282.
11. Meltzer B. *The Inner Circle.* https://www.goodreads.com/quotes/tag/life-decisions. Accessed February 8, 2017.
12. Brody H. *The Healer's Power.* New Haven, CT: Yale University Press; 1992:38–39.
13. Shea SC. *Improving Medication Adherence: How to Talk with Patients About Their Medications.* Philadelphia, PA: Lippincott Williams & Wilkins; 2006.
14. Ellison JM. Enhancing adherence in the pharmacotherapy treatment relationship. In: Tasman A, Riba M, Silk K, eds. *The Doctor–Patient Relationship in Pharmacotherapy.* New York, NY: Guilford Press; 2000:84.
15. Weiden PJ. The adherence interview: better information, better alliance. *Psychiatr Ann* 2011;41(5):280.
16. Ahmed I. Psychological aspects of giving and receiving medications. In: Tseng W-S, Streltzer J, eds. *Culture and Psychotherapy: A Guide to Clinical Practice.* Washington, DC: American Psychiatric Publishing; 2001:131.
17. Weiden PJ. The adherence interview: better information, better alliance. *Psychiatr Ann* 2011;41(5):280.
18. Frankl V. *Man's Search for Meaning.* https://www.goodreads.com/author/quotes/2782.Viktor_E_Frankl?page=10.
19. Gordon T, Edwards WS. *Making the Patient Your Partner.* Westport, CT: Auburn House; 1997.
20. Weiden PJ. The adherence interview: better information, better alliance. *Psychiatr Ann* 2011;41(5):280.
21. Barrett JE, Barrett JA, Oxman MD, et al. The prevalence of psychiatric disorders in a primary care practice. *Arch Gen Psychiatry* 1988;45(12):1100–1106. doi:10.1001/archpsyc.1988.01800360048007.
22. Spitzer L, Williams JB, Kroenke K, et al. Utility of a new procedure for diagnosing mental disorders in primary care, the PRIME-MD 1000 study. *JAMA* 1994;272(22):1749–1756.
23. Ansseau M, Dierick M, Buntinkx F, et al. High prevalence of mental disorders in primary care. *J Affect Disord* 2004;78(1):49–55.
24. Kroenke K, Spitzer RL, Williams JB, et al. Anxiety disorders in primary care: prevalence, impairment, comorbidity, and detection. *Ann Intern Med* 2007;146:317–325.
25. Rivelli SK, Shirey KG. Prevalence of psychiatric symptoms/syndromes in medical settings. In: Summergrad P, Kathol RG, eds. *Integrated Care in Psychiatry: Redefining the Role of Mental Health Professionals in the Medical Setting.* New York, NY: Springer Publishing; 2014:5–27.
26. Kessler RC, Berglund P, Demler O, et al. Lifetime prevalence and age-of-onset distributions of DSM-IV disorders in the National Comorbidity Survey Replication. *Arch Gen Psychiatry* 2005;62(6):593–602.
27. Summergrad P, Kathol RG. *Integrated Care in Psychiatry: Redefining the Role of Mental Health Professionals in the Medical Setting.* New York, NY: Springer Publishing; 2014.

CHAPTER 10

Choice Triad Redux: Caring for the Patient

"In general, things either work out or they don't, and if they don't, you figure out something else, a plan B. There's nothing wrong with plan B."[1]

Dick Van Dyke
WINNER OF MULTIPLE EMMY AWARDS

In the last three chapters, we have delineated a variety of specific techniques for exploring the three steps of the Choice Triad. But, before proceeding to Part 3 of our book, "Specialized and Advanced Techniques for Enhancing Medication Interest," it is worth returning to the Choice Triad one more time. As we do so, we will add some final, yet vital, polish to our skills in navigating it, including some tips on enhancing our educational skills when communicating information to our patients regarding the pros and cons of specific medications. In addition, we will examine various methods for both the optimization of Plan A and effective ways for nondefensively acknowledging that a Plan B may be in order. It is often our patients that are the first to know that a Plan B is needed. This chapter provides interviewing techniques that can help us to become more quickly aware of our patients' insights.

We will focus our attention not on our initial appointment with our patients, but on the nuances in play during follow-up med-checks. As important as our initial meetings with our patients might be, the enhancement of the medication alliance is a long-term affair. The use of a medication is not a single choice, it is an ongoing choosing. Like a garden, if not attended to longitudinally, and with genuine care, the results can be disappointing.

As we reexamine the Choice Triad, we will once again see that *collaborative exploration is the transformative engine of the MIM*. It is our collaborative exploration, reflected by our shared decision making, that communicates our sense of caring to our patients. We will discover that it is during our ongoing med-checks that some of the most treacherous waters may lie when navigating the Choice Triad. This chapter is about how to navigate those rough seas with both grace and compassion.

Exploring the Choice Triad: The Importance of Sequence

Generally speaking, to be fully motivated to continue with a medication, patients tend to embrace the three steps of the Choice Triad in sequential order. Although the logic and importance of this process seems at first glance to be self-evident, I have found it to be all too easily missed as clinicians deal with the hectic time constraints of clinics and hospital units. Indeed, one of the most common stalemates that I have seen in supervision occurs when I find a clinician vigorously attempting to convince a patient that a medication's pros outweigh its cons when the patient is not yet convinced that there is something significantly wrong in the first place (Step 1 of the Choice Triad).

As we mentioned in an earlier chapter, in the patient's mind there can be no pros if there is nothing wrong. To push the point of the "pros" of the medication with such a patient will seem, at best, annoying, and, at worst, disengaging, for the patient will feel that "this guy just doesn't get it." It will also appear illogical to the patient for a simple reason. It is.

We are left with the following interviewing principle: *Do not engage in frivolous attempts to secure patient interest in any step of the Choice Triad until the previous steps have been reasonably secured.* Let's see how this principle is applied in the real world of a hectic clinic.

We had mentioned that it is useful in the initial interview to ascertain the patient's "diagnostic passport." For whatever reason, sometimes this passport check is not done. Even when it is undertaken during the first appointment, the patient's passport information may change over the course of treatment.

With regard to the latter circumstance, patients may come across misleading information regarding their disease (or become convinced they have a different disease) from their wanderings on the web. Or, because of their unconscious hopes that there isn't anything serious going on, they may distort the information provided by Dr. Google, convincing themselves that the dangers from a specific disease are not really that bad (not uncommon with asymptomatic diseases such as hypertension, hyperlipidemia, and early diabetes when the costs of taking medications seem to be overly burdensome for a disease that "isn't really bothering me").

If, during ongoing therapy, a clinician comes to feel that a patient's belief in Step 1 is waning, it is important to find out. Ultimately, the likelihood of strong medication follow-through is dictated by the robustness of the patient's belief that there is, indeed, something seriously wrong that could cause him or her significant pain and/or death. When one is suspicious that a patient's belief in Step 1 has weakened, it is generally best to remember an admonition that has served us well: *Assume nothing. When in doubt, ask directly in a sensitive fashion*:

TIP 58 Gauging Step 1 of the Choice Triad

"Jim, do you really believe, deep in your heart, that you have [whatever disorder is present]?"

or

"Jim, in your gut, do your really feel that your high blood pressure could kill you if we don't treat it?"

or

"On a scale from 1 to 10, with 1 being 'I'm not really sure I still have seizures' to 10 being 'I'm totally convinced my seizure disorder is still active' where would you place yourself?"

or

"On a scale from 1 to 10, with 1 being 'I'm not really sure my high cholesterol will give me a heart attack or a stroke if untreated' to 10 being 'I'm totally convinced we need to get my cholesterol down or I may very well get a heart attack or stroke and that really frightens me' where would you place yourself?"

Sometimes a patient's ambivalence quickly dissipates when the interviewer subsequently provides clarifying information. At other times, the patient's doubts may require a gentle, yet persistent, collaborative education on the dangers and/or presence of the disease in question.

If Step 1 has been secured, it is equally important to secure Step 2 before proceeding to Step 3. With regard to ascertaining whether or not the patient has embraced Step 2 of the Choice Triad (the patient feels that a medication can help deliver relief from the identified disorder, symptom, situation), in my experience, gentle directness once again will do the trick:

TIP 59 Gauging Step 2 of the Choice Triad

"Ben, I've noticed that you seem a little bit hesitant about the medication, do you actually think it will help you or are you having some doubts about that, and I really want to know, because if you have some doubts perhaps it might not be the right fit for you?"

Regarding Step 3: A Couple of Tricks of the Trade for Helping Patients to Weigh the Pros and Cons

Duane DiFranco, a physician attending one of my MIM workshops, shared that he has found it to be useful to literally share the metaphor of using a scale with which to weigh the pros and cons. He feels that there is a power to making the implicit model of "weighing the pros and cons" explicit. I have found this to be true. Although Duane's technique is often first utilized in the initial appointment, it is often an image that the patient and his or her physician, nurse, or other provider can return to again and again during ongoing med-checks. It also emphasizes that ultimately, it is the patient who calls the shots on whether to take a medication or not:

TIP 60 The Scale Metaphor Brought to Life

"One of the things I can do is to make suggestions of what medications and dosages might be useful in helping you. It's almost like I'm pointing out weights that you can place on a scale. I can help you know what weights you ought to place on the scale, and your job is to decide how much each of those weights weigh. You are the person who decides how much the medication weighs on the pro and the con sides of the scale for you personally. As you share this information with me, together we can look at these pros and cons, and you can decide what is best for you."

I have found that this visualization of a collaborative scale is a compelling and memorable image for many patients. You can try it out for yourself. I sometimes like to draw the image of a scale on a sheet of paper or on a whiteboard. In addition, there are many excellent images for scales on the web that you can download and make into a laminated card. Such a card will then be readily available for use with your patients. Some clinicians may even prefer to make a small poster utilizing the downloadable image. And as Duane suggests, it is a powerful image that can be referred to by both parties for the rest of the care of the patient.

In the weeks or months following an initial prescription, our patients must decide whether to continue with the prescribed medication – their metaphorical committee must vote yay or nay. The scale will tip one way or the other. Our goal is to help the patient's internal committee (the patient's varying opinions regarding beliefs and feelings regarding all three of the concerns being weighed in Step 3 of the Choice Triad – efficacy, cost, and meaning) to make the wisest decision. Sometimes it is wisest to continue a medication. Sometimes it is not.

The following principle from Chapter 9 comes to mind: *Invite the patient's committee to vote inside your office not outside it by asking specific questions concerning the patient's emerging views of the pros and cons of the medication* ***during each*** *medication evaluation. Once again, assume nothing.* The questions we delineated in Chapter 9 were designed to accomplish this task – uncover exactly how the patient's committee is about to vote. But there is a catch.

Effectively employing some of the interviewing techniques from Chapter 9 will allow us to directly hear from our patients their unique beliefs and fears, but it does *not* guarantee that we will hear how they will, ultimately, weigh their beliefs and fears. The techniques discussed in Chapter 9 do not ensure that the "committee" will vote in front of us – that the patient will make his or her final decision during the office visit itself. Our next task is to increase the likelihood that such a finalized, albeit potentially reversible, vote will take place in front of us, for only then can we offer our feedback, education, and opinions. The following interviewing technique, in its differing variations, is an effective tool for prompting a patient to collaboratively weigh the pros and cons before us so that he or she can arrive at a decision with us:

TIP 61 Tipping the Scales

a. "We've reviewed some of the pros and cons of the medication; now that you've been on it for a while, what do you honestly think about the medication so far?"
b. "Do you really like this medication?"
c. "Do you feel that the relief you are getting from your medication is outweighing its side effects or any of the problems they are causing, you know, like the sleepiness the medication is causing in your classes?"
d. "At this point in time, do you feel that the pros are outweighing the cons with this medication? Remember, I'm counting on you to let me know, because you are the only expert here on how the medication feels to you. I'm not taking it, you are."

It is important to note not only what the patient says when utilizing Tipping the Scales but also how the patient is saying it. Nonverbal evidence of hesitancy may be the only indication that a more deeply rooted concern lies just below the surface of a patient's half-hearted, "Yeah, yeah, it's okay I guess." Such a response can be usefully explored by a simple, "You sound a little hesitant, Judy, what are some of your concerns?"

A Compassionate Nuance: Working With the Cognitively Impaired

As we mentioned in the opening comments of this chapter, compassion is an essential ingredient for our success in exploring all three steps of the Choice Triad, but the following tip is not about the Choice Triad per se. It is a somewhat miscellaneous tip, yet it seems to fit this chapter in a paradoxical fashion, for, ironically, some of our patients may not even remember that they made a choice to begin with. For some patients, the Choice Triad can become an indecipherable shadow of the past. Dementias are ubiquitous and will be even more ubiquitous in the decades to come as the baby boomer generation ages.

There are many other patients, often much younger in age, who are also suffering from severe brain damage. Indeed, there are few misfortunes more painful to watch than a patient whose life has been massively changed for the worse by the few seconds involved in a car accident with a drunk driver, or experienced by a one of our vets whose foot has inadvertently landed on an IED, or an adolescent who is coping with the aftermath of an uninvited biologic invasion such as meningitis. It is with these patients, suffering from organic brain damage, that our compassion is often most intensely needed. And, yet, it is with these exact patients that our patience can become strained – if we our honest with ourselves – by the annoying behaviors that such patients may display triggered by their disease processes.

The confusion and fears of these patients sometimes complicate their ability to take the very medications they need to find relief. Their obstinacy, and their occasional belligerence, can be frustrating. It is not unusual for patients with severe cognitive deficits to be unable to even remember why they are taking their medications, and consequently, they may become – quite appropriately – frightened or agitated when asked to take them. In such situations, staff sometimes choose to follow such patients around with the medication in tow, often perceived by the confused patients as an attempt to be "forced" to take something they do not even remember they need.

Such actions may neglect the patient's sense of personal space while making it more difficult for the patient to have the needed time or space to reprocess why he or she needs the medication and what might be the damaging results for the rest of the day if the medication is missed or the patient becomes upset about the issue of taking the medications. Of course, some patients, as a result of their deficits, can never make these distinctions. They are merely left in a state of terror that they are being drugged or simply being forced to do something that they do not want to be done.

The "chasing" of such patients with their medications often results in the outright refusal of the medications by the patient, an increase in agitation by the patient, or the use of physical restraints on the patient. This scenario is often followed by a breakdown in trust and the generation of feelings, in the patient, of being wrongfully accused by the staff of noncooperation.

While providing a MIM workshop in Whitby, Ontario, Canada, I had the privilege of receiving a very insightful tip. The tip was provided by Katherine Cherrington, a nurse working at the Whitby Mental Health Centre Corporation at the time. It is a tip that really helped me to better understand how I, and other staff, could minimize the occurrence of the problems described above. The tip is meant to be of use with patients suffering from an organic brain insult, who still retain some memory and cognitive abilities to plan. For the tip to be viable, the patient must also still retain an ability to hold a limited conversation. It is a bit of a longer tip, but well worth our attention, and I shall let Katherine describe it in her own words as best I remember them:

TIP 62 Making the Best of a Tough Deal of the Cards

"With patient's coping with tough organic brain damage, I find it valuable to try to uncover, and maximize, whatever cognitive skills remain. It can be surprising to discover that even fairly severely damaged patients may have the ability to 'cut a deal' if one has the patience to hold a quiet conversation with them, clearly and simply delineating the details of the deal, and gently reminding the patient of the deal throughout the day (this last part being an important prerequisite for success).

"More specifically, I will sit down with the patient (and sometimes other staff are also present) and we will arrive at an agreed-upon deal with the following three agreements:

1. He/she will take the medications in question.
2. He/she will remain calm.
3. He/she will talk to the assigned staff about any concerns.

"Because of memory impairment the patient will be gently reminded of these shared goals at least daily *(generally multiple times throughout the day depending on the degree of memory impairment)*. Because of the multiple reminders throughout the day, there are no surprises for the patient when the medications are offered, for the patient is expecting them.

"If for some reason the patient refuses the medications, my approach is simply to remind the patient of our shared goals (which have been written down on paper for just such moments of sharing). I gently remind the patient that this is solely his choice and what the consequences might be depending on his choice. I will then let him know that I will be at the medication room in 15 minutes, and that I hope that he makes the right decision that will help him to make the best gains for the rest of the day.

"If he has started to feel a bit agitated, I remind him that it is not too late to turn things around and make sure the rest of the day goes great, and I'll see him in 15 minutes at the med room. Done with a reassuring calmness and lack of 'forcefully pushing the meds,' I find that this approach has often been very successful."

I have little to add here. One would be hard-pressed to find a more beautiful example of the twin MIM principles of collaborative exploration and moving with the patient on the Agreement Continuum.

Ongoing Med-Checks: How to Enhance the Medication Alliance

The Art of Collaborative Negotiation

Side effects are problematic and are often dose related. As a patient weighs the pros and cons, the severity of the patient's side effects at recommended doses may outweigh the benefits, a fact of life we described in our last chapter. A patient may simply say, "I can't take this medication at this dose."

At such times, it is important to remember that during medical and nursing training, we are often examining bell curves and statistics that purport to tell us what the "minimum effective dose" for any medication may be, but these parameters are not necessarily true for all patients. Some people, such as slow metabolizers, lie outside our bell curves and may respond to a medication at lower doses than the recommended dose. Such patients are also more likely to suffer problematic dose-related side effects even at the lower end of the recommended dosage range. We don't always know which patient is going to respond in which way to a medication dosage. Sometimes this situation can provide creative openings to try surprisingly low dosing levels with patients suffering from what would be otherwise intolerable side effects. *If the following can be done safely from a medical standpoint*, it offers a way to collaboratively employ a lower dose:

TIP 63 Collaborating on How Much and When

"Mrs. Mack, it looks like the dizziness is just not going to go away, and I totally agree that it is a side effect that simply is too problematic to tolerate, despite the fact that we are getting some good control of your blood pressure.

I have an idea. Some people can still get good effects from medications at lower doses. I suggest we try your medication at a lower dose than it is usually given, and see if it still helps with your blood pressure while also seeing if the dizziness goes away. It might not work, but we can at least try it and see what happens. I know that you are uncomfortable with the current dose and I can see why."

A nurse in one of my MIM workshops, Cindy Carey, suggested adding the following phrase to the technique of Collaborating on How Much and When, "I'm wondering, what dose of this medication might you feel comfortable taking, say for the next week or two to see what happens?" I have found this to be a wonderful closing question. It epitomizes the MIM principle of moving with the patient on the Agreement Continuum.

If the patient's requested dosage is reasonable and safe, a trial can be tried. I find that patients are often pleased that their own input is so valued by the prescriber. In some instances, the lower dose proves inadequate, but I have been pleasantly surprised at how often a lower dose provides good relief with an acceptable side-effect profile.

From a forensic standpoint, if you choose to try a dose lower than recommended, be sure to document in your note exactly why you are doing so. If the lower dose proves to be inadequate, the prescriber will need to search for another appropriate medication or try to see whether there are unexplored ways of helping the patient tolerate the side effects at the necessary higher dose. In some cases, a CAM therapy might be an effective replacement.

We can see that our techniques for enhancing medication interest, during ongoing med-checks, mirror the types of techniques we used in writing our first scripts for a patient as described in Chapter 6. Indeed, they are derived from the same interviewing principles highlighting the value of moving with the patient as opposed to moving against the patient. For instance, a similar strategy to the technique of Collaborating on How Much and When can be useful when starting any new medication with a well-known patient, especially if the patient appears wary of the dosage of the medication. In such instances, the clinician can suggest starting at a very low dose, telling the patient:

TIP 64 You Call the Shots

"Let's start really low. See how you feel after a couple of weeks, and I think you will feel pretty good, at which point you can decide to raise the dose to the normal level. It's up to you; you call the shots. And next time we meet we'll see how things are going at whatever dose you're on and decide our next step to getting you maximum relief."

This strategy maximizes the patient's sense of control. I find that patients frequently return having raised the dose to the desired level.

You might also recall from Chapter 6 (see page 93) that we have already delineated a similar technique (Feel Free to Discontinue), which was designed for those situations in which the patient seems particularly hesitant about starting a medication. It too works by maximizing the patient's sense of control. *If it is safe to abruptly stop the newly prescribed medication* the clinician can add: "We have really covered the side effects carefully and hopefully you won't get many or any. But if for some reason, before our next appointment, you feel concerned about a side effect and you can't reach me or one of my staff by phone or e-mail, feel free to stop the medication immediately. You can give me a call afterwards and we can see if we can come up with a better fit at our next appointment". Both techniques are examples of paradoxically gaining control by yielding control. And both techniques show the continuity of the spirit and principles of the MIM from the very first prescription to the very last.

Returning to our exploration of the challenges and solutions inherent in providing ongoing med-checks, sometimes a patient simply cannot remember to take a medication at a certain "ideal time." For instance, a patient taking a medication t.i.d. (*ter in die* – Latin for "three times a day") may consistently miss the midday dose. Once again, although the recommended t.i.d. dose is most effective, one can sometimes try a b.i.d. (*bis in die* – Latin for "twice a day") dosing, with slightly increased dosage at the b.i.d. doses as partial compensation for the missed middle dose. Obviously, the smoothness of blood level will be affected, but the medication regimen may still be effective. Indeed, this b.i.d. dosing, that the patient enthusiastically embraces, is bound to be more effective than the recommended t.i.d. dose that is almost always missed, and which the patient eventually stops altogether, "because Dr. Shea told me it only works if I take it three times a day." Once again, an ideal treatment plan that the patient cannot do is not ideal. It is a failure.

Paradoxically, failure is also a real possibility when we have already found success. I am referring to those situations in which we have found that a medication is working well, but it will need to be maintained indefinitely to keep the disease in remission or the patient's symptoms under control. When we tell a patient that it will be necessary to be on a medication for life, the news is often difficult to digest, especially if the medication has major side effects and long-term risks, such as liver disease or kidney disease. It is only natural for a patient to balk at such a disconcerting picture of the future. The cons of the medication have just skyrocketed, despite its success.

Linda Cunning, a physician from one of my MIM workshops in Wisconsin, has come up with a psychologically savvy fashion of working with patients on this issue. The trick is to be the first one to acknowledge the difficulties inherent in agreeing to take medications (such as steroids, other immunosuppressive agents, antihypertensives, antihyperlipidemic agents, and antimanic medications such as lithium) indefinitely, with phrasing such as the following:

TIP 65 Negotiating a Short-Term Contract

"You know, Mr. Johnson, it really isn't reasonable to commit to taking a medication for the rest of your life. I couldn't do it. Life is complicated. Things change. I know that. On the other hand, because this lithium is so valuable for you in helping you control your bipolar disorder, let's try something in much smaller steps, something that is reasonable and practical. Why don't we contract that you will take the lithium for just a year. At the end of that year, we will see how it is helping and then we can contract for another year if you think it is working well for you. One year at a time. Now that length of time is much more manageable for making a contract. What do you think?"

Nice touch. The technique fits the MIM perfectly, with the patient and clinician jointly recognizing the difficulties of maintaining medication interest over time. Together, once again with the patient calling the final shot, a mutually reasonable contract is created.

The Delicate Art of Collaborative Discontinuance

If, during follow-up visits, a patient spontaneously raises concerns about a side effect, it is usually important to explore this side effect thoroughly. *A spontaneously raised side effect often suggests that it is causing enough problems that the patient may be considering stopping the medication.* In my experience, if a side effect is spontaneously raised several times, this medication is probably heading for the back shelf of the medicine cabinet. If the clinician has any questions about the intensity of a patient's misgivings, here is the time to ask and here is an effective way to do it.

TIP 66 Probing for Impending Discontinuance

"Mary, we've been trying to decrease this side effect, but I know it's still a problem. What kind of thoughts, even fleeting in nature, have you had about maybe stopping the medication?"

After using this technique, patients sometimes describe serious misgivings about the medication in question. This disclosure opens the door for a productive discussion of what to do for the side effects and whether to continue the medication without there being any shame or guilt for the patient about having had such thoughts. Once again, we are doing everything we can that will decrease oppositional feelings between our patients and ourselves.

Another way of nipping this problematic process in the bud – patients being hesitant to suggest discontinuance because they fear the clinician will be upset with them – is to remind the patient that we, too, are aggressively on the lookout for side effects. As mentioned in an earlier chapter, part of our goal is to be a watchdog that alerts our patient when it may be best to stop a medication because the side effects are outweighing the benefits.

I have found no better way to convince a patient of my vigilance regarding side effects than to be the first one to suggest stopping a medication. When patients repeatedly raise a problematic side effect, one that could easily lead them to stop the medication, a response such as the following can go a long way toward reassuring them that we, too, share their concerns:

TIP 67 Proactively Recommending Discontinuance

"Jim, I just don't like the problem we are having with this side effect. If we can't get it under control, I really think we may need to stop this med, even though I know it's also helping too. I'm just worried that the pros of using it are being outweighed by the cons. What do you think?"

Having addressed the issue of stopping a medication, the next obvious question is, "How do we approach suggesting a new medication to our patients?" Truth be told it is not as simple a process as one might think. Frustration, shame, and guilt can once again raise their heads. Their appearance, especially when numerous medication trials have proven to be ineffective, can be deadly to the medication alliance.

As our patients struggle with their symptoms and side effects, many become both frustrated and demoralized. They can grow tired of a seemingly endless stream of medications that appear to go nowhere and sometimes create more problems than they solve. Their reaction is both logical and natural. It is frustrating for us as well.

A subtle deterioration can creep into the ongoing medication alliance at these junctures, if we are not careful. Some patients may feel a gnawing guilt that they have lost motivation to try new medications, and, if they have a particularly strong alliance with us, they may develop damaging feelings of guilt and shame, as if they are letting us down. Such feelings can generate a withdrawal of the patient from the therapeutic alliance, reflected by occasional "no-shows," less animated sessions, and a less open discussion of the patient's frustrations and concerns.

A child and adolescent psychiatrist at one of my workshops in Waco, Texas, shared a finely worded statement that immediately allies the physician or nurse clinician with the patient's own feelings of frustration; it is a statement that is made to a patient, who has just had a series of medication failures and is now being started up on "yet another drug."

TIP 68 Aligning with the Patient's Frustration

"You know what? What we want with this new medication is not just the same old same old. What we want is something that is better, not just different. We want you to feel better. If we just get different, then we have to take another look at our plan. We will keep working together till we find something that helps and really helps, and I think we will."

Fine-Tuning the Art of Patient Education

As we draw closer to the end of our chapter, we must address one last cornerstone of effective person-centered interviewing as it portends to helping patients navigate the Choice Triad. If one thinks about it, when patients are weighing the pros and cons in the third step of the Choice Triad, their ability to effectively perform their benefit/risk analysis is dependent on the quality of the information that we have made available to them. One might think that if a clinician has communicated clearly, then the clinician's job is done. Research suggests otherwise.

Studies have demonstrated that 40% to 80% of the medical information communicated from providers to patients is forgotten immediately.[2]

If that were not bad enough, almost half of what is retained is incorrect.[3] It's difficult to wisely weigh the pros and cons if you do not know what they are. These data are rather startling. It's troubling to think how many patients with whom well-intentioned providers felt they had successfully communicated, in reality, had been the participants of successful miscommunication.

These miscommunications can arise from both sides of the stethoscope. Clinicians may not take the time to effectively communicate information, may use terms that confuse the patient, might miss cues that the patient is not comprehending the information, or may not provide enough time for questions. Other clinician factors arise from the massive workloads and hectic paces of clinic and hospital practices. For instance, clinicians may distort or delete important information (sometimes because they have provided the information so many times over the years that they are not concentrating on their presentation for they are merely acting from habit). Similarly, almost any experienced clinician can attest that sometimes one is seeing so many patients with the same diagnosis on a single day that it becomes easy to forget what one said and to whom.

From the patient's side of the stethoscope, it is important to match the sophistication of the educational language to the intellectual and educational levels of the patient, for patients can vary greatly in this regard. In addition, patients are often hearing complex information for the first time while in a state of anxiety, fear, and, sometimes, even shock (when hearing bad diagnostic or prognostic news). Needless to say, anxiety and fear are not conducive psychological states for learning and retention.

A variety of methods for addressing and transforming these challenges exist. Let's start by taking a look at one of my favorites.

The Teach-Back Method

Perhaps the single most important take-home principle from this section is, "*The **only** way to know if patients have understood and retained educational material is to ask them to repeat it back to you in their own words.*" This principle and its resulting interviewing techniques have been around for a while. It is best known as the "teach-back method" but is also known as the "show-me method" or "closing the loop."[4] The University of North Carolina at Chapel Hill has a wonderful site regarding tips for enhancing patient education, including excellent material on the Teach-Back Method from which much of this section was adapted.[5] You can also find many excellent demonstrations of it on YouTube.

Let us begin by looking at several examples of the Teach-Back Method that are directly related to medication education, followed by several other examples of the method that demonstrate its wide applicability to patient education using diabetes as an illustration:

TIP 69 Teach-Back Method

a. "I want to make sure I was clear about the potential side effects of this medication, could you tell me in your own words what some of its most common side effects might be?"
b. "I want to make sure I was clear about some of the more serious side effects of this medication, even though it is very unlikely you will get any of them, could you tell me in your own words what some of its most serious side effects could be?"
c. "I want to make sure I was clear about all the ways I think this medication might help you. Could you, in your own words, tell me how [name of medication] is going to help with your heart disease [name of disease in question]?"
d. "I want to make sure I was clear about all the ways I think this medication might help you. Could you, in your own words, tell me how [name of medication] is going to make your life better?"
e. "I want to be sure that I explained your medication correctly. Can you tell me how you are going to take this medicine?"[6]
f. "We covered a lot today about your diabetes, and I want to make sure that I explained things clearly. So let's review what we discussed. What are three strategies that will help you to control your diabetes?"[6]
g. "We covered a lot today about your prediabetes, and I want to make sure that I explained things well. Can you tell me how you would describe it to a friend?"[7]
h. "I want to be sure that I clearly described some of the steps you can take to prevent type 2 diabetes. Is there one thing you can do this week to get started?"[7]

If the patient cannot teach-back the information in his or her own words, the provider can repeat the information, taking care to make sure the information is being provided in an easily digestible manner adjusted to the patient's educational level. The provider can then repeat the teach-back request until the information has been learned and consolidated. Visual aids can be useful, as well as the use of reading materials to help with consolidation after the patient returns home. *Reading materials are only useful if written at an appropriate reading level. Keep in mind that about 10% of the American population is essentially illiterate and many more can only read at the level of early grade school.*

Generally, it is important to use the teach-back method after a relatively brief section of material, for patients will not retain long "didactic monologues." Indeed, if the patient is having trouble repeating information, it is often because the educator has provided too much information in one passing or is using language that is too complicated.

Also note that phrases such as, "I want to make sure that I explained things well" and "I want to make sure I was clear about . . ." are critical to the success of the approach. They decrease defensiveness in the patient by metacommunicating that the patient is "not being tested" or "taking an exam"; rather, the clinician is making sure that he or she taught effectively and was clear regarding teaching points.

The term "Show-Me Method" refers to the idea that if the patient is supposed to do something behaviorally, one can only know if the patient is capable of doing so by watching the patient perform the task. Various processes can interfere with behavioral tasks especially in the elderly including cognitive deficits, vision deficits, and tremors or muscle weakness. We have already seen the Show-Me Method recommended with regard to an important medication-related issue. In Chapter 9, I mentioned that one way of lowering costs for patients was to prescribe medications in pills that could be cut in half, for higher dose pills are often only fractionally more expensive than pills manufactured at lower doses. If you will recall, I said that if one is suggesting this practice, it is wise to ask the patient to actually cut a pill in front of you to ensure that the patient can effectively make the cut (especially important with elderly patients).

In addition to the University of North Carolina's outstanding Health Literacy Site mentioned earlier, the interested reader can find excellent material on the Teach-Back and Show-Me Methods, as well as other patient education materials on websites such as the Iowa Healthcare Collaborative and Health Literacy Consulting.[8,9]

As a final note, it is important to remember that depending on how much medical information is being conveyed, time will necessitate that you limit the amount of teach-back you can employ. Decisions will need to be made regarding what material is the most important material to be retained, which brings us to our next topic.

The Importance of Primacy and Recency Effects When Teaching Patients

Clinicians often find themselves providing long lists of information to patients. Such lists can include lists of side effects, lists of dosing directions, lists of patient instructions (such as what to do, or not do, if you miss several doses of a medication), lists of abnormal symptoms or sensations that may indicate the emergence of serious adverse reactions, and lists of who to call when. The problem with lists is that they are hard to remember. And, when made into written lists, they get misplaced or lost. A psychologist, Katherine Vestevich, PhD, attending one of my MIM workshops provided the following useful insights regarding retention optimization when providing lists. Here they are in her own words as best I can remember them:

> **TIP 70 Utilizing Primacy and Recency Effects**
>
> "Anytime I am providing a list of information to a patient, I find the following principles from learning studies in cognitive psychology to be useful. The concept of 'primacy effects' suggests that people will tend to remember best the first few items (in a cluster) at the beginning of a series. 'Recency effects' occur at the opposite end of the list, where people will tend to remember the last few items mentioned the best. Thus, the first and last cluster of items tend to be retained the best in a long list.
>
> "This suggests that if you are giving a patient some information, and some of the information is more critical to retain than other information, it is often wise for the clinician to consciously place this more critical information first and/or last. It's a slick trick that works well."

Regarding common patient education lists, such as lists of side effects and serious adverse reactions, it makes sense to place the most important side effects and adverse reactions at the beginning or ending of their respective list. The most important patient directions, subsequent to the patient's decision to try a medication, should also be mentioned at the beginning or ending of a list of instructions (as well as being written down).

Thus, if one wants to emphasize that if a patient misses multiple doses of digoxin he or she should *not* try to catch up by taking a bunch of doses all at once, this information should be at the beginning or ending of a list of instructions. A trick of the trade that I have found to be useful is to mention particularly critical information at the beginning of a list as well as repeating it at the end for re-enforcement purposes. The principles of primary and recency effects can also guide us in determining which pockets of information warrant the use of the Teach-Back Method if time constraints limit its use as they essentially always do in today's hectic clinics.

A Final Tip on Patient Education: Asking Questions About Questions

Our final tip is short and sweet, but I have found it to be surprisingly useful. A maxilla-facial surgeon taught it to me. When he would make evening rounds on his patients the night before surgery, as he was closing the conversation (which was often only a quick 5 minutes or so), he would always ask, "Do you have any questions about the surgery tomorrow?" Generally speaking, patients asked few questions. He assumed that this paucity indicated that he had done such a nice job of patient education the weeks before the surgery that there was little left on his patient's minds.

One evening, for no particular reason, he inadvertently asked his typical question differently, "What kinds of questions do you still have about tomorrow's surgery?" His patient paused, then asked, "Should I be talking with my family members tonight in case I don't make it tomorrow?" The surgeon was shocked by the intimacy of the question and the fear it reflected. The question resulted in 15 minutes of frank yet reassuring conversation. As he got up to leave, his patient commented, with a genuinely relieved affect, "thanks for taking the time to talk tonight."

The surgeon told me he was puzzled, for in the weeks preceding the surgery, the patient and he had discussed the pros and cons of the surgery in detail, including serious adverse outcomes. Nevertheless, from that point onward, he always asked his question with an assumption that patients the night before major surgery would almost always have questions. They did. Oftentimes, the questions were related to concerns, misperceptions, and fears.

I have found the process to be similar with my patients regarding medications. As we have seen, patients retain surprisingly limited amounts of information when talking with health care providers. Many times, when we are talking, our patients are only half-listening, for their anxieties and feelings of vulnerability are preoccupying their minds. Consequently, I have found that the majority of patients have questions about their medications after already agreeing they want to take them. I don't ask, "Do you have any other questions about this medication?" Instead, I use the following technique:

TIP 71 More Questions? Almost Always

"Jim, we're sort of wrapping up about using this medication. I think it's a great idea, but we've covered a lot of ground, I'm wondering what other questions you might still have about using it, from side effects to how it might help. Any question is a good question?"

If the patient genuinely does not have any other questions, I sometimes, if time permits, use this as an opportunity to use the Teach-Back Method as related to what I perceive to be one of the most critical bits of information that I had passed on. I might add something like this, "Jim, if you don't have any other questions, I've got one more for you, just to make sure I made the importance of this point. If you miss several doses of this medication, what are you going to do the next time you remember to take the medication?"

Concluding Comments

At this juncture, we have come to the end of our return visit to the Choice Triad. Hopefully, we have added some polish to our skills in applying the interviewing techniques designed for its navigation and for providing sound patient education. We have seen, as Dick Van Dyke suggested in our opening epigram, several nice examples of negotiating "Plan Bs" as when renegotiating doses, dosing schedules, and jointly considering discontinuance of a medication.

In our next chapter, we will see that Plan Bs sometimes involve the collaborative decision to utilize an alternative therapy rather than traditional medications. In other instances, Plan Bs entail the introduction of a new traditional medication replacing one that did not accomplish its desired task. In yet other instances, Plan Bs consist of adding a new medication to whatever medications are already on board that were not providing adequate relief.

You will recall that in Chapter 6 we examined interviewing techniques that were of value in prescribing a medication for a new patient during an initial appointment. In our next chapter, we will address the challenge of starting a new medication in a patient well known to us. This process of starting a new medication creates a perfectly timed bridge for a transition to Part III of our book, "Specialized and Advanced Techniques for Enhancing

Medication Interest," for our next chapter is entitled, "Starting, Switching, and Adding Medications."

In Chapter 11, the techniques we will discover can be of value during a first visit or in a visit occurring after 20 years of work together. In fact, introducing a new medication is an everyday occurrence with many of the patients well known to us, not only because we might need to switch medications for an ongoing illness (Plan B), but because we often will find ourselves – unfortunately, as our patients age – needing to introduce a medication for a newly emerging illness. In either case, there is an art to doing this shared decision making well. The secrets of this practical art are seldom addressed in the literature. In our next chapter, we will do just that.

REFERENCES

1. Van Dyke D. February 8, 2017. https://www.goodreads.com/quotes/tag/plans?page=3. Accessed February 24, 2017.
2. Kessels RP. Patient's memory for medical information. *J R Soc Med* 2003;96(5):219–222.
3. Anderson JL, Dodman S, Kopelman M, et al. Patient information recall in a rheumatology clinic. *Rheumatol Rehabil* 1979;18(1):18–22.
4. Schillinger D, Piette J, Grumbach K, et al. Closing the loop: physician communication with diabetic patients who have low health literacy. *Arch Intern Med* 2003;163(1):83–90.
5. North Carolina Program on Health Literacy. "*NC Health Literacy.*" Chapel Hill, NC: University of North Carolina. http://www.nchealthliteracy.org. Accessed July 20, 2017.
6. North Carolina Health Literacy Free Teach-Back Tool Kit. *The Teach-Back Method.* http://www.nchealthliteracy.org/toolkit/tool5.pdf. Accessed July 20, 2017.
7. National Institute of Diabetes and Digestive and Kidney Diseases. *Use the Teach-back Method.* Bethesda, MD: National Institute of Diabetes and Digestive and Kidney Diseases (NIDDK). http://www.niddk.nih.gov/health-information/health-communication-programs/ndep/health-care-professionals/game-plan/talk-with-patients/teach-back-method/Pages/index.aspx.
8. Institute for Healthcare Improvement. *Always use teach back!* Cambridge, MA: Institute for Healthcare Improvement. http://www.ihi.org/resources/Pages/Tools/AlwaysUse-TeachBack!.aspx. Accessed on July 20, 2017.
9. Health Literacy Consulting. http://www.healthliteracy.com. Accessed July 20, 2017.

PART THREE

Specialized Topics and Advanced Techniques for Enhancing Medication Interest

CHAPTER 11

Starting, Switching, and Adding Medications: Finding Collaborative Solutions

"We must adjust our plans to succeed in light of the changes that have occurred."[1]

Andrea Goeglein, PhD
APPLIED POSITIVE PSYCHOLOGIST

Introduction to Part 3

In Part 2, we explored many of the intricacies that arise when we are talking with our patients about their medications. We approached this challenge by creating metaphorical toolboxes. Each toolbox contained a variety of potential interviewing techniques from which we could create flexible approaches. The diversity of available techniques allows us to create approaches that fit the unique needs of any given patient.

In Part 3, we will examine a set of toolboxes that address some of the more daunting topics that the reader will undoubtedly meet in the hectic world of clinical practice. We will explore specialized challenges and answer provocative questions not yet addressed. For instance, "Do patients lie about how they are taking their medications?" and if so, "Are there interviewing techniques that can help us to uncover the truth?" (Chapter 12); "How important are cross-cultural influences on medication interest?" and "Are there interviewing techniques that can help us to better understand and move with these cultural currents?" (Chapter 13); and "Do family and friends ultimately dictate our patients' medication interest and follow-through?" and "Are there questions designed to uncover these familial and interpersonal beliefs/biases?" (Chapter 14).

Before addressing these questions, let us return in this chapter to the art of introducing a new medication, whether we are doing so with a patient new to our practice, a well-known patient for whom we are switching medications, or simply adding a new medication to a list of medications that have proven to be ineffective at providing adequate relief or healing. Much of the key to success in these situations will lie in our ability – as Andrea Goeglein so matter-of-factly intones in our opening epigram – to nondefensively, and in a truly collaborative fashion, change plans midstream if the stream dictates that we must do so.

In this regard, I have found that I must consistently remind myself that my ultimate goal is not to "make" the initial plan work; it is to collaboratively develop a plan – whether it be Plan B, C, or D – that actually does work. The clinician's investment should always be in changing the initial plan as necessary, not in stubbornly trying to prove its worth to oneself and/or to the patient, when – despite everyone's best intentions – it has proven to be inadequate.

The Art of Collaborative Medication Selection

Working with Preconceived Biases

Patients do not always arrive at our offices with a "clean slate" regarding what medications they want us to prescribe. Their biases may be toward or against a medication that we feel is the most indicated. Many times, these opinions are based on input from family members and/or friends (the focus of Chapter 14), as well as being the result of "direct to consumer" advertising by pharmaceutical houses. At other times, Dr. Google has alerted the patient to the "correct prescription" for "what ails ye," it is only necessary for the dufus in the white coat (that's you or me) to write the correct prescription. In the patient's eyes, we need not even take a history.

Fortunately, in many instances, patient's preconceptions are in agreement with our opinions as well. And, in some instances, the patient has an idea that may very well be better than our own. Occasionally, Dr. Google is pretty smart.

In any case, during one of my MIM workshops, Mark Bernstein, a physician, provided a simple suggestion that I have found to be surprisingly useful:

TIP 72 Asking for the Patient's Med Recommendation First

"Do you have a medication in mind that you might want to try for your asthma [whatever disease is in question]?"

If we are in a situation where we are switching out and replacing a medication that has proven to be ineffective, a slightly different twist can be given to the above question. In those instances, where I had originally reviewed a variety of potential medication choices, I might add, "Raj, earlier I had shared a variety of medications that might be useful for your multiple sclerosis. Are there any medications that we talked about back then that you think you might like to try now?"

When one is simply discussing the initial choice of a new medication, whether with a new or a well-known patient, I think you will find Asking for the Patient's Med Recommendation First to be useful in many ways. The apparent simplicity of this tip betrays a wealth of complexities. This question – an inviting gateway into shared decision making – immediately places the patient's opinion where it ought to be, at the forefront of the prescribing clinician's mind. The patient may have excellent ideas as to which medications may be effective, or the patient may have some misinformation about specific medications that can be easily corrected.

The patient's answer may also, indirectly, open the door to an understanding of influential "committee lobbyists," to whom we alluded earlier, ranging from family members to pharmaceutical houses to Webmasters, who may have been the originators of the patient's interest or disinterest in a particular medication. Such biases, if left undetected, could be the determining factors as to whether a medication ever leaves the inside of its bottle even when the patient leaves our office in apparent agreement with the prescription. If such a patient, on returning home, encounters renewed peer pressure against the medication, such interpersonal pressure may well prevail. Better to be aware of this pressure, and address it, before the patient leaves the office. We will address specific interviewing techniques for uncovering such pressures in Chapter 14.

In a similar vein, if patients are not assertive enough to spontaneously suggest medications that they have their "hearts set on getting," they may leave our office disappointed with their prescriptions. Such prescriptions have an uncanny knack of ending up in wastepaper baskets. The previously described tip ensures that such a hidden disappointment cannot occur. Ultimately, we might *not* prescribe the medication requested by the patient (if we feel it is inappropriate) but at least we will have been able to discuss our reasoning and, in the process, modeled a method of shared decision making.

This tip also raises the value of uncovering a valid, not sugar coated, idea of the patient's initial gut feelings about taking a newly prescribed medication. No reason exists for us to not be privy to this vital information regarding medication interest before the patient leaves our office because all we need to do is ask. Shared decision making cannot occur unless there is a genuine sharing of opinions. Once again, the very act of asking for the patient's opinion metacommunicates that we value it. Such interviewing techniques continue to underscore our desire to be an ally with the patient against his or her disease not an opponent against his or her beliefs.

I sometimes precede the above question with the even broader question, "What do you think might help with your symptoms?" Such a question allows the patient to suggest approaches from CAM (exercise, dietary changes, acupuncture, yoga, etc.), which may, indeed, be excellent first choices for intervention with some problems and for some patients.

Our patients' views are not always the result of interpersonal or cultural pressures, good or bad. At times, the patient's views are shaped by the patient's knowledge of family history. In fact, by the end of an initial H&P, we may have forgotten or missed a relevant bit of family history. In such instances, the patient may be the best "interviewer" in the room. In this regard, Edward Fasolino, a physician, provided an excellent tip in a MIM workshop over 10 years ago:

TIP 73 "Got a Relative" Inquiry

"When first introducing a medication from a class of medications for a specific disorder, such as high blood pressure, I often ask, 'Is there anyone in your family who is taking a medication for high blood pressure?' If the patient responds affirmatively, I ask, 'Do you know what it is called?' If he or she does, I ask, 'Does it seem to be working well for that person?' If the patient feels that it is (and I think it would be a reasonable medication choice), I ask, 'Would you like to try that medication to see if it might help you too?' I find that many patients respond very well to this approach."

Creating Collaboration by Providing a Medication Menu

While giving a workshop in Ohio, Joseph Holtel, a physician, offered a useful method of nurturing a collaborative relationship when prescribing a new medication. Many diseases have various medications or alternative methods – which may be reasonable therapeutic options – ranging from medication classes with differing options within them (antihypertensives, antidepressants) to nonmedication interventions for diabetes and heart disease (exercise, diet, etc.).

In these instances, Holtel suggests that instead of making a medication recommendation, the clinician shares some information about the pros and cons of a sampling of the possible medications, including specific pros (rapidly helps with sleep, particularly good with anxiety) and specific cons (may cause sleep disturbance, may impair sexual dysfunction). The clinician then asks the patient which one he or she might like to try.

Joseph feels that this approach had proven to be useful for three reasons:

a. It optimizes the patient's ability to wisely select his or her own medication. Patients seem to tolerate side effects better if they helped to choose the medication themselves.

b. It metacommunicates that there are many alternative medications available if the selected medication proves to be less than optimal in relieving symptoms.

c. It provides a platform for the patient to describe in his or her own words to family members and friends why a specific medication is being used when the patient's family and friends may have had preconceived ideas of which medication should be used.

The above tip introduces yet another avenue that clinicians can pursue in creating a collaborative medication alliance. It can be useful to more deeply pursue the patient's personalized (sometimes idiosyncratic) concerns about *potential* side effects in greater detail when delineating the list of potential medications as suggested above. This tip was provided in a MIM workshop by Melinda Cobb, MD:

TIP 74 Personalizing Potential Side-Effect Choice

"I often let patients know about the key side effects of several medications that might help them. After doing so, I actively seek input from the patient over which side-effects may be the most concerning to him or her personally as illustrated by either of the following questions: (1) 'If we were to use one of these medications, is there a potential side effect that you would most want to avoid?' or 'Considering the potential side effects of these medications, which medication do you find the most appealing to try?'"

This technique also emphasizes an important aspect of side effects that we mentioned back in Chapter 7, but is worth highlighting again. Namely, patients may vary on how problematic a particular side effect is to them. One patient may find a side effect to be a mere inconvenience (dry mouth for an accountant), while another patient may find the exact same side effect to be highly problematic (dry mouth for an actor or grade school teacher). In my own practice, I have sometimes been surprised at a patient's thoughts on side effects, having assumed that a patient was viewing a specific side effect as very bad when indeed, for him or her, it was "no big deal" or vice versa.

I particularly remember a woman in her mid-30s, who had been suffering from a fairly severe depression with some accompanying suicidal ideation. We began an antidepressant that worked quite well. For months, she seemed very pleased. I then noted several sessions in which she seemed more withdrawn than usual and seemed less at ease with me than before. At the next session, I discovered, to my surprise, that she had stopped the antidepressant several weeks earlier without telling me.

Apparently, she had been having an extramarital affair for almost half a year and had stopped the medication because of its sexual side effects. For her, it was worth risking the return of her numerous distressing depressive symptoms – including frightening suicidal thoughts – than risking the sexual robustness of her ongoing affair! If I had employed the technique of Personalizing Potential Side-Effect Choice, I believe there is a very good chance this setback in care (and in the therapeutic alliance, for she felt uncomfortable not sharing her affair nor her concerns with the medication's side effects with me) might have been avoided.

Let me share one more example of the collaborative power of sharing a medication menu with a patient when first deciding on a medication of choice. It was a tip provided by an allergist when I was giving a MIM workshop in Charlotte, North Carolina. John T. Klimos shared with participants that after having reviewed some of the potential common side effects of the various approaches that could be taken, he would ask the patient, "How much better do you want to be? (pause) Let me explain what I mean." He would then continue:

TIP 75 Letting the Patient Set the Goal of the Intervention

"Tabisha, we have different types of things we can do to try to help you to get relief from your allergies. And each one, as we have seen, can have its own pros and cons. They also will have limitations on how much relief you can get. Our goal is to help you to find the approach that suits you best and that you are most comfortable with while getting you the degree of relief that you want.

Let me describe what I mean. If you simply try to avoid the allergen that is causing your bad allergy, I believe we will be able to get you to about 10% to 15% improvement. If we try some of the medications we have been talking about, I think we'll be able to achieve about 50% to 60% improvement. And if we use the allergy shots, I bet we get to about 80% to 90% improvement. Now that you know the side-effects of each approach and the potential benefits, how much relief do you think you want to try for? I can use whatever approach seems best for you and we can always change the approach in the future if you want to. Whichever approach you want to try, I can give you some more details to help you know even more about it."

Initial Acceptance: How Can You Tell if a Patient Is Planning to Take the Medication After He or She Walks Out the Door?

Sometimes patients, because of their own anxieties, social hesitancies, or feelings of being rushed, don't really "come clean" with their ambivalent feelings about a new medication. If they walk out of our office, and these vague fears have not been addressed, even though they may outwardly have agreed to take the medication, they have often inwardly decided not to. The result may well be a "no-show" at the next appointment or a patient who, indeed, shows up, but shows up without the prescribed medication in his or her bloodstream. The clinician can use any one or more of the following questions (or come up with a new inquiry) to directly uncover such potential ambivalence:

TIP 76 "I Really Want to Know" Inquiry

a. "Jenny, now that we're getting close to starting up on this medication, in your gut, do you have any hesitancies about it. I really want to know, so that we can make sure that we pick the very best medication for you."
b. "What are your thoughts about starting up on this medication?"
c. "Now that I've talked about all of the benefits and potential common side effects, what are your thoughts about whether or not you think this medication is worth a try?"
d. "What concerns, if any, do you have about trying this med?"

All of the above questions are direct in their approach. If you prefer a more indirect approach, I have found the following question to be revealing, "What's most appealing to you about trying this medication?" If your patients cannot quickly come up with an answer, their hesitancy speaks loads about their intent to follow-through with the prescription. In addition, you will often be able to gauge your patients' genuine enthusiasm by the greatest of all truth detectors – their body language. Whether direct or indirect in your approach, the trick is to get the patient's ambivalence "out on the table" rapidly, before any final decision is made. I have been consistently pleased by the openness of patients to share their opinions on these critical matters, if I take the time to ask.

Moreover, I have sometimes found that the patient's advice is sound, and my initial choice of a medication was not a good one. I remember an articulate woman who was a bank manager suffering with a depression. She presented with jet-black hair cut in a sophisticated fashion. Her dress was that of a sharp business woman, a gray three-piece business suit and newly polished shoes, heels neither too high nor too low. Despite her apparent confidence in the business world, she had a deeply imbedded need to please, part of the reason she had appeared for therapy.

True to form, as I described the antidepressant I was recommending, she thoughtfully nodded her head and seemed politely interested. But when I asked, "What are your thoughts about starting up on this medication?"

she commented, "I think it sounds like a pretty good idea, but both my mother and sister tried that medication and got horrible nausea from it. They hated it. But I guess I'll try it, if you think it will help."

Clearly, this was not the best first choice of an antidepressant for this patient. I probably never would have heard this information, unless I had asked the question that I did. She knew this was not the right medication for her. Now, I did.

It is of note that this valuable information could also have been revealed through the use of the "Got a Relative" Inquiry described earlier in this chapter. Note that both techniques can help fix errors of omission, for I should have gathered this family information earlier in the interview, but, when time pressures are heated, I find it all too easy to forget to ask pertinent questions. One of the immense benefits of the MIM is that the use of any one interviewing technique, or several of them, during a single appointment can lead to valuable, sometimes invaluable, information. All of the MIM techniques encourage the sharing of information. All enhance the foundation stone for forging a powerful medication alliance – trust.

Nevertheless, even when we have developed a robust sense of trust with our patients, miscommunication about their intent to follow-through may unintentionally happen. Despite genuine medication interest, the patient's motivation may be undercut by having expectations that the medication simply cannot meet. Because of our familiarity with our medications, we may inadvertently assume that the patient holds the same knowledge base as we do about their potential limitations. Even if we have clearly spelled this information out, the patient's hopes – sometimes desperate in nature – can lead him or her to "not hear" what we are saying. One answer to this dilemma was provided by Linda Cunning, DO, in one of my MIM workshops. As we have so often seen, simplicity and a gentle directness are often the best solution:

TIP 77 Uncovering Hidden Expectations

"What would you like this medication to do for you?"

I have found this to be such a powerful tip – and the answers it reveals often so unexpected – that I recommend making it a habit in your practice.

In addition to maximizing the likelihood of patient follow-through, the technique of Uncovering Hidden Expectations has an added bonus. With some patients, the sophistication of their answer, the reasonableness of their logic, and the intensity of their belief – reflected by their tone of voice when answering – can provide useful information on the patient's intellectual functioning, cultural biases, genuine interest in the medication, and even personality style. It also serves as an immediate checkup on the effectiveness (or ineffectiveness) of one's previous educational efforts regarding the medication. Uncovering Hidden Expectations, in some instances, almost functions as an informal variation of the Teach-Back Model from our last chapter.

As we wrap up our survey of techniques for gauging our patient's motivation level when starting a new medication, let us look at an interviewing technique that can only be utilized with a patient well known to us, with whom we have developed a relaxed and comfortable bond. These are the delightful types of relationships we forge where humor and laughter play a refreshing counterpoint to our trials and tribulations as we jointly battle against the patient's long-term illness. With such patients, we often develop a keen sense of intuition for them and they of us.

If after you have discussed a new medication and a patient agrees to take it, but nonverbally the patient doesn't seem to be jumping up and down with enthusiasm about the medication, just ask, candidly, what he or she intends to do:

TIP 78 The Humor of a "Nonstarter"

"You know, Mike, I'm getting the feeling that you are just a bit hesitant to start this medication. Which is okay, but I just have a hunch here (well-timed pause) you're not going to take this thing, are you?"

Said with gentle wryness, and with absolutely no tone of condemnation, this technique, if the clinician's intuition is on the mark, often results in a smile from the patient, not unlike the smile of a kid caught with his hand in the cookie jar. Once the patient's misgivings are out on the table, productive shared decision making can resume.

Not Pushing the Initial Prescription

Occasionally, the first time we raise the possibility of using a medication, the patient is flooded with both new information and ambivalence, and, consequently, it may not be wise to press for commitment at such moments. Sometimes we are discontinuing a medication trial that has failed and are suggesting a new medication. With these patients, especially if they have experienced the intense disappointment of a series of "med failures," it is no wonder that they are hesitant. Although the hectic pace of such clinics often pressures us to make rapid interventions, in these situations, it is often best to not push a patient to make up his or her mind.

The axiom that we have previously emphasized about treatment plans in general, we can now apply specifically to medications: An ideal medication that a patient does not want to take is not an ideal medication, it is a foolish one. It is a medication that is doomed to never leave the confines of the patient's medicine cabinet.

We can now concretize these observations into the following interviewing principle. *If you have suggested a medication, from oral hypoglycemic agents, anticoagulants, and antihypertensives to birth control pills and antidepressants, and the patient looks hesitant to begin it –* ***even after you have spent considerable time exploring the patient's concerns*** *– it may be wise to give the patient more time to contemplate the decision.* Any application of pressure, when first suggesting a new medication, may feel oppositional to the patient. Such pressure flows counter to the principles of the MIM.

Nothing is worse for long-term medication interest than to have a patient halfheartedly agree to start a medication and then, once home, decide it is not such a "hot idea" to start "this thing" or, if started, to stay on it. Once deciding not to take a medication or to stop taking one, it is very hard to convince a patient to restart because, as we noted in an earlier chapter, if a patient restarts a medication, the patient must first admit that he or she was wrong to stop it in the first place, hardly a fun thing to do. These "restarted" patients are highly prone to once again stop the medication in order to prove the correctness of their initial decision. The following technique from Raphaelle Butler, a MIM workshop participant, can be effective at giving patients the needed time to make a well-informed decision with which they are comfortable. Raphaelle gives the patient a medication sample commenting:

TIP 79 Taking the Heat Off the Decision to Start a Medication

"I think your hesitation makes good sense. It's smart to weigh the pros and cons. I know I would. Here is a small sample of the medication that I think might help. You can go home and think about what we have been talking about and perhaps go to the web and check out information on the medication. If you decide you want to give it a try, then you can start it up yourself the way we discussed and see how it goes."

Raphaelle reports that patients vary on what they do, but always seem pleased with the lack of a push from the prescriber. He reports that some of his patients check the medication out on the web and decide not to try it. Others check it out on the web and subsequently start it up on their own. Others have questions at the next appointment, and if satisfactorily answered, proceed to use the medication.

When using the technique, Raphaelle recommends providing specific websites. I very much agree with this idea. In this regard, the clinician can inventory his or her most commonly prescribed medications. The clinician can subsequently create cards (particularly nice if laminated) that list appropriate initial sites for investigation by the patients. In doing so, I would choose sites in which the creator of the site has "no horse in the race" in the sense of the site creator having either a financial or a personal reason for the viewer to use or not use the medication in question. By contrast, a random search by the patient may lead the patient to potentially biased pharmaceutical sites, who may rave about their own product, or to equally biased sites in which the creator of the site is highly opposed to the use of any medication. After visiting more balanced sites, patients can better explore other sites effectively, making their own informed decisions about the quality of the information they find.

As we have discussed earlier, one of your most frequently prescribed medications, if you enter primary care or psychiatry, will be antidepressants. Be aware that the web is loaded with strongly antipsychiatry sites. In this regard, it is best to initially steer the patient to more balanced sites avoiding those sites that have strong personal biases (antipsychiatry) or, at the other end of the continuum, have equally strong financial interests (pharmaceutical sites). After visiting the balanced sites on your list, the patient can continue his or her own web search where he or she will undoubtedly come across these more potentially biased sites. As noted above, armed with balanced information, the patient will be in a better position to make his or her own decision about the usefulness of the information found in them (there may be both useful and not useful information on sites from both ends of the continuum).

Some clinicians, when using the technique of Taking the Heat Off the Decision to Start a Medication, prefer providing a prescription instead of a sample to ensure that adequate medication will be available before the next session. Note that a prescription alone (no sample) will require the patient to make a trip to the pharmacy and to spend some money to boot (both of which could function as deterrents). By contrast, a sample, if available, makes it easy to start the medication if one desires to do so.

Perhaps the most effective approach to this technique is to provide both a small sample and a prescription – the best of both worlds. In any case, you can flexibly adapt this strategy to best suit the needs of your patient and the resources of your clinic.

In essence, the above technique and the following two techniques are examples of gaining by yielding. All three emphasize the collaborative concept of moving with the patient in a concrete fashion; that it is the patient who is in control. It is the patient who is making the choice. Of course, in the final analysis, it *is* the patient who has total control. We are not yielding anything. The patient will decide what pill goes into his or her mouth, thank-you very much! But how we present our recommendations – with a sensation of "pushing" or a sensation of "yielding" – may very well ultimately determine whether our recommendation is embraced or rejected.

In the following tip, from another MIM workshop participant, Gabrielle Beaubrun, the sensation of yielding is impeccably metacommunicated almost to the point of paradox. I have found the technique to be curiously effective with patients who seem particularly hesitant about starting a medication. I'll let Gabrielle delineate the tip in her own words as I best remember them:

TIP 80 The "Give Me a Call" Offer

"In situations, when there is a non-urgent need to begin a medication, and especially with patients who have multiple questions/doubts about a medication, I have found the following strategy to be useful (particularly with patients who like to use the web or like to read about medications). In the appointment, I focus on, and emphasize, the ways that I think the medication will help. Then I surprise the patient by *not* giving a prescription immediately, instead, I say the following:

> *'I want you to be sure about this decision. Read up about this medication and give me a call if you decide you want to give it a try.'*

"I proceed to give the patient the name of the medication on a piece of paper with some of the benefits and side effects listed as well as possible web resources for learning about the medication. In my experience, almost all of these patients contact me within a week asking for the prescription to be called in to the pharmacy. Now that the patient is asking me for the medication, based on his or her own research, I find that there is a much higher likelihood that the patient will not only try the med, but will also be more interested in sticking with it despite side effects."

One can even take the practice of creating a paradox one step further. One can emphasize that you do *not* want the patient to make a decision now or even before the next appointment.

TIP 81 "Not Now" Paradox

"You know, Mike, I can sense you are still a little hesitant to start up on this medication. That's fine. It's smart too. You should take time to weigh the pros and cons of any medicine before you try it. In fact, I don't want you to make your decision today. I think it's much smarter to give it some thought, talk it over with your wife or friends if you want to, and next time we'll review the pros and cons again. If you are still having some concerns, then we'll discuss them and see if we think it's a good idea to try the medication or not. Remember, if you don't like how it is working, you can always stop it.

"I have a good gut feeling you will really like how you feel on it. I have had some excellent luck with this medication with a lot of patients. But there is absolutely no reason to rush into a decision. Here is some more information on it; you can read it and see what you think. And here are some good websites as well that, I think, give a nice balanced view of the possible benefits and side effects of this particular medication. In my opinion it is very important that you personally be comfortable with a medication before you start it. Does that sound like a good plan to you?"

With all three of our techniques in this section, the bottom line is a simple one. One of the key ways to enhance medication interest – when patients appear ambivalent about starting up a medication or switching to a new one – is to give them the time to make their own decision at their own pace. If we rush a prescription onto a patient, potentially creating a sensation of "push," we are likely typing a prescription for a patient who will not be filling it.

We have concluded our survey of the principles and techniques that can help us to initially start up medications and/or perhaps switch medications if, as Andrea Goeglein commented in our opening epigram, "we must adjust our plans to succeed in light of the changes that have occurred," in short, treatment failure. Our treatment failures can often be transformed into treatment successes depending on our flexibility and the unique wisdom that is unleashed by genuine clinician-patient collaboration, the essence of shared decision making.

REFERENCE

1. Goeglein A. www.goodreads.com/quotes/tag/adjust. Accessed November 3, 2017.

CHAPTER 12

Why Patients Hide the Truth About Their Medication Practice and How to Help Them Share It

"My reality is blurred by the mists of words."[1]

Oscar Wilde
VICTORIAN PLAYWRIGHT AND AESTHETE

INTRODUCTION

Over a century ago, Oscar Wilde – known for his wickedly witty social commentary – was wryly noting that spoken words were not necessarily the spoken truth in Victorian times. Even today, it can be a rude awakening to primary care clinicians or specialists – especially if they are particularly good at establishing sound therapeutic alliances – that their patients are distorting material or frankly lying to them. This dilemma most frequently presents itself when clinicians are exploring the type of obviously sensitive/taboo material discussed daily in a typical primary care clinic (such as substance abuse, suicidal ideation, intimate partner violence, and incest), but it also presents when exploring material that is not as obviously sensitive such as missing medication doses or unilaterally discontinuing medications (the topics of this chapter).

A century after Oscar Wilde made his observations, one of our most pithy of contemporary wits and social commentators, Stephen Colbert, reminded us that today, there is still a problem with this "truthiness" thing.

Indeed, whether it is when we are exploring obviously sensitive areas such as domestic violence or thoughts of suicide or less obviously sensitive areas such as a lack of medication follow-through, we do not know for certain what is going on in our patients' minds. We never will. The delicate arabesques of the mind cannot be easily transferred from one person's brain to another's. Even direct conversation is, at best, a second-generation copy of internal experience, brimming with data dropout, distortion, and all the other problems associated with second-generation copies. As Oscar Wilde intimates in our opening quotation, our patients' words often weave only mists.

Not infrequently, when physicians, nurses, physician assistants, clinical pharmacists, and case managers are trying to uncover the actual medication practices of their patients (e.g., how often is the medication truly being taken in contrast to how it was prescribed), these clinicians are traveling through such mists. Research has shown that patients do not usually voluntarily tell their clinicians that they do not intend to use a medication as prescribed (or are already not doing so).[2–6]

For instance, in the Laplane study, a disturbing 83% of the adult patients surveyed over six U.S. states indicated that they would *not* tell their prescribing clinician if they had no intention on filling the prescription that they were holding in their hands as they walked out of the clinic door,[5] an example of what has been termed "primary nonadherence."[7] With regard to antipsychotics specifically, patients were hesitant to share their changes in medication practice to their clinicians because they feared being viewed as bad patients and as such might be reprimanded or lectured (Weiden's damaging "obedience mode" from Chapter 6), a patient fear that can be seen, in my opinion, across essentially all medication categories.[8]

Moreover, studies have demonstrated that clinicians consistently overestimate the degree to which their patients are taking medications as prescribed.[9–11] Research by Steele and colleagues showed the troubling fact that only 12% of their patients spontaneously mentioned anything about how they were actually taking their medications during a clinic visit.[12] As we have seen so many times before in this book, if one wants to know, one has to ask. Steele's research demonstrated that when physicians did ask, how they asked about missed doses played a significant role in whether valid answers were forthcoming. We will be examining some of the useful techniques delineated by Steele and colleagues shortly, but before we do, it is of value to better understand why patients are prone to lie about their medication practices.

The Truth Behind the Deceit

The first truth is that when patients provide us with unreliable information about missed medications, they are not necessarily intentionally distorting the truth or being deceitful (an act that requires an intentional decision to not tell the truth). Some patients are trying to communicate the truth but are not able to do so.

One variant of this phenomenon can be seen with patients who simply, psychologically speaking, do not require an overly accurate way of interpreting life experiences nor reporting such experiences. For such patients, there is no psychological drive "to be precise." They just don't place a premium on this quality nor are they hard-wired to do so. In essence, it's "enough to be close-enough" in relating history and behaviors. For those of us that put a premium on precision, this approach can drive one to distraction, but it is important to realize that there is no malice or conscious intention behind such faulty reporting.

If such a patient misses a dose or two a week, that's close enough to "what the doctor ordered." Consequently, when asked, the patient will respond without a moment's hesitation that he or she is taking the medications "as prescribed." For some medication schedules, although not ideal, such an inconsistent medication follow-through may be okay (an anti-hypertensive regimen for mildly increased blood pressure), for others not so much (birth control pills, an AIDS regimen, or antiplatelet medications post cardiac stent surgery). In a subsequent section of this chapter, we will see some techniques that may help such patients to provide more accurate reporting.

A different example of a patient, who is not intentionally distorting or lying when underreporting missed medication doses, is much more common – patients dealing with the memory problems related to cognitive dysfunction or dementias. Similarly, some of our younger patients may be handicapped by overwhelming life stresses and/or mental disorders that impact on their cognition and memory.

The second truth is that when patients provide us with unreliable information about missed medications – and they are *intentionally* doing so – it is seldom for nefarious or malicious reasons. Rather they are simply being human, and like all of us, they don't like to do the wrong thing. Moreover, it is important to them to be perceived by others (in this instance, you and I, their prescribing clinicians) as doing the right thing. No one wants to be viewed as "being a bad patient" who has "obedience issues." Two paradoxes arise in this regard.

As we already know, some patients miss doses because they choose to miss them. In short, they lack belief in one or more of the steps of the Choice Triad. Consequently, they either want their doses decreased or they want their medication stopped. Another set of patients have chosen to take the medication (are comfortable with all steps of the Choice Triad), but are having problems with medication follow-through per se (can't remember to take the medications, can't afford the medications, can't get to the pharmacy to procure the medication, etc.).

It is here that we find our first paradox, for both types of patients – those patients who chose to omit doses *and* those who had no intention of missing doses – may be hesitant to share that they "are not doing what the doctor ordered." Even those patients who have intentionally chosen to miss doses, as we have seen earlier in our book, may still have considerable trouble telling their physician or nurse clinician that they have lowered the dose unilaterally. In point of fact, many patients who have stopped taking their medications are hesitant to "own-up" to their discontinuance, for fear of being reprimanded or being viewed as a "bad patient."

This internal pressure to please a respected prescribing clinician or case manager engenders our second paradox. Curiously, the more the patient likes the health care provider – the more important it becomes to please that provider. In such instances, because the patient is particularly embarrassed that he or she is not taking the medication as prescribed, it becomes even more important to deceive the provider! This is why clinicians who routinely have great rapport are, not infrequently, oblivious to the fact that some of their patients are providing inaccurate information regarding missed doses, for "I have great relations with my patients." And they do. *That's the problem.*

This does not mean that we should not strive to create powerful therapeutic alliances with our patients. It simply means that even when such alliances are formed, we should always be aware that the truth may be harder to uncover than meets the eye. Put from the perspective of Stephen Colbert, truthiness may still be a problem even when there is great trustiness in the relationship.

Setting the Stage for Truthfulness: An Invitation of Sorts

At first glance, it may appear that we are in a bit of a bind: the more powerful the therapeutic alliance, the more sheepish patients may be to admit that they are "not doing what they are supposed to be doing." The way out of the bind is to make the covert overt early in the relationship. Namely, we put it "out on the table" for all to see that it might be hard to tell the truth about missing doses. We make the element of truthfulness, and its acknowledged difficulty, a part of the alliance negotiation itself.

The first step is to admit to ourselves, and to our patients, that there is a trust issue here related to deceit. The second step is to share with the patient that the problem does not reflect badly on either the patient or ourselves, for it is a simple reflection of human nature. As we delineated above, people are going to miss doses for both intentional and unintentional reasons. It is to be expected. If we are truthful with ourselves, even physicians, nurses, physician assistants, and other providers sometimes monkey, indeed are notorious for monkeying, with the medications prescribed for their own disorders, a situation of which I have been guilty myself. It highlights the age-old axiom that it is best, in this instance, for patients to do as we say not as we do.

As noted in an earlier chapter, the fashion in which patients, in reality, take medications as opposed to how they are prescribed is referred to in the clinical literature as their "medication practices." If we have followed the principles of shared decision making while discussing our prescribing practices toward medications during the first appointment (as discussed in Chapter 6), we will be well on our way to setting the foundation for truthfulness about these medication practices in later appointments. We will have established that we are not "pill-pushers." Quite the opposite, we will have demonstrated, via our words and actions, that we are collaborative consultants who genuinely listen and who genuinely care.

Having set this collaborative stage, some clinicians find it wise in subsequent appointments to repeat the message that they are interested in hearing about patient side effects – as well as any information on missed doses – especially if the dosing schedule is inconvenient or hard to remember. Some clinicians find it useful, and surprisingly effective, to simply ask the patient about his or her medication practices from the past as follows:

TIP 82 The Medication Practice Question

"Mr. Jenkins, as we work together, and I feel we are really off to a very good start, I always like to get a better picture of how my patients worked with previous doctors and nurses. In that light, many of my patients have told me that they have sometimes lowered or increased the doses of their medications on their own, you know, without first talking with their doctor or whoever was prescribing the medication for them. Have you ever found yourself doing that, perhaps for a very good reason?"

The gentle frankness of the question is often appealing to patients. And when said with an equally gentle tone of voice – sometimes with a bit of an "I bet you have" smile or eyebrow raise – one often not only gets the truth from the patient but also a chuckle. And here the alliance deepens. The "bad thing" is prospectively now out on the table and does not necessarily have to be a bad thing that is inevitable.

Depending on the patient's answer one can continue, "I hope you will always feel free to talk with me about any concerns with your medications. And if you have missed some doses just let me know. Just about everyone misses doses now and then. And it's always better for us to talk openly and work together to find the right medications for you. Is that a deal?" Approaches like this one can unlock the door to hearing about our patient's medication practices from the very earliest stages of our work together.

Curiously, sometimes months or years later, this door will have insidiously shut itself again, requiring yet another key. In such instances, I think that you will find that the following technique can function as an effective key, and it works whether the patient is unintentionally missing doses or purposefully doing so:

TIP 83 Unlocking the Door on Missed Doses

"You know, Marcellus, many of my patients find it easy to keep missing doses of their medications perhaps because it's hard to remember to take them or perhaps they feel uneasy about taking them. In either case I really want to know how you are feeling about the medication, for we have to find the right one for you and that's different from patient to patient. In any case, the more you can accurately tell me about missed doses, the more useful information I can provide about what we should do next whether we might decrease, increase, or even stop your medication. I never want you to feel hesitant to share that you missed some doses or even stopped the medication for whatever reasons. So, getting back to your [name of medication] I was wondering roughly how many doses do you think you might have missed in the past 2 weeks?"

This technique is useful when a clinician has become suspicious down the road that a patient has been withholding information about missed doses.

The question arises, "Are there techniques that might be ***more routinely*** proactively used that may prevent even the need for employing Unlocking the Door on Missed Doses?" The answer is yes.

VALIDITY TECHNIQUES: TOOLS FOR UNCOVERING SENSITIVE AND TABOO TOPICS

Cutting Through the Mists: An Introduction

It was back in the late 1990s that the term "validity techniques" was first coined in the field of clinical interviewing.[13] By definition, validity techniques are statements and/or questions designed specifically to help patients share difficult or taboo material. The wording of each technique is behaviorally described and each technique is given a specific name, much as we have done throughout this book with our MIM techniques. When first introduced, there were merely a handful of validity techniques. During the ensuing decades, over 15 validity techniques have been described by experts in the field of clinical interviewing.

These techniques are useful in uncovering any topic that may prove difficult to share including drug and alcohol abuse, taking a sex history, intimate partner violence, child or elder abuse, incest, homicidal ideation, suicidal ideation, financial difficulties, infidelities, crimes, bullying at schools or the workplace, sexual intimidation, minimization or exaggeration of medical symptoms, hesitancy to share psychiatric symptoms, as well as the topic of this chapter – problematic medication practices. As such they are of particular practical utility in primary care and specialist settings being of use with just about every patient who walks through the clinic door. As one might expect we can use them to great advantage when trying to unravel our patient's medication practices.

But before we can effectively apply them to uncovering problematic medication practices, it is useful to understand their definitions and to see their practical applications in a more generic sense. It is outside the purview of this book to examine most of the many validity techniques nor can we explore their use outside of uncovering our patient's medication practices in detail. *Nevertheless, because of their immense utility in primary care and nursing, I will provide several samples of their use outside of medication practices as I define them.* Interested readers can find all of the current validity techniques described in detail – many of which are subsequently demonstrated by streaming video – in one of my previous texts from which the following definitions have been adapted.[14]

Normalization

In this technique first delineated in 1998, the interviewer uses a phrase – often at the beginning of a question – that metacommunicates to the patient that it is safe to talk about the subject in question, for the clinician has heard other patients frequently describe it.[13] When used effectively, the patient realizes that he or she is not the only person who has ever experienced the behaviors or problems under scrutiny. Normalization can be very useful in raising essentially any sensitive or taboo area. It is particularly useful with patients who seem to be guilt ridden or filled with social anxiety that they are somehow odd or doing something bad. Normalizations often begin with words such as, "Many of my patients have told me that . . . " or "Sometimes people who have . . ."

Let's look at a couple of examples to see how normalization can be applied for uncovering secrets regarding a variety of sensitive topics starting with missed medication doses. In the following examples, the normalization is italicized:

a. "*Many of my patients tell me that it is easy to forget their medications, especially if they are taking them twice a day like you are.* Have you found yourself missing any doses in the last couple of weeks?"
b. "*Sometimes when people get really angry they say things they later regret.* Has that ever happened to you?" [gently opening the door to an exploration of potential domestic violence with a patient suspected of being a perpetrator]
c. "*It's not unusual when there has been a lot of drinking in a family, like you told me your dad was doing when you were growing up, for there to be some violence.* Did your dad ever hit you or your mom or brothers and sisters?" [sensitively broaching the topic of child abuse with an adult you feel may have been abused]
d. "*Sometimes when people are as depressed as you've been, they find themselves having thoughts of killing themselves.* Have you been having any thoughts like that?" [sensitively raising the topic of suicide]
e. "*Sometimes when people are in as much pain as you are describing, they find themselves taking more pain meds than are prescribed.* Have you

had any thoughts like that?" [raising the topic of substance abuse, as might be found with prescription opioids]

Note that as demonstrated with the above illustrations, when using normalization appropriately, the interviewer, at first, will always allude to someone outside of the office thus metacommunicating to the patient that it is safe to talk about this topic for the interviewer has heard it before. You may have noticed that the technique of Opening the Door to Missed Doses, described earlier in the chapter, begins with a nicely phrased normalization (e.g., "You know, Marcellus, many of my patients find it easy to keep missing doses of their medications perhaps because it's hard to remember to take them or perhaps they feel uneasy about taking them.").

Gentle Assumption

With this technique, the clinician, using a gentle tone of voice and nonaccusatory wording, *assumes* that a suspected behavior is occurring instead of asking *if* it has occurred. The technique was first developed by sex researchers Pomeroy, Flax, and Wheeler,[15] who discovered that questions such as, "How frequently do you find yourself masturbating?" were much more likely to yield valid answers than "Do you masturbate?" If the clinician is concerned that the patient may be "put off" by the assumption, it can be softened by adding the phrase "if at all" as with, "How often do you find yourself masturbating, if at all?" I have found very few patients to be bothered by the use of gentle assumptions, *if previous engagement has gone well and the tone of voice used with the gentle assumption is nonjudgmental*.

The definition of a gentle assumption can be clarified by contrasting this technique with questions that are *not* examples of gentle assumption. Any question that asks whether or not a patient engaged in a given behavior (e.g., often beginning with words such as "Have you ever . . .") is by definition *not* a gentle assumption. Directly pertinent to our interests, instead of asking a patient "Have you found yourself missing any doses over the past couple of weeks," the clinician would ask, "How many doses do you think you've missed over the past couple of weeks?"

Gentle assumptions are frequently used to hunt for other entities in a list after a sensitive topic has already been raised. For example, if the topic of suicide has been raised and a method explored, the clinician might hunt for other methods by saying, "Anne, what other ways have you thought of killing yourself?". Let us now examine some other examples of using a gentle assumption in a primary care setting. We will once again lead with an inquiry into missed medications:

a. "In the past 2 months since I've seen you, how often do you think you may have missed more than a couple of doses in a single week, just roughly?"
b. "Roughly speaking, Jim, what percentage of the times that you and your wife are having intercourse do you have problems with your erections?" [helping a patient who is complaining of erectile dysfunction to give a more accurate picture of the frequency of the problems]
c. "What other problems with the law have you ever had?" [continuing to explore a list in this case regarding illegal activities]
d. "Who else has complained about your drinking?" [attempting to procure a better list of people troubled by a patient's drinking that may better reveal the extent of the patient's drinking and the resulting social damage it has caused]

Symptom Amplification

The two validity techniques that we have examined thus far offer promising avenues for helping patients to more openly admit to missing medication doses. But they do not address the equally important question, "How many doses are being missed?" When it comes to missing doses, we need to have the most accurate picture of how many doses are actually being missed in order to make reasonable recommendations to our patients as to how to proceed.

If a patient is missing an inordinate number of doses, it may indicate that significant obstacles may have arisen preventing effective medication follow-through such as forgetfulness, inconvenience, or problems traveling to and from the pharmacy, many of which can be resolved if their presence is made known. On a potentially more problematic note, the missed medications may indicate a significant hesitancy in one or more of the steps in the patient's Choice Triad reflecting imminent discontinuation. Another problem arises from a phenomenon that we touched on earlier. We saw in Chapter 1 that patients sometimes miss many doses of a medication between appointments, but start taking them correctly directly before meeting with the clinician or having bloodwork performed (the white jacket phenomena).

No matter what the cause, serious problems may arise in our treatment recommendations if the patient, intentionally or unintentionally, underreports the number of doses being missed. For instance, it may appear that the patient's symptoms have not shown adequate response at the prescribed dose (which is not being taken) resulting in a suggested inappropriate increase in dosage by the clinician.

Such miscommunications can result in various problems as with the patient subsequently taking the medication at too high a dose or, more likely, deciding to discontinue the medication altogether. All the while, the therapeutic alliance is taking a hit, for the patient is no longer feeling comfortable secondary to his or her own ongoing deceit. The result is an ensuing corruption of therapeutic trust – a problem of which the clinician is not even aware.

Unfortunately, patients, being all too human, frequently downplay the frequency or degree to which they have engaged in any behaviors that might reflect negatively on them, a process well known to us from our everyday experiences, as minimization. In primary care and specialty clinics, such behaviors may include obvious candidates for minimization such as drinking behaviors, gambling activities, and acts of domestic violence (fear of being viewed as a "bad person") to less obvious candidates including medication practices that differ from those prescribed (fear of being viewed as a "bad patient").

Symptom amplification, first delineated in 1998,[13] allows a clinician to bypass such distorting mechanisms without disengaging the patient, a disengagement that might otherwise have occurred if the interviewer had directly challenged the patient's minimization. In fact, with the use of symptom amplification, the clinician deftly allows the patient to naturalistically use his or her minimization as a defense while still uncovering a better estimate of the patient's amount of activity in the proscribed behavior.

This face-saving psychological sleight-of-hand is accomplished by setting the upper limits of the quantity in question at such a high level that when the patient downplays the amount, the clinician is still aware that there is a significant problem. No confrontation or challenge to the patient's minimization occurs, yet more valid data results. For a question to be viewed as symptom amplification, the clinician must suggest an actual number in the question, set it high, and proceed to advance the number to even higher amounts.

For instance, a clinician suspicious that he or she is in the presence of a heavy drinker can, once the topic of drinking has been raised, ask about the extent of the drinking behavior as follows, "How much liquor can you hold in a single night, a pint, a fifth?" When the patient responds "Oh no, not a fifth, I don't know, maybe a pint," the clinician is still alerted that there is a problem despite the patient's minimization.

Here are some other examples of symptom amplification with missing medication doses as our first illustration:

a. Jim, in the weeks since we last met, how many doses of your [name of medication in question] do you think you might have missed, just roughly: 10 doses, 15 doses, 20 doses?"
b. How many times have you actually struck your wife in your entire marriage: 20 times, 40 times, 60 times? [uncovering the extent of intimate partner violence once a patient has admitted to it]
c. How many bags of heroin might you go through in a day: a bag, five bags, a bundle? [uncovering the extent of use once use is uncovered]
d. On your very worst days, how much time do you spend thinking about killing yourself: 8 hours a day, 12 hours, 15 hours? [helping to uncover the extent of suicidal intent]

We have arrived at a sophisticated understanding of three core validity techniques. Now let's see how we can mix and match them to optimize our ability to uncover missed doses.

Validity Technique Combinations for Uncovering Missed Doses: Doublets and Triplets

As I mentioned earlier, Steele and colleagues discovered in their research that the words used by clinicians had a distinct impact on improving the validity of their patients' self-reporting on missed doses.[12] Specifically, they found that the secret lay in combining the two interviewing techniques we call "normalization" and "gentle assumption" into a doublet. Thus, they used a gentle assumption but always softened it first by employing a normalization as follows:

TIP 84 Normalization/Gentle Assumption Doublet for Missed Medications

"Mr. Jeffers, many patients tell me that it can be easy to forget to take their medications at times (normalization). In the weeks since we last met, how many doses do you think you might have missed, just roughly (gentle assumption)."

I have found this interviewing doublet, delineated by Steele and colleagues, to work extremely well. You will have to see how it works for you, but I have a suspicion that you will be very pleased. I have seen clinicians inquire about missed doses with questions such as, "Have you missed any doses?" or "You've been taking your medications as we discussed?" and receive assurances that all medications are on board. A second clinician, during a later interview, will uncover a number of missed doses with the same patient through the use of the Normalization/Gentle Assumption Doublet for Missed Medications. I am reminded of the famous words of the social scientist Thomas Kuhn, "The answers you get depend upon the questions you ask."[16]

Not surprisingly, the technique seems to be even more effective if one adds a symptom amplification at the end, creating a triplet as follows:

TIP 85 Amplifying Triplet for Missed Medications

"Mr. Jeffers, many patients tell me that it can be easy to forget to take their medications at times (normalization). In the weeks since we last met, how many doses do you think you might have missed, just roughly (gentle assumption): 10 doses, 15 doses, 20 doses? (symptom amplification)"

At one of my workshops on advanced interviewing techniques, methods for effectively uncovering missed medication doses arose as a topic for discussion. The following technique was shared by Gerda Van Alst, a physician. Dr. Van Alst's suggestion introduces a validity technique we have not mentioned yet called shame attenuation of which there are many useful variations.[14]

Like normalization, shame attenuation was designed for raising taboo topics in a sensitive fashion. Unlike normalization, shame attenuation metacommunicates that it is safe to talk about the ensuing topic not by metacommunicating that the interviewer has heard it from other patients. Instead, the safety is metacommunicated by indicating that the interviewer truly "gets it." He or she understands the amount of pain or difficulty the patient must be experiencing and recognizes that the resulting problematic behavior is understandable. In short, it attenuates (decreases) the shame of the patient resulting in an increased likelihood of sharing:

TIP 86 Shame Attenuation/Gentle Assumption Doublet for Missed Medications

"Mr. Jeffers, I know it is hard for you to take these medications (shame attenuation), how many of them did you manage to take this past week? (gentle assumption)."

There is a quiet elegance to this very sophisticated question. I like the way the question communicates empathic understanding with the opening phrase, "I know that it's very hard for you to take these medications" (shame attenuation). In addition, I think that inside the next phrase we may discover the real secret to the question's effectiveness by Dr. Van Alst's use of the word "manage," a word choice that subtly acknowledges the fact that it would be reasonable for anyone to find it difficult to take the medication while implying that credit is due for those times when it is taken as recommended. No doubt part of the elegant effectiveness comes from the way in which the interviewer does not ask about a negative (how many doses missed) but, instead, asks about a positive (how many doses were taken).

I think you will find that the Shame Attenuation/Gentle Assumption Doublet for Missed Medications is a wonderful question to utilize with patients whose medication regimen requires them to take a multitude of medications and/or are being asked to ingest medications that are unpleasantly large in size as sometimes seen with chronic illnesses such as AIDS as we discussed in Chapter 9. In such instances, patients may find themselves gagging as they try to take their medications.

THE SHAME CYCLE: A CURIOUS YET PROBLEMATIC PHENOMENA

Let us look at the problem of shame in a little more detail. As we have already emphasized, people forget to take medications. It happens, even to the most motivated of patients. How often it happens is related to both internal factors (how prone the patient is to forgetfulness, the presence of disorders such as adult attention deficit disorder and dementia) and external factors (frequency of dosing, the pace of the patient's workday). Both internal and external factors combine to determine how inconvenient, and thus easily forgotten, taking a medication becomes for any given patient.

In many instances, forgetting a dose or two is no big deal, but for some patients it can escalate into a much more problematic phenomena, known as the "shame cycle," that not only plays havoc with drug levels, but can damage the therapeutic alliance to the point that a patient may even drop out of care. As we saw earlier in the chapter – when discussing why patients are prone to lie about their medication practices – this type of therapeutic rupture, paradoxically, is most commonly encountered and is most destructive with clinicians who are particularly good at engaging patients. It also unfolds insidiously, essentially being invisible to the treating clinician and hence beyond intervention.

The shame cycle occurs more frequently in patients who have low self-esteem as seen with patients who have been abused, live with belittling partners, have poor life-skills resulting in a steady diet of failures, or are cruelly shamed as being physically unattractive in their cultures. In short, the shame cycle is prone to occur in a lot of our patients encountered in everyday primary care practice.

Such patients often have an intense need to be liked and are exquisitely rejection-sensitive. Pleasing their clinicians – to be perceived by them as "good patients" – is unusually important for such patients, even more so than we have already discussed. When such a patient finds a warm and engaging clinician, he or she quickly bonds.

To the treating clinician, all seems to be going well; the clinician likes the patient, and the patient likes the clinician. The appointments are a pleasure for both parties, until . . . . . until one of these patients, perhaps a patient with more than a fair share of forgetfulness, begins to miss doses. These patients then experience shame and/or guilt. The frequency of this new psychological cost – feeling shame and/or guilt – will be directly related to the frequency with which medications are missed.

Each time such a patient comes into a clinician's exam room, the patient is fearfully anticipating a question from the clinician along the lines of, "Mrs. Phillips, have you been taking the medication the way it is prescribed, you know, twice a day, once in the morning and once at night?" No matter how warmly this question is proffered, the patient is now faced with a dilemma – tell the truth and risk losing the respect of the clinician or lie and risk losing self-respect for one has become a "liar." It is a lose-lose proposition. Not infrequently the perceived risk of being viewed as a bad patient is so intense that the patient opts for the latter – lying – to save face. This path further stokes the shame cycle, because the patient subsequently experiences a new shame related to his or her ongoing acts of deception.

For these patients, there ensues an insidiously unpleasant association occurring when "seeing Dr. Shea," despite the fact the patient views Dr. Shea as warm and caring. As more and more doses are missed, the shame cycle intensifies. These situations – the medication is being taken erratically – are bad enough but something much more damaging is about to happen. These patients are about to stop coming to their appointments.

Patients who stop do so because the intensity of their shame and guilt is too big a price to pay. For these patients, the psychological cost of the inconvenience related to missing doses has now become too high, and it is no longer "worth it to them to take this drug." When the next appointment day comes, it is all too easy to rationalize, "I've got a lot I need to do this week. I just have to get to the grocery store. I just don't have time to go today. I'll go to the next appointment." A missed appointment means more shame, more lying, more guilt, and more missed appointments. The shame cycle worsens. Soon enough our patient is a permanent "no show."

What is particularly frustrating is that the clinician often has no idea that any problem is arising, and, consequently, can do nothing to transform it. The following strategy can be useful in short-circuiting this shame cycle. I often implement it in the first couple of appointments, especially if I intuit that the patient may be prone to shame and guilt. It goes like this:

TIP 87 Short-Circuiting the Shame Cycle

"It is very easy to forget to take a dose. If you notice yourself doing that, please note whether there is anything inconvenient about the timing of the dose. If there are any missed doses, we can put our heads together to see whether we can figure out a better time or an easier way to remember. The bottom line is that I really think this medication can help you, but I want to find a way that is easiest for you to remember to take it. Can you promise to let me know about any missed doses? And we'll see what we can come up with to make sure taking the medication is easier to remember. Is that something that you think you can do?"

What a nice antidote to the shame cycle. No shame here. Patients often model whom they think they are by whom they think we think they are. If when a patient misses doses, the clinician's tone is one that conveys displeasure, the patient will often adopt the image that he or she is at fault, that is, a bad patient.

When using the technique of Short-Circuiting the Shame Cycle, there is none of that. The prescriber views the inconvenience of the scheduling as the "bad guy" and the patient as the "good guy," whose input is vital. The patient is viewed not as the problem but as the solution. The strategy is a wonderful example of an effective application of the MIM's core principles.

At the next session, the prescriber asks, "Did you notice any problems with the doses being inconvenient or find yourself missing any of them?" With such words the discussion of missed doses opens up gracefully without a shred of shame or guilt. Sometimes patients have even kept a list of the missed doses. Such meticulous tracking can be positively reenforced with, "You've done a great job of keeping track of the missed doses. It will really help us to find a convenient time for you to take the medication."

Suddenly, a patient who – without the use of our strategy for short-circuiting the shame cycle – would have been experiencing a negative experience for missing doses is – with the use of the strategy – having a positive experience for responsibly reporting the missed doses. The potentially oppositional field seen in the shame cycle has been completely reversed.

By the way, a lot of slick ways can be used to help forgetful patients remember doses. Naturally, plastic pillboxes, in which the day's doses are placed in separate compartments, can really help, and they have the added advantage that one can readily see when a dose has been missed – the pills are still in the case!

Some of my favorite memory triggers rely on making the presence of the medication bottles hard to miss by associating them with something that the patient never misses doing:

1. If the patient brushes his or her teeth daily, then the provider can suggest placing the medication bottle right between the patient's toothbrush and toothpaste tube. It is hard to miss a dose with this technique, especially if the provider emphasizes that the patient should take the medication before brushing his or her teeth.
2. Placing the medication bottle directly beside morning vitamins is also very effective. Care must be taken if children are in the house that no confusion can occur, nor should potentially dangerous medications be out in such instances.
3. Yet another technique that some of my patients claim has worked nicely is to place the medication bottles on top of the pillow on the bed or on or near their alarm clock, two places that must be encountered every night before sleeping.
4. It is also useful to brainstorm with the patient's family on any novel ideas they may have on how to remind the patient. Unique, creative, and, more importantly, very effective reminders sometimes come from such family brainstorming.
5. Reminders conveyed by smart phones or smart watches can be very useful.

Conclusion

As we wrap up, I would like to offer one more strategy for gaining more valid material regarding the medication practices of our patients. It is not an interviewing technique per se, but clinicians, from prescribers (physicians, nurse clinicians, physician assistants, and clinical pharmacists) to nonprescribers (nurses, case managers, and family members), have found it to be of use for many decades. Specifically, it can be invaluable to ask patients to bring their medication bottles with them to their appointment or to ask to see them if you are doing a home visit. This practice allows health care providers to directly see how many pills are left in the bottles.

This request can serve a second purpose as well. I believe that you will find that, pursuant to your request, some of your patients will present with parcels of medications so large that they will remind one of a bewildered Santa Claus, sans snow and reindeer, toting a sack full of toys when entering your office. They will seem equally bewildered when asked for what condition or symptoms each of the myriad of medications has been prescribed.

I have found that such encounters can serve as a jarring, yet useful, reminder to me of how many medications are being prescribed by myself and other clinicians, a fact that does not register as strongly when I am reviewing a chart or an electronic health record. Something about sorting through these immense bags of "who knows what" serves as a cogent reminder to make sure that I am prescribing as few medications as are necessary to help the patient find relief. These medication-laden Santas are deliriums just waiting to happen.

In closing, we have explored a variety of excellent interviewing techniques and strategies for helping patients to more easily share the truth about their medication practices. I have not meant to convey that any particular technique is right or wrong, nor more or less effective than others. Instead, they have been offered as jumping-off points for the reader to become familiar with what techniques are available for flexible use. By subsequently employing them, you will quickly be able to choose those techniques with which you feel most comfortable. Or perhaps, in some instances, the chapter will have spurred the reader to uncover new techniques not described in these pages. At a minimum, the chapter provides a new toolbox from which we can pull the interviewing techniques that potentially best suit the needs of any specific patient.

We have also seen in this chapter the various reasons that patients may understandably withhold information about both their hesitancies concerning a medication and why they may be hesitant to share missed doses. But we have not exhausted the subtleties of this dilemma, for we have not yet come to grips with one more set of influences that can impact on the whole process – the clinician and the patient may come from different cultures.

REFERENCES

1. Pearson H. *Oscar Wilde, His Life and Wit.* New York, NY: Harper & Brothers Publishers; 1946:129.
2. Britten N, Stevenson FA, Barry CA, et al. Misunderstandings in prescribing decisions in general practice: qualitative study. *BMJ* 2000;320:484–488.
3. Donovan JL, Blake DR. Patient non-compliance: deviance or reasoned decision-making? *Soc Sci Med* 1992;34:507–513.
4. Gordon K, Smith F, Dhillon S. Effective chronic disease management: patient's perspectives on medication-related problems. *Patient Educ Couns* 2007;65:407–415.
5. Lapane KL, Dubé CE, Schneider KL, et al. Misperceptions of patients vs. providers regarding medication-related communication issues. *Am J Manag Care* 2007;13:613–618.
6. van Geffen EC, van Hulten R, Bouvy ML, et al. Characteristics and reasons associated with nonacceptance of selective serotonin-reuptake inhibitor treatment. *Ann Pharmacother* 2008;42:218–225.
7. McHorney C. The adherence estimator: a brief, proximal screener for patient propensity to adhere to prescription medications for chronic disease. *Curr Med Res Opin* 2009;25(1):215–238.
8. Day JC, Bentall RP, Roberts C, et al. Attitudes toward antipsychotic medication: the impact of clinical variables and relationships with health professionals. *Arch Gen Psychiatry* 2005;62(7):717–724.
9. Nakonezny PA, Byerly MJ, Rush AJ. Electronic monitoring of antipsychotic medication adherence in outpatients with schizophrenia or schizoaffective disorder: an empirical evaluation of its reliability and predictive validity. *Psychiatry Res* 2008;157(1–3):259–263.
10. Davis MS. Variations in patients' compliance with doctors' orders: analysis of congruence between survey responses and results of empirical investigations. *J Med Educ* 1966;41:1037–1048.
11. Goldberg AI, Cohen G, Rubin AH. Physician assessments of patient compliance with medical treatment. *Soc Sci Med* 1998;47:1873–1876.
12. Steele DJ, Jackson TC, Gutmann MC. Have you been taking your pills? The adherence-monitoring sequence in the medical interview. *J Fam Pract* 1990;30(3):294–299.
13. Shea SC. *Psychiatric Interviewing: The Art of Understanding.* 2nd ed. Philadelphia, PA: W. B. Saunders; 1998.
14. Shea SC. Validity Techniques for Exploring Sensitive Material and Uncovering the Truth. *Psychiatric Interviewing: The Art of Understanding.* 3rd ed. London, England: Elsevier, Inc.; 2017:149–185.
15. Pomeroy WB, Flax CC, Wheeler CC. *Taking a Sex History.* New York, NY: The Free Press; 1982.
16. Bayles D, Orland T. *Art & Fear.* Santa Barbara, CA: Capra Press; 1993:93.

CHAPTER 13

Pills and People: Assessing Cultural Beliefs About Medications

". . .understanding the symbolic functions of medications is as important as knowing their elimination half-lives or suggested dosing regimens."[1]

Jonathan Metzl, MD, PhD
Michelle Riba, MD

INTRODUCTION

Quietly sitting in its bottle, a medication can appear to be a simple inanimate "thing" defined by the parameters of its color, shape, and size. But a pill is more than a mere thing. It is a thing animated by the culture in which it lives. The surrounding culture, whether it be Hispanic, Black, White, Asian, or Native American, gives each medication its meaning, power, and appeal. In this sense, it behooves the prescriber – whether nurse practitioner, nurse clinical specialist, physician, physician assistant, clinical pharmacist, or other provider – to determine the "cultural address" of the medication about to be prescribed. With each patient, this cultural address will be unique and distinctive.

In Chapter 9, where we examined our toolbox for helping patients to navigate the third step of the Choice Triad, we examined the impact of the Cluster C factors (psychological/symbolic meanings arising from the use of a specific medication). We found that medications often acquire symbolic meanings to patients which can be, at times, determinative factors in their weighing of the pros and cons. Our focus was on the *personalized* symbolic associations generated by taking a medication on issues such as self-esteem, fear of personal weakness, and concerns of biologic dependence.

In this chapter, we will expand on these issues, exploring the impact of more *generalized* cultural influences as they impact on the patient's weighing of his or her pros and cons. Such cultural nuances may also impact on the quality of communication between the prescriber and the patient. Achieving effective cross-cultural communication may be more elusive than first meets the eye. I am reminded of the sage words of the playwright George Bernard Shaw who quipped, "The single biggest problem communicating is the illusion it has taken place."[2] One of the greatest creators of this illusion is cross-cultural misunderstanding. When such misunderstandings occur, the clinician thinks he or she is at the right cultural address but, unfortunately, is walking on the wrong side of the street.

To create an effective toolbox for identifying the correct address and communicating clearly with patients from cultures different than that of the prescriber's culture, our chapter is divided into three parts: (1) assessing the influence of other healers, (2) uncovering cultural beliefs about medications, and (3) problems with generics related to pill size, shape, and color. It should be noted that it is impossible in a brief chapter to effectively address the immensely important topic of culturally adaptive interviewing in the broader sense of creating a sound therapeutic alliance. For the interested reader, I have addressed this topic in a comprehensive, yet concise, monograph elsewhere.[3]

Part 1: Assessing the Influence of Alternative Healers

Working with Culture-Specific Healers

When we work with our patients, it is often a mistake to think we work alone. Whether patients inform us or not, they are frequently seeing other healers associated within the matrix of their current culture or culture of origin. Sometimes, the healers are specific to a given culture (shamans in the Hmong or First Nation peoples). Other times, they are a generalized movement that crosses many cultures (practitioners of complementary and alternative medicine [CAM]). In any case, the healers that are simultaneously seeing our patients speak to them with a powerful voice.

These healers may voice strong views about our medications both for and against their use. I can think of no occasion in which it is not wise to find out what is being said by them. In most cases, I have found them to be of great value in ongoing care. Occasionally, there is a problem. In either instance, it is important to find out what these other influences are for a given patient. Whatever the case, the following interviewing principle guides the practice: *Ask your patients, in an open and interested fashion, if they are seeing other healers who are either particular to their culture (as in a shaman) or generic across cultures (such as a practitioner of CAM).* The following technique provides several ways in which to put this principle into practice regarding culturally specific healers:

TIP 88 The Shaman Questions

"Do you visit or use a shaman?"
"Have you talked to your shaman about our work together?"
"What is your shaman's view about our work together?"
"What do you think he (or she) will think about you starting up on a blood pressure medication (substitute whichever class of medications is relevant)?"

If the patient has not already done so, I subsequently suggest that the patient should ask his or her shaman about the use of the medication. As we saw in Chapter 6, such coordinated care can be critical to success. Also note that the term for the healer must be adjusted for the cultural heritage of the patient including religious/spiritual background, familial beliefs, and geographic locale. Thus, the healer might be called a sorcerer, a medicine man, priest, rabbi, or faith healer.

Working with Practitioners of CAM

To avoid confusion, it is worthwhile to briefly address the definition of CAM. According to the Mayo Clinic,[4] "CAM" – the most popular term in clinical parlance at the time of the writing of this book – refers to wellness and health interventions that are not viewed as being typical of conventional Western medicine and nursing (although the acronym CAM is quite popular in the clinical literature and academic classroom, I find that patients seem to be more comfortable using terms such as "alternative healer," "holistic healer," or "new age practitioner").

In the acronym CAM, the term "complementary" refers to those healing practices that are used in conjunction with traditional Western medicine. By contrast, the term "alternative" refers to the use of nonconventional therapies *instead* of traditional Western interventions. For the interested reader, extensive and valuable information on CAM is available at the website for the National Center for Complementary & Integrative Health (NCCIH).[5] NCCIH is the U.S. federal government's lead agency for scientific research on medical and health care systems, practices, and products that are not generally considered part of conventional medicine.

In CAM, there is a heavy investment in a holistic approach to medical care that focuses on physical, emotional, and spiritual health (in Western medicine, this exact principle is part and parcel of what is now called patient-centered medicine and person-centered medicine). CAM practitioners employ a variety of practices that emphasize mind-brain interaction. Such practices include modalities (such as meditation, tai chi, qigong, acupuncture, and yoga), manipulative and body-based approaches (such as massage therapy and spinal manipulation), and natural products (such as herbs and dietary supplements).

Interestingly, in the past several decades, many Western-trained physicians, nurses, and physician assistants have become adept at using interventions from both traditional mainstream medicine and nursing with the best evidence-based approaches from CAM. Such combined approaches to patient care are often referred to as "integrative medicine."

With regard to collaborating with practitioners of CAM, when I first ask – and I make an effort to ask all of my patients – if they are currently seeing a practitioner of CAM, I often soften the initial inquiry with a normalization (one of the validity techniques from our last chapter) because many patients falsely assume that medical and mental health providers have a built-in bias against alternative medicine. Some do. I don't. Whether you do or you don't, the following technique can help you to assess the presence of an alternative healer:

TIP 89 Normalizing the Use of a CAM Healer

"It is not uncommon for some of my patients to be seeing a practitioner of alternative or holistic medicine while they are working with me, and it's always useful to know of such efforts so that we can work effectively together. Are you by chance working with anyone else on your diabetes (substitute whichever disorder is relevant)?"

I believe that the discussion between ourselves and our patients over the concurrent use of traditional and alternative healing practices is both so common and so important that it is worth more of our attention. Some patients will come to the initial H&P already seeing a CAM practitioner. You will find that some of these patients will spontaneously share this information. Many will not, for fear that the clinician will disapprove. Consequently, as mentioned above, I make an effort during the medication history to ask about the topic of alternative and holistic approaches.

In other instances, patients become interested in CAM treatments long after we have begun our relationship, often prompted at the suggestion of friends, family members, or from wanderings on the web. Whether it is within the initial appointment or during a subsequent appointment, I tend to use the same approach: an open and nonjudgmental interest in what the patient is doing.

The topic of CAM, if not handled properly, can become a major trip wire into an oppositional relationship instead of a partnership. As noted above, some patients are so convinced that their physician, nurse, or other health care provider is going to be opposed to CAM approaches that they simply do not bring them up, even though they are concurrently seeing an herbalist, acupuncturist, or chiropractor. Such a lack of openness and trust does not bode well for a long-term partnership between a prescriber and a patient.

When patients encounter an unexpected openness to their interest in CAM, it can reassure them that we are not opponents – we are trusted allies. If by any chance, in subsequent discussions, the provider feels that the patient's choice of an alternative approach may be damaging, it is easy enough to warn the patient of this concern, and, openly discourage its use. If I have approached the general topic of CAM interventions with a collaborative openness, I have found that most patients will *not* find my concern about a specific CAM's potential for problems as being oppositional in nature. Indeed, they are appreciative of my genuine concern.

Interestingly, to date, I have seldom encountered the problem of a CAM presenting a danger. Instead, the issue of danger to the patient more often presents as the patient being told by an alternative healer to *not* follow my recommendations. This relatively rare, but real, problem can be gracefully addressed, as we shall soon see in the next tip below.

In any case, if a patient unexpectedly, in ongoing care or during his or her initial appointment, comments that he or she is trying an herbal remedy or some other CAM practice, I ask with a genuine warmth and curiosity, "Oh, do you think it is helping?" If the patient says it is – and I am comfortable the CAM is a safe intervention – I enthusiastically comment, "then by all means you should keep using it." Patients are genuinely pleased by this unanticipated response on my part. I then proceed to share the following:

TIP 90 Expressing Interest in CAM Treatments

"Some people think that all physicians (supply the name of your particular discipline) are highly opposed to alternative medicine. This is simply not true. I feel certain there are many things that we will learn about healing from many different systems. Indeed, digitalis, a great heart medication, was first used as an herbal remedy centuries ago. I myself have found that acupuncture can be helpful in certain pain conditions and St. John's wort in some depressions.

"My only cautionary note is that, in some instances, only a standard medication will, in my opinion, provide the necessary relief or cure. In these instances, it is critical not to stop the medication. I will always give you my best medical advice on whether you should try a specific alternative technique. That's my job as your clinician. Also, always let me know if you are thinking of starting on any vitamin or herbal supplement, because these agents occasionally can interact with medications, sometimes causing unwanted side effects.

"I am also very eager to talk with your alternative specialist to share what I am doing and how it is helping, and to hear the same about his or her approaches. There are several alternative specialists in the area with whom I have a very good working relationship.

"One final thing. As you can see from my openness to alternative methods, I believe that good healers have a keen interest in what other healers are doing. If you bump into an alternative specialist that in any way begins to knock my medications or what I am doing, beware of them. They clearly are not open healers. Their bad-mouthing of my methods should alert you to go elsewhere, so that we can find someone who wants to join our team, not someone who wants to destroy it, because we've got a great team going here."

I have never had this approach backfire. On the other hand, I have had some patients switch CAM healers because they did not like the healer's attitudes toward me. As we can see, this nonoppositional approach, which fosters an ongoing collaborative feeling, has transformed a potentially oppositional trap into an opportunity for an even stronger alliance.

Part 2: Uncovering Cultural Beliefs About Medications

Shrinking Worlds, Cross-Cultural Challenges, and the Rise of Ethnicpharmacology and Ethnopharmacology

Cultures can bias people either toward the use of traditional medications or away from them. In resonance with the MIM, the clinician's goal is always to work with the patient to collaboratively find an approach to healing with which the patient is comfortable. Oftentimes this comfort level is predetermined by the patient's culture. At all times, it is incumbent of the clinician to try to understand the patient's health and illness views as sculpted by the patient's culture, ethnicity, and familial matrix. It is also important to be cognizant of any alterations in the patient's physiologic handling of a specific medication related to genetic factors.

With regard to the use of indigenous agents and medications, the addressing of these factors – from cultural, ethnic, and sociologic to biologic – is sometimes referred to as "ethnicpharmacology,"[6] and, as such, it represents a subdivision of the larger field of cross-cultural medicine and nursing. Note that definitions of this field and its relationship to the field of *ethno*pharmacology vary. For instance, the field of *ethno*pharmacology is commonly distinguished as focusing on indigenous, natural, and folk remedies. The International Society for Ethnopharmacology (a rich resource for the reader on such remedies) describes ethnopharmacology as being the "information and understandings about people's use of plants, fungi, animals, microorganisms and minerals and their biological and pharmacological effects based on the principles established through international conventions."[7] In this section, we will be focusing on the insights to be gained from ethnicpharmacology regarding the use traditional Western medications across differing cultures.

Before doing so, it is important to note that the general field of cross-cultural medicine and nursing is filled with exciting changes, newly minted concepts, complicated nuances, and a certain degree of urgency. The urgency arises from the shrinking of our world – the result of multiple factors including voluntary emigrations; escapes from terrorism, genocide, and war; the ever-increasing extent and influence of the web; and the growing penetration of online and telecommunication material into our lives from different parts of the world via televisions, computers, tablets, and smart phones. The bottom line is simple: Physicians, advanced practice nurses, physician assistants, and clinical pharmacists are going to be prescribing for patients – whether in person or through the web (via web chat or applications such as Skype or FaceTime) – who are frequently from different cultures, races, ethnic groups, religious backgrounds, political beliefs, sexual orientations, ages, worldviews, and socioeconomic classes than the prescriber.

As clinicians, we too come from a variety of races, cultures, and geographic regions. We may be Latina/o, Black, White, Asian, Indian American or Native American, or have been born and educated in the United States, Africa, South America, Japan, France, India, Malaysia, and so on. For the contemporary clinician, this diversity creates a fascinating arena for clinical interaction when prescribing. It also creates the potential for the type of miscommunications of which George Bernard Shaw was alluding earlier.

In Part 2, we will examine some of the key topics related to ethnicpharmacology that can be of use for avoiding such miscommunications and, if unavoidable, transforming them. This introduction is merely that – an introduction. It can be followed up by accessing the many resources currently available in the clinical literature and on the web, where you will find excellent reviews on quite specific topics such as the role of ethnicpharmacology in enhancing medication interest and follow-through in the elderly[8] to practical resource centers on the overarching topics of ethnicpharmacology and ethnopharmacology as can be found on the transcultural website of Campinha-Bacote.[9]

Direct Cultural Prohibitions: What's in This Thing?

Let us begin our exploration by directly addressing the interface between religious belief and medication use. In an insightful book chapter, Iqbal Ahmed describes a variety of specific beliefs that can negatively impact on medication interest and use.[10] Religious issues regarding diet can present medication interest problems that can catch an unsuspecting clinician off guard. Muslims may decide against using a liquid medication if they find that it contains alcohol. Similarly, a Jewish patient may stop using a medication if it is found to have porcine products as part of its binding agent. Outside of religious factors, but in a similar vein of concerns, a vegetarian may very well refuse a medication if it contains animal-derived products and an animal rights activist could easily refuse any medication that was developed using animal experimentation.

In the past, many of these roadblocks to medication interest would have gone undetected by patients. With the advent of the web, such information is just a click away. Having discovered some information about their medication that causes cultural concern, as we noted in our last chapter, these patients may stop their medications abruptly without alerting their clinicians for fear of being viewed as bad patients.

Indirect Cultural Concerns: Problems with Dosing Schedules and Routes of Administration

Specific religious and cultural restrictions on the use of certain medications (or products used to bind the active components of a medication) are not the only reason that a patient may appropriately be hesitant to use a medication. Sometimes cultural beliefs and religious practices may interfere with the use of medications because the use of the medication is at cross-purposes with more generic customs and traditions.

Perhaps one of the best examples of such a process occurs with Non-Muslim practitioners working with Muslim patients during the sacred month of Ramadan.[11] During this month, between dawn and sunset, Muslims will abstain from eating, smoking, and intercourse. The fasting also prohibits taking oral medications. The practices of Ramadan are designed to allow Muslims to improve their spiritual and physical relationships with God. Although Ramadan allows those Muslims with medical conditions to continue medications or food intake as is deemed necessary for safety, a study by Salti and colleagues showed that most patients with type 2 diabetes (86%) and close to half with type 1 (43%) would choose to fast in an effort to comply with standard Ramadan practices.[12]

One can easily see that a clinician who inadvertently ignores the religious traditions of these patients – not only misses a rich arena for shared decision making – but risks arriving at the false assumption that his or her patients will continue their pre-Ramadan diabetes regimen. Such an assumption is problematic at best and, at worst, dangerous. Somewhat surprisingly, a study by Ali and colleagues showed that only 34.1% of providers asked their Muslim patients with diabetes whether they would be fasting.[13] It would be my guess that some of the clinicians, who did not ask, felt that they had previously communicated the dangers of not taking diabetic medications so effectively that their patients would surely continue with their medications and normal eating habits during Ramadan or raise the issue if they intended not to do so. A better example of George Bernard Shaw's dictum, "The single biggest problem communicating is the illusion it has taken place," would be hard to find.

Fortunately, although a bit tricky, a variety of approaches to managing diabetes during Ramadan have been found.[14] But to utilize these strategies, one must first be aware of the patient's religious traditions enjoining the patient to fast during Ramadan and, second, be savvy enough to ask directly about the patient's intentions to proceed with such fasting. In this Ramadan example, we see that the cultural conundrum has nothing to do with direct prohibitions or hesitancies about the medications per se and everything to do with the fact that the use of the medication will break a revered fasting tradition.

In a similar fashion, cultural beliefs may impact on a patient's preferred route of administration. For instance, patients from various cultures may differ dramatically not only on how comfortable they may feel in discussing their sexuality – and what they consider to be their "private parts" – they may also vary on the degree to which they feel comfortable touching these regions whether sexually or not sexually.

For example, in some Islamic and African cultures, women who have yeast infections may prefer oral medications to vaginally inserted medications.[15] If such is the case, it may behoove a prescriber to suggest an oral preparation first (or at least offer one as a possibility), even if it was technically less efficacious than the vaginal preparation. As we have seen frequently in our book, an efficacious medication that remains inside a bottle or a tube is not efficacious, it is useless. A less efficacious medication that finds itself inside the patient's body is clearly a superior intervention.

When first prescribing a medication or during ongoing care, if one becomes suspicious that a patient has developed cultural concerns about a medication, a clinician can sometimes unmask such concerns using the following technique:

TIP 91 Cultural Taboo Tap

"Besides side effects, do you have any concerns about this medication such as how it was made, how it looks, or how we are using it or anything that might not seem like a good fit for your culture or religious beliefs, anything at all, no matter how small it may seem?"

The Cultural Taboo Tap can be useful in uncovering both direct cultural prohibitions (such as problems with animal additives to the medication matrix) and indirect cultural concerns (such as problems with dosing schedules and routes of administration).

Direct, Yet Subtle Concerns: Too Much of a Good Thing

Sometimes cultural bias shows itself as a gentle yet pervasive hesitancy about taking any medications as opposed to concerns about a specific medication, as illustrated above. In Indochina, patients often believe that medications should be taken only during the acute phase of an illness, being at considerable risk for dropping a medication quickly after becoming asymptomatic. They may also fear that chronic use will result in drug dependence.[16]

Sometimes the hesitancies are related to specific illnesses. Asian Americans occasionally find diabetes to be a peculiar illness to understand, for diabetes is less common in their countries of origin. The relationship between abstract blood glucose levels and the use of medications to alter these levels, as well as restrictions in diet, may seem foreign to some. Indeed, the concept of dietary requirements does not fit in nicely with the Asian way of thinking about food.[15]

As another example of a subtle, yet very real, bias against any medication use among Asian patients, research by Horne involving 500 undergraduate students from the United Kingdom demonstrated such a generalized hesitancy.[17] The students self-identified themselves into two groups: students with a European background or students with an Asian background. The Asian students perceived medications as intrinsically harmful agents, perhaps even as addictive substances that should be avoided. These same students were less likely to endorse the benefits of modern pharmaceuticals.

This study also demonstrates that young adults not infrequently, unbeknownst to themselves, unconsciously adopt the belief systems current within their culture, whether determined by folk-custom passed from generation to generation or the latest website or video that has gone viral. No matter what age, reluctantly or not, people often absorb the beliefs of their parents or immediate family, although many adolescents and young adults would be loath to admit it. Thus, younger patients may more readily describe a hesitancy about a medication stemming from such subtle, yet deep-rooted beliefs, if one invites the patient to describe first his or her parents' beliefs before describing his or her own.

It is an indirect way to enter an adolescent patient's belief system through a backdoor of sorts:

TIP 92 Parental Backdoor Question

"I'm always interested in seeing how different cultures and generations view medications. Do your parents have particular beliefs about medications, such as whether or not they are useful or how often people should take them?"

This unassuming backdoor approach sometimes leads to unexpected answers as well as gateways for productive collaborative exploration with an adolescent or young adult. The ensuing conversations occasionally present rich opportunities for enhancing medication interest.

I will illustrate this point with a prototypic adolescent/clinician interlude involving the potential use of an antidepressant. As noted in a previous chapter, primary care clinicians, combined with other nonpsychiatric clinicians, prescribe more antidepressants than psychiatrists. It is a trend that will only continue, for the organizational process of systematically integrating psychotherapists from various disciplines such as clinical psychology, social work, and counseling directly into primary care clinics is the wave of the future.

Readers who eventually become primary care clinicians (as well those who become specialists) will probably be handling the psychotropic medications of many of the patients being seen concurrently with these integrated therapists. Psychiatrists will probably be seeing primarily those patients with more challenging presentations or who proved to be unresponsive to initial medication trials. In short, nonpsychiatric physicians and nurse clinicians will probably see an even greater uptick in prescribing antidepressants in future years.

We will see the effective use of the Parental Backdoor Question as it unfolds in the following dialogue involving a young Asian American graduate student, whom we shall call Steve, who has been seeing an embedded therapist at the school's university health center. Although well engaged in psychotherapy, Steve's depression has worsened, and he has been referred for a potential trial of an antidepressant. We will pick up the conversation shortly after the physician had shown a patient education video on the web, regarding the possible role of neurotransmitters in depression, after which the physician has recommended the use of an antidepressant:

Pt.: Do you really think this medication might help me with my depression?

Clin.: Yes, I think there is a good chance of that, although I can't give any guarantees. But I am certainly hopeful it can and, if not, we will try to find one that will. (pause) . . . Is there something specific that makes you a little hesitant?

Pt.: Not really, I just don't know. I'm just feeling sort of off-balance now, and I'm not sure what I should do.

Clin.: Perhaps a medication might not be right for you. (moving with the student's concerns along the Agreement Continuum) I see that you've been in therapy with Susan Draper (fictional name) for several months, and she's great by the way, and, as you know, she was thinking that a medication might give you a gentle advantage right now with your depression. (patient shakes his head up and down reflectively but not convincingly) You know, Steve, I'm always interested in getting a read on how different cultures, and even generations within single cultures, vary on their opinions on medications. You're a sociology grad student and you might find this interesting as well. (Steve perks up a bit) Tell me a little bit about how your parents view medications like antidepressants. They're still back on mainland China, aren't they? **(Parental Backdoor Question)**

Pt.: Oh yeah, and they're pretty traditional if you know what I mean.

Clin.: In what sort of ways?

Pt.: My Dad is really big on Taoism. You know, all that yin and yang kind of stuff. He thinks my depression is caused by an imbalance of sorts.

Clin.: What do you think?

Pt.: I don't really know. I'm not real into that stuff, but I have a healthy respect for it.

Clin.: I think you should. Some feel it is related to acupuncture which I feel can be an excellent therapy for various pain syndromes. I'm not entirely certain how it fits into our understanding of depression, but there are some real similarities here between that kind of model and what we are looking at with using an antidepressant.

Pt.: How do you mean? (seems genuinely interested)

Clin.: We think the neurotransmitters we talked about earlier normally have a very delicate balance between them just like we saw on that web video. Although we are far from understanding how the antidepressants truly work, we do know that depending on what circuit they are in and where their axons land on other neurons, they can function as either excitatory or inhibitory. I think in your dad's language they would be viewed as yang or yin forces, active versus passive. This antidepressant is designed to reset that natural balance. There may be much more to it than this simplistic view of balancing neurotransmitters, but, in my opinion such balancing probably plays a part in at least some depressions.

Pt.: Hmmm. That's interesting. If it gives me bad side effects, can we stop it?

Clin.: Of course. You can stop it any time you want. In fact, unless my patients have a serious depression that keeps returning, I don't tend to recommend long-term use of antidepressants, for there is mounting evidence that long-term use can have some complications, which we will discuss in a little bit. But we would be using them judiciously in the shortterm, with your psychotherapy with Dr. Draper, to see if we can get you some faster relief, especially since you have some pressures on you to get your dissertation done. In addition, if you don't mind, we will move the dose quite slowly (**Mini-Dose Recommendation**, see pages 82) to see if we can better find your reset amount, to find the right balance for your particular brain, with the minimum of side effects (clinician intentionally emphasizes the concept of finding a balance).

Pt.: (perkier now) You know, on second thought, it sounds pretty sweet. I don't see what I can lose, as long as we can stop it anytime I want, and I still feel pretty depressed. I've really been worrying that I'm not going to have the energy to finish my dissertation. Let's see if we can reset the biochemistry. I like that idea.

This prescriber has used the Parental Backdoor Question quite effectively. Notice how smoothly one can weave it into the conversational flow. Also note that although Steve doesn't completely accept the cultural legacy bequeathed by his father (Taoist medicine), the beliefs still reside comfortably within his soul. In retrospect, the presence of his father's beliefs was probably leaked by his earlier comment, "Not really, I just don't know. I'm just *feeling sort of off-balance* now, and I'm not sure what I should do." The word "off-balance" may well be an echo of the Taoist belief in illness being related to an imbalance of the universal forces of yin and yang.

Moreover, by listening astutely with an open mind to Steve's response to the Parental Backdoor Question, the interviewer recognized a window for creating cultural resonance between two widely disparate disease models (Taoist medicine and empirical neurophysiology). By opening the window, the interviewer transformed an initial roadblock to medication interest into a bridge toward culturally inspired motivation. As a consequence of the clinician's deft use of interviewing techniques, the son could unconsciously honor his father's Eastern philosophy while trying something on the cutting edge of Western medicine.

Recognizing Unique Illness Beliefs and Culturally Preferred Treatments

In Taoist and other Asian orientations, the importance of balancing yang (active) and yin (passive) forces can also be understood as balancing hot (yang) and cold (yin) energies. Some Latina/o cultures hold a similar belief in the necessity of maintaining a "hot-cold" balance with regard to wellness and health.[18] Certain diseases are viewed as hot or cold disorders. Examples of hot diseases are diabetes mellitus, gastroesophageal reflux, peptic ulcer disease, hypertension, and *Bilis* ("bile," rage). Pregnancy, although not a disease, is viewed in Latina/o culture as a hot condition. Cold diseases include cancer, colic, headache, pneumonia, upper respiratory infections, and conditions such as menstrual cramps.

In both the Asian and Latina/o cultures, it is often viewed that hot-cold imbalance can foster disease. In addition, "hot diseases" should be treated by cold remedies and "cold diseases" by hot remedies. Clinicians can resonate with these beliefs by learning about traditional remedies that represent the correct balancing agents as well as recognizing that specific prescribed Western medications may be viewed as hot or cold. The patient's resulting medication interest may be significantly impacted by the patient's belief that the prescribed medication is of the correct temperature balance.

The complexity of these cultural health and illness beliefs raises a point that we have not discussed yet. No one can be expected to be culturally literate about all the potential cultures that we encounter as clinicians and case managers. It is reassuring to know that cultural competence is not necessarily to be found in such a profound cultural literacy. Cultural competency is more often exemplified by an attitude of cultural awareness, openness, and willingness to adapt flexibly to the beliefs one encounters. Warmth, cultural interest, and a willingness to learn from patients is often much more important than actual cultural literacy (which is clearly useful and with which you will become more and more familiar as you continue to practice in any specific community). Indeed, I have seen clinicians who were quite culturally literate but not particularly culturally competent and vice versa.

Also, if you are entering a new clinical rotation, or are beginning to practice in a new location in which patients may come from unfamiliar cultures – in addition to reading about local health and illness beliefs – a clinician's best source for information is often to pick the brains of colleagues who are familiar with the culture. In this regard, consider asking specifically about what cultures will be encountered, what the health and illness beliefs of the culture are, and, specifically – regarding the topic of this book – what are the culture-specific beliefs about the use of medications, their dosing, and their administration.

After exhausting these collegial resources and readings, always remember that indigenous healers can provide a remarkable depth of cultural knowledge. Moreover, if a patient presents with a cultural belief previously not encountered by you, a genuine interest in learning about it can be invaluable as with, "Najib, I'm not completely sure I've heard about that belief before, can you tell me a little more about it?" I have found that a genuine curiosity, and a willingness to admit a lack of knowledge, is often highly valued by patients. I am reminded of one of my favorite axioms voiced by the Renaissance physician and alchemist, Paracelsus, "Every physician must be rich in knowledge, and not only of that which is written in books; his patients should be his book, they will never mislead him."[19]

Language itself can play a role in miscommunication between the prescriber and the patient. Sometimes the two are not talking about the same disease while using the same name for a disease. At other times, the two participants may have distinctly different ideas about the nature of a disease. In either case, the resulting confusion can impact on both medication interest and medication follow-through.

A particularly good illustration of this discordance can be found with the popular term "high blood."[18] For many patients, "high blood" is a slang term for hypertension but not for all patients. In the southern United States, among some Blacks, it can refer to the belief that there exists a disease in which there is thick or excessive blood. It is further believed that this disorder will come and go. Consequently, patients holding this definition for "high blood" will feel that treatments for the illness should be intermittent and time-specific to the experience of the symptoms.[20] One can see how a clinician, unaware of this belief, could easily miss the fact that a patient viewing "high blood" in this fashion will probably not stay on antihypertensives over long periods of time. It would not be logical to do so.

The risk of miscommunication can become even more likely when one considers another slang term "*high*pertension," whose presence can be determined only by spelling, a situation once again found in some southern Black cultures. In this condition, it is believed that there can be temporary, sudden rushes of blood to the head.[20] Once again, if a patient feels that this is the condition for which the high blood pressure medication has been prescribed, then it would make sense to stop the medication between episodes. Such a belief would be particularly easy to have, for it would seem to make sense that the rush of blood to the head would be more likely when one's blood pressure numbers were high.

One could see how the provider and the patient could merrily misperceive that they are on the same page about the same disorder when they are not even in the same book. Indeed, one study found that patients who had this understanding of their hypertension (as opposed to the meaning within traditional medicine) were 3.3 times less likely to have follow-through with their medications as prescribed.[20]

Problems With Generics Related to Pill Size, Shape, and Color

Generics supposedly possess bio equivalency (same efficacy at the same number of milligrams) when compared with brand name medications. For whatever reason, this does not always prove to be the case. Whether related to manufacturing errors or to a decrease in placebo effect, some generics do not work as well as the brand name version with specific patients.

In this regard, when switching from a brand name to a generic, it is important to reassure the patient that the medication, generally speaking, should have the same beneficial results while costing the patient significantly less money. At the same time, it should be added that if, for any reason, the results are not as good, then the brand name can be reinstated (although it must be acknowledged to the reader that one may need to battle an insurer to do so, but it is a battle worth waging).

We now come across another fascinating cultural variable, related, somewhat unexpectedly, to the appearance of the pills that we are prescribing. Generic medications will generally vary in appearance (both shape and color, but especially color) from the brand name pills they are replacing, as well as from each other. (Note that different pharmacies in the same city may use differing generics.) Thus, anytime one switches from a brand name to a generic, there is often a change in the appearance of the pill itself. Such changes may also occur if the patient changes pharmacies or the pharmacy changes distributors.

Research spearheaded by Aaron Kesselheim revealed some rather startling results regarding the impact on medication interest related to these changes in appearance.[21] Kesselheim looked at patients whose seizures had been stabilized on a specific brand name antiepileptic medication and were subsequently switched to a generic brand. The research found that if the generic pill was a different color from the brand name pill, the adjusted odds of a color change having occurred immediately before a prescription was stopped was 53% greater than in controls in whom there was no discontinuance.

Stated more simply, a large number of patients stopped their medications if the generic was a different color than the originally prescribed medication.

Kesselheim has postulated that the finding might be related to several factors, including (1) the patient's fear that the pharmacist has made a mistake, (2) the breaking up of a patient's routine for taking a medication, and (3) the patient is experiencing a *nocebo* effect. If the patient had acquired a positive *placebo* effect, based on the appearance of his or her medication, the change in color might subsequently create the opposite effect. The patient now fears that "this new medication" may not work. The following interviewing principle is pertinent here: *When switching to a generic prescription, forewarn the patient about possible changes in appearance of the medication while reassuring him or her that this change is normal and generally should not decrease the effectiveness of the medication.*

At the next appointment, if I remember to do so, I ask the patient how much the generic pills cost, for I positively reenforce any decrease in cost. Such a reenforcement of one of the new pros of the medication (lower financial distress) can help the patient to keep this important factor in mind when weighing the pros and cons of taking the medication in Step 3 of the Choice Triad. I find that this moment in the appointment is an opportune time to add the following:

TIP 93 Color Tab Question

"I'm just curious, Stephanie, like we discussed last time, is the pill a different color or shape?"

If different in appearance, one can ask the patient if that was okay or if he or she was surprised. Because of the large amount of information thrown at them in each session, it is easy for patients to forget bits of information. Some patients may have already forgotten the previous discussion about potential changes in pill appearance with the use of generics. If so, one can once again reassure the patient that all is well and is as expected.

Concluding Thoughts

As we close, we have seen how cultural traditions, customs, biases, and expectations can generate problems with both medication interest and follow-through. From the knowledge gained from this chapter, we have also discovered that there are interviewing techniques and clinician attitudes that can often attenuate such problems. We began this chapter with a quotation by Metzl and Riba. We will end it with another one, for they summarize nicely what we have accomplished:

> . . . this literature (clinical literature on culture and medication use) teaches the importance of recognizing the multiple, often conflicting meanings of medications in clinical interactions. Attention to these complexities can provide important avenues of communication between doctors and patients. Lack of such attention increases the chances of a miscommunication in which the doctor and patient incorrectly think that they are talking about the same thing when discussing medication.[1]

Despite our more sophisticated understanding gained in this chapter, there remains one more aspect of the patient's culture that we have not yet touched on, the role of input from family, friends, and media. This interpersonal and unique aspect of the patient's culture may be last in our attention but first in importance.

REFERENCES

1. Metzl JM, Riba M. Understanding the symbolic value of medications: a brief review. *Prim Psychiatry* 2003;10(7):45–48.
2. Shaw GB. Cincinnati, OH: Transcultural C.A.R.E. Associates. www.transculturalcare.net/favorite-sayings/. Accessed June 8, 2017.
3. Shea SC. Culturally Adaptive Interviewing: The Challenging Art of Exploring Culture, Worldview, and Spirituality. In *Psychiatric Interviewing: The Art of Understanding.* 3rd Ed. London, England: Elsevier, Inc.; 2017:e66–e159.
4. Mayo Clinic website. *Tests and Procedures: Complementary and Alternative Medicine.* http://www.mayoclinic.org/tests procedures/complementary alternative-medicine/basics/definition/prc-20021745. Accessed on June 8, 2017.
5. National Center for Complementary & Integrated Health (NCCIH). Bethesda, MD: National Center for Complementary & Integrated Health. http://nccih.nih.gov/about. Accessed June 8, 2017.
6. Minority Nurse Staff. Ethnopharmacology: what nurses need to know. In: *Minority Nurse.* New York, NY: Springer Publishing Company. http://minoritynurse.com/ethnopharmacology-what-nurses-need-to-know/. Accessed June 8, 2017.
7. Heinrich M. Journal of Ethnopharmacology: An Interdisciplinary Journal Devoted to Indigenous Drugs [editorial]. Available at www.ethnopharmacology.org/ISE_journal.htm. Accessed October 10, 2017.
8. Chia LR, Schlenk EA, Dunbar-Jacob J. Effect of personal and cultural beliefs on medication adherence in the elderly. *Drugs Aging* 2006;23(3):191–202. doi:10.2165/00002512-200623030-00002.
9. Campinha-Bacote J. Cincinnati, OH: Transcultural C.A.R.E. Associates. www.transculturalcare.net/ethnic-ethno-pharmacology/. Accessed June 9, 2017.

10. Ahmed I. Psychological aspects of giving and receiving medications. In: Tseng W-S, Streltzer J, eds. *Culture and Psychotherapy: A Guide to Clinical Practice*. Washington, DC: American Psychiatric Publishing; 2001.
11. Grindrod K, Alsabbagh W. Managing medications during Ramadan fasting. *Can Pharm J (Ott)* 2017;150(3);146–149. doi:10.1177/1715163517700840.
12. Salti I, Benard E, Detournay B, et al. A population-based study of diabetes and its characteristics during the fasting month of Ramadan in 13 countries: results of the epidemiology of diabetes and Ramadan 1422/2001 (EPIDIAR) study. *Diabetes Care* 2004;27(10):2306–2311.
13. Ali M, Adams A, Hossain A, et al. Primary care provider's knowledge and practices of diabetes management during Ramadan. *J Prim Care Community Health* 2016;7(1):33–37. Also available at http://journals.sagepub.com/doi/10.1177/2150131915601359. Accessed June 6, 2017.
14. Ibrahim M, Magd MAA, Annabi FA, et al. Recommendations for management of diabetes during Ramadan: update 2015. *BMJ Open Diabetes Res Care* 2015;3(1):e000108 . doi:10.1136/bmjdrc-2015-000108.
15. Grissinger M. Cultural diversity and medication safety. *Pharm Ther* 2007;32(9):471–472.
16. Kroll J, Linde P, Habenicht M, et al. Medication compliance, antidepressant blood levels and side effects in Southeast Asian patients. *J Clin Psychopharmacol* 1990;10:279–282.
17. Horne R, Graupner L, Frost S, et al. Medicine in a multi-cultural society: the effect of cultural background on beliefs about medications. *Soc Sci Med* 2004;59(6):1307–1313.
18. Juckett G. Cross-cultural medicine. *Am Fam Physician* 2005;72(11):2267–2274. Also available at http://www.aafp.org/afp/2005/1201/p2267.html. Accessed June 8, 2017; page 6 of 8.
19. Jacobi J. *Paracelsus: Selected Writings*. Princeton, NJ: Princeton University Press;1995:50.
20. Centers for Disease Control (CDC). Health beliefs and compliance with prescribed medication for hypertension among black women – New Orleans 1985–1986. *MMWR Morb Mortal Wkly Rep* https://www.cdc.gov/mmwr/preview/mmwrhtml/00001793 .htm Accessed on 11.10.17.
21. Kesselheim AS, Misono AS, Shrank WH, et al. Variations in pill appearance of antiepileptic drugs and the risk of nonadherence. *JAMA Intern Med* 2013;173(3):202–208. doi:10.1001/2013.jamainternmed.997.

CHAPTER 14

Medication Interest: The Impact of Family, Friends, and the Digital World

"The loved ones of the patient may not have a medical license or healthcare background, but their voice and presence matters in the hospital room."[1]

Brian Boyle

SURVIVOR OF A NEAR-FATAL CAR WRECK REQUIRING MONTHS OF CRITICAL CARE HOSPITALIZATION

Prescribing Medications: A Family Affair

The Challenge and the Opportunities

The Importance of Hearing the Family's Voice and Acknowledging Its Presence

From the perspective of person-centered medicine and nursing, we can view the patient as a cascading series of unique moments in time, in which the biologies, psychologies, intimate relationships, family dynamics, cultures, and spiritualities of our patients intersect to create the person before us. It is an ever-shifting matrix of which we are a part as soon as the patient enters our examination room. But though we may be physically alone with our patients we are never psychologically alone with them. We are always joined by the patient's internalized perceptions of the opinions, fears, and hopes of his or her loved ones.

In some instances, the loved ones may be sitting in the examination room or hospital room with us. In all instances, the patient is judging our words through the lens of his or her preconceived views about medications – which are often powerfully shaped by those very same loved ones whether they are in the room or not. The truth is that we don't so much prescribe for a single patient as we prescribe for a single family. The opinions of the patient's nuclear family, spouses/partners, parents, and siblings sometimes sway the patient more than our opinions as physicians and nurses.

It is a two-way street. For as much as family members impact on our abilities to prescribe, our prescriptions have a major impact on the lives of these family members. The impact of our prescriptions on the patient's loved ones is frequently for the good (relieving the pain of their family member – the patient – or even saving his or her life). On the other hand, if we are frank, the impact is sometimes not so good (our medications create intolerable side-effects whose impact on the patient's functioning and mood negatively reverberate throughout the family). Worse yet, sometimes our medications kill. It is all quite complex. In this final chapter of our book, we will try to simplify these complexities while uncovering interviewing techniques that can maximize our ability to bring healing to both our patients and those who love them.

In recent years, the importance of input from family members has been increasingly emphasized in the medical and nursing literature as reflected by terms such as "person-centered medicine," which, as we have seen, emphasizes a holistic approach to treatment planning that includes biological, psychological, familial, cultural, and spiritual factors. The importance of family members as partners in the collaborative treatment team is also nicely captured in the phrase "patient- and family-centered care" (PFCC).

The field of pediatrics (as well as obstetrics), where family members are critical components of both treatment planning and medication follow-through, have pioneered the concept of PFCC. A growing literature highlights that many factors, including patient satisfaction, family satisfaction, improvements in patients' health outcomes, faster recovery times, decreases in emergency room visits, and decreases in the overuse of health care resources as well as increases in clinician satisfaction, seem to be correlated with the effective implementation of PFCC.[2–7] From the perspective of medical and nursing training, efforts have been made to innovatively introduce the principles of PFCC into training programs.[8,9] For the interested reader, an excellent introduction to this rapidly advancing field can be found at the Institute for Patient- and Family-Centered Care.[10]

What Family Members Bring to the Table

In a traditional sense, family members can improve the quality of care for the patient in many ways. For instance, hospital errors remain disturbingly high, with a sizeable chunk of those errors being related to medications, ranging from patients receiving the wrong medication to inappropriate dosing or scheduling.

The electronic health record – despite promises of being an advance in record keeping – has actually, in some instances, resulted in more errors, for some clinicians are busy madly typing away instead of carefully listening to patients. Consequently, as patients relay their medical histories and their past/current medication regimens, clinicians miss information or inaccurately record critical data as they rush to be a listener, writer, transcriptionist, and clinician simultaneously. Moreover, it is often the first and last roles that are short-shrifted in the process.

In addition, miscommunications among physicians, nurses, and other providers can be surprisingly high in hospitals and clinics partially caused by the intense time pressures and understaffing present in today's clinical environment. In any case, considering the additive impact of the above factors in creating a clinical milieu conducive to medication errors, I have found family members to be wonderful guardian angels, who often can catch these communication errors before they become clinical mishaps.

Family members can also function as valuable "lobbyists," in the good sense of the word. As noted earlier in the chapter, a family member's words may be significantly more convincing than our own to a patient who is weighing the pros and cons of a medication. By taking the time to openly discuss the reasons for the use of a medication, as well as its side effects, a family member may become a powerful advocate for the use of the medication.

In the clinic setting, our patients' decisions to continue or to not continue a medication often happen between appointments. At such critical moments, we will not be by their side. Family advocates for the use of our prescribed medication – if we have taken the time in the clinic to meet with them, hear their concerns, and provide them with accurate information – will be present to voice support for the use of the medication. There is no more important member of the clinical team, at that moment, than the aforementioned family member.

Considering the above advantages to effectively including family members in medication discussions and decisions, we can see that – although there is a time cost to involving family members – the benefits can be enormous with regard to fostering medication interest and follow-through with patients. Moreover, the time lost when a patient relapses secondary to medication discontinuation may very well be much larger than the time it would have taken to effectively converse with the family member in the first place.

Along these lines, family members may ask questions – challenging medical recommendations – that may point out potential problems of which the harried clinician, who is often caring for multitudes of patients, might be unaware. By contrast, family members are only caring for one patient and may see things that we can easily miss. I am reminded of the old adage, "No one will care more about your money than you." Similarly, no one will care more about a loved one than the people who love that person. I have come to view family members as extraordinarily valuable resources. Indeed, I'm disappointed if the patient, unfortunately, has no family members invested in his or her care.

With regard to medication interest and follow-through, there remains one more advantage brought to the table by the presence of family members in a clinic setting. Patients, who have concerns about side effects – or are indeed stuck at any one of the three steps of the Choice Triad – may be more likely to share such concerns while sitting at home chatting with their families than during a clinic-based med-check. As we have discussed before, when in the presence of the health care provider, many patients will feel a need to be a "good patient."

Further enhancing the effectiveness of family members as agents for uncovering valid information regarding the patient's genuine medication interest is the simple fact that, compared with clinicians, they are more familiar with the patient's nonverbal behaviors and mannerisms. This familiarity may enhance their ability to uncover a patient's hesitancy about a medication more quickly than the clinician. Bottom line: Family members can provide excellent information on a patient's true medication interest and follow-through that may have, without their input, been unavailable.

A recent piece of nicely implemented research by Benjamin, Cox, and colleagues provides some empirical support for the above assertions.[11] On today's wards, readers of this book may encounter a relatively new clinical practice known as "family-centered rounds" (FCRs). In FCRs, family members are invited to round with the clinical team and are encouraged to ask questions, many of which will inevitably be related to medication use. Benjamin, Cox, and colleagues studied 150 children and their FCRs, which were videotaped and analyzed. Three hundred forty-seven FCRs were studied. Eighty-three (55%) of the 150 families *simultaneously* asked questions about their child's medications. The most common topics were medication scheduling (24%)

and adverse drug reactions (11%). Staff and family members found the resulting conversations to be satisfying in a personal sense and practical as well (both clarifying scheduling and enhancing medication follow-through after discharge). But to me, the most striking finding was the following: In 8% of the discussions, the family's input resulted in changes in the child's medications deemed as valuable by the treating clinicians.

On a final note regarding the value of conjoint treatment planning with family members regarding medications, let me add one more sidebar. It is certainly not a point that is as important as improving patient care; it is, nevertheless, something that is both real and pertinent. Put succinctly: a good relationship with a patient's family is, arguably, the best malpractice insurance a clinician can ever have, especially if the issue is malpractice related to a patient's death.

There is only one person who will file a malpractice suit if a patient dies – a family member. And family members who feel that a clinician has genuinely cared about their loved one, did the best that he or she could, and took the time to include them in their family member's care are, in my opinion, significantly less likely to institute court action. Indeed, even if a clinician makes an inadvertent, yet costly, mistake, a family member who feels a powerful bond with that clinician may very well decide not to pursue legal action. On the other hand, even if a clinician has provided a reasonable standard of care, but has ignored family members, antagonized them by tersely communicating with them, or otherwise made them feel dismissed or irrelevant, then that clinician is basically asking to be sued following a patient's death.

One final caveat remains. Regarding confidentiality, the patient must be comfortable with the sharing of any clinical knowledge with any specific family member. Moreover, part of our clinical expertise involves an awareness that, unfortunately, some family members may be detrimental to care, as can be seen if a family member is antagonistic to the patient and/or is abusive to the patient. In such situations, the treatment team will need to discuss among themselves, and with the patient, the degree with which a specific family member will be actively involved in treatment discussions. Naturally, if intimate partner violence, child abuse, or elder abuse is suspected, the team should take appropriate actions for the patient's safety.

What Clinicians Bring to the Table for Family Members

Too often, in my opinion, an important point is not emphasized enough in the training of health care providers. Our goal, whether we are physicians, nurses, physician assistants, clinical pharmacists, or case managers, is not limited to relieving the pain of the identified patient. We should also be dedicated to relieving the pain of those who love the patient. As alluded to earlier, our medication recommendations not only impact on our patients. They have major impacts and consequences for family members.

On an obvious level, if we save the life of a loved one, we will have done enormous good for those who love the patient. This is true of everything from prescribing effective oncologic medications to providing a life-saving surgical intervention or preventing a suicide in a patient coping with severe depression or bipolar disorder. On a less obvious level, collaboratively arrived upon medication decisions – as reflected in models such as person-centered medicine, the shared decision-making model, and the medical home as well as in the MIM itself – can indirectly decrease the suffering of family members. They do so by decreasing the familial concerns and stresses related to providing ongoing care for the patient once home. In this sense, it really is true that we are prescribing not so much for patients as we are for families.

By way of example, a wise decision on the medication regimen for a patient coping with the debilitating sequelae of congestive heart failure, diabetes, multiple sclerosis, or a stroke can have major ramifications for family members who are "on-call" 24/7 and are wrestling with compassion fatigue. They will be truly grateful if their load is decreased by increasing the mobility and functioning of their loved one. By contrast, poor decisions on medication regimens resulting in a deterioration of the patient's functioning, or an increase in the patient's pain or side effects, will have powerful ramifications for those family members functioning as caretakers. In short, one of the reasons for including family members in medication decisions is the fact that they truly have "skin in the game."

It is important to remember that family members experience appropriate, and genuine fear, about what is going to happen "when we get home" whether the patient is being discharged from a hospital or is leaving a clinic appointment. Including family members in shared decision making can go a long way toward relieving these fears.

This fear sometimes manifests most intensely when a prescriber is seeing a patient, with a complicated history of medication cocktails for the first time as a transfer. Family members may have encountered frustration as previous prescribers have "monkeyed around with my son's meds right off the bat!" Having finally found – sometimes after years of trial and error – a medication combination that has brought the best relief to date, one can imagine the magnitude of family members' fears that a new clinician is going to monkey around again with the patient's medications. Truth be told, sometimes clinicians – without consulting first with the patient's caretakers – do just that on first seeing a transferred patient.

During such initial appointments with transferred patients, I have found the following to be of great value in decreasing the fears of the patient's family members when the patient is living at home and is being directly cared for by them:

TIP 94 Don't Worry, I'll Consult You First Statement

"One of the most foolish things a physician (use whatever your discipline might be) can do is to change medications before talking with parents (use whatever family member is involved in the patient's care) and the patient about what is working. Your input is vital. I have no intention of making a recommendation regarding your son's medications until after we talk in detail. No one knows the history of your son's responses to medications better than you and your son. By the way, if your son agrees, I would like to always try to talk with you and get your thoughts about any potential major medication changes. What is your opinion about his current set of medications?"

Of course, the other reason to consult with the family member first is simply because the above is true – family members can provide invaluable information. Electronic health records can be notoriously sparse on the comparative impacts of differing medication regimens and even more sparse regarding the clinical thinking of previous prescribers. Families often, not always, are well aware of which medication combinations have worked or failed and why.

Another caveat to keep in mind is that just because a recent journal article has trumpeted a new approach to a particular disorder, it does not mean that such an approach is best suggested during an initial transfer if the patient has room for improvement but is currently stabilized. The reception of the family and the patient may be significantly more positive if one waits a few appointments until the therapeutic alliance with both has been better established before trying a new "state of the art" drug.

Finally, as we have touched on in previous chapters, it is during those moments when our medications fail – no medications are available to decrease the patient's symptoms nor provide a cure – that our roles as prescribers are perhaps most tested. At such times, patients and family members are frequently desperate for our skills as listeners, comforters, and trusted allies. Both patients and family members not infrequently fear that once it is determined that our medications will not work, prescribers and other health care providers will view their roles as being done. As noted earlier, patients, and their loved ones, can often fear abandonment at such times.

The role of the prescriber is not limited to writing prescriptions; indeed, our role is to be there when there are no more prescriptions to be written. I have found that a simple comment to family members (as well as to the patient) such as, "Just so you know, Jane, I'm going to be involved in Mack's care to the very end, and I'll do everything I can to help things go as well as we can for both you and Mack. You haven't seen the last of me, trust me on that," when followed with a gentle smile, can be hugely reassuring. In this sense, we can see that that the values of PFCC and person-centered medicine provide a guiding compass for how we can enhance both medication interest and follow-through in both the patient and his or her family members.

Techniques for Engaging Family Members in Medication Decisions and Follow-Through

Indirectly Tapping Family Opinions

It is ideal to directly ask family members for their opinions, but they may not have accompanied the patient nor be immediately available by phone. Nevertheless, we have seen that we are never truly alone with the patient, for the patient brings his or her psychologically incorporated family opinions regarding medications into the examination room. When looking at the patient, we can imagine that there are bleachers behind the patient populated by fathers, mothers, brothers, sisters, and children (if the patient is elderly). On those bleachers, we may see family members cheering on the decision to use medications or booing wildly against their use.

If we have garnered family support, one can hardly imagine a more powerful voice in the patient's ears. Such support bodes well for enhanced medication interest and eventual follow-through with our medication recommendations. Of course, the reverse is also true. A family member who is opposed to the use of a medication is a powerful, often insurmountable, force toward medication discontinuance. To not consciously, and intentionally, address the medication interest of key family members when prescribing is to invite treatment failure.

Our guiding interviewing principle becomes one of: *Try to remember to always ask patients what they anticipate their family members will say about the medication. Similarly, in follow-up visits, ask what they have actually said.* Oftentimes, time constraints and practicality make such inquiries difficult. Fortunately, most patients are more than willing to fill us in on the opinions of their social supports, if we know what questions to ask:

TIP 95 Anticipating Family Response Question

"How do you think your spouse (partner, brother, sister as indicated) will feel about you starting up on an antidepressant (substitute medication in question)?"

A not uncommon reply is, "To tell you the truth, Charlie doesn't really believe in this kind of thing." Depending on the methods by which Charlie expresses this opinion – ranging from mild discouragement to abusive anger – we may have uncovered a critical roadblock to medication interest.

I chose an antidepressant as an example, for family members not infrequently will have strong opinions about the use of antidepressants as well as any other psychotropic medications. Despite the intense time pressures of a primary care setting, when prescribing psychoactive medication it is, in my opinion, *very important* to remember to use techniques such as the Anticipating Family Response Question for opposition to such medications in the home-front is common.

Truth be told, family members often have strong reservations about the use of various medications from anticoagulants and anti-inflammatories to agents for reducing lipids or blood pressure. Sometimes these fears arise from anti-medication blogs they may have seen on the web or they may arise from hearing the litany of adverse reactions listed at the end of DTC advertisements.

In other instances, family members have friends who have had particularly unpleasant side effects or serious adverse reactions to the medications we are prescribing. No doubt, they will, appropriately so, warn their family member about these secondhand disturbing experiences in no uncertain terms. In some instances, the family member himself or herself has had marked problems with the prescribed medication (such information may also be important, if it is pointing toward a genetic reason to not prescribe the medication in question).

In addition, some family members will have a generalized bias against medications, preferring the use of interventions from complementary and alternative medicine (CAM). Such patients may be sitting on our imagined bleachers intensely booing our treatment recommendations. These "bleachers" may be an imaginative metaphor, but there is nothing imaginary about the intensity with which a family member may voice his or her opposition to a medication once the patient has returned home. Of course, in the long run, the best solution to the problem is to directly ask pertinent family members their opinions while actively involving them prospectively in the shared decision making.

Every family member will need to move through the steps of the Choice Triad in the exact same fashion that we have described for our patients in the previous pages of this book. In keeping with the spirit of the MIM, when a family member strongly opposes the use of a specific medication, he or she is not viewed as being resistant or oppositional. Instead, family members are viewed as having a genuine concern about their loved one arising from one of the following beliefs: (1) that there is nothing wrong with their loved one that would warrant intervention, (2) that a medication is not the best first choice for help if there is, indeed, a problem, or (3) the cons of the medication outweigh the pros, and their loved one will be hurt by the use of the medication.

In short, the family member has a belief from which it is logical to oppose the use of the medication. It would be illogical to support its use. Once again, we see that if we, personally, held the same belief about a medication being prescribed for one of our own family members, we too would advise our own loved one to not use the medication in question.

As we have seen, family member input can be invaluable in choosing the best medication for the patient, for sometimes they are correct – the proposed medication is a bad choice. We are reminded of the study by Cox and colleagues on FCRs in which 8% of the family members' spontaneous input led to changes in the treatment plan.

Directly Tapping Family Opinions

The first trick is to get the family member into the examination room. One of the earliest opportunities for accomplishing this task can be easily missed because the hectic pace of clinic practice can make a clinician simply not think of it. Bottom line, in many first appointments, someone (often a family member) has transported the patient or accompanied the patient. Considering that many first prescriptions are never filled and that patients often discontinue medications within several weeks of starting them, we cannot afford to wait indefinitely to have contact with a family member (especially if that uncontacted family member is going to be opposed to the patient's use of the prescribed medication). Consequently, the opportunity presented by a family member accompanying the patient to his or her first appointment is too valuable to miss, which leads us to the following simple yet highly effective technique:

TIP 96 "Who Brought You to the Dance?"

"Tyra, I'm curious if anyone came with you today and is out in the waiting room?"

If the answer is "yes," then one can follow up with, "Would you be at all interested in having her (him) join us while we talk some more about possible treatment options?" It is very important regarding confidentiality to make sure the patient genuinely wants his or her family member involved. Any, even subtle, hint that the patient is hesitant requires that a careful exploration of the patient's concerns be done, and the family member should only be invited if the patient is totally comfortable with the idea.

Several points are worth mentioning. There should be no pressure on the patient to include the accompanying family member. Indeed, how the patient responds may give hints as to whether the accompanying family member is trusted by the patient (keep in mind that family members can be antagonistic to the patient or even abusive). On the positive side, generally, I believe you will find that family members who have accompanied a patient on a first appointment are often good support systems.

Sometimes, when answering the Who Brought You to the Dance Question, we will discover that the person who provided the ride (or is present as an accompanying support system) is a friend not a family member. Patients may or may not want this person involved, and clearly the clinician will follow the patient's lead.

I think you will generally find that the best time to ask the Who Brought You to the Dance Question is after you have initially discussed treatment options with the identified patient so as to ferret out the patient's personal views first, without any possible biasing by the family member. If the patient-clinician dyad has decided for whatever reason that medications are not the first choice (perhaps CAM interventions or no treatment at all are the best fit for this particular patient), it is still useful to meet with the family member to address the patient's preferences in a positive fashion while beginning to build an alliance with the family member.

If the clinician disagrees with the patient's preferences, it is seldom, if ever, a good time in a first appointment to try to see if the family member can provide support for the use of the medication to the patient. Such an initial encounter will put all persons involved (patient, clinician, and family member) in an awkward and potentially oppositional relationship that may never be transformable.

If a family member joins the session, the following types of questions, as time permits, can be of use:

TIP 97 "Family Member's Health Care Beliefs Exploration"

a. "What are some of your thoughts on what is going on with Rohan (your son, your husband, etc.)?"
b. "Do you have any ideas about what might be valuable in helping Rohan?"
c. "Did you have much contact with Rohan's previous physicians, nurses, or other providers?"
d. "How much contact would you like to have with us as we work together to help Rohan?"

After such questions, the clinician can explain how he or she sees the patient's problems, can share the patient's diagnoses, and can describe the pros and cons of the medication in question and why it was chosen. If the family member is a parent intimately involved in ongoing care, it is also a moment, if deemed to be valuable, to utilize the Don't Worry, I'll Consult You First Statement at which point the clinician can begin a more direct exploration of the family member's support or concerns about the proposed medication for his or her loved one:

TIP 98 "Direct Family Member Inquiry on Patient's Meds"

a. "How do you feel about our current plan?"
b. "Do you know anybody who has been on this medication, or have you ever been on this medication?"
c. "Do you have any concerns about the medication?"
d. "What are your hopes about what this medication might be able to do for Rohan?"

If the patient is living with the accompanying family member and/or the family member is responsible for the ongoing care of the patient, the above questions can provide a nice jump start to building a sound medication alliance that moves with the family member on the Agreement Continuum, regarding medications for the identified patient. It is also an excellent time to provide and consolidate information on dosing schedules and administration.

As we have discussed before, to check how much of this critical information has been retained by the caretaker, it can be useful to use the Teach-Back technique described earlier for use with patients in which the clinician asks, "To make sure I was clear, can you, in your own words, tell me how Rohan should be taking his medications and how often?" Obviously, this information should also be written down for all involved.

This is a good time to remind ourselves of a very important point discussed in Chapter 9 but well worth re-addressing here. As is true with the previous interviewing tips discussed in each chapter of this book, the reader will never be able to use all of these tips with family members in any single appointment with a patient. In fact, because of the extremely tight time considerations encountered in the real world of hectic clinics and hospital units, with any given patient, only a couple of tips from all of the chapters in this book will be used in any given appointment. Many times, the reader will be lucky to have enough time to use more than one or two in a single appointment.

On the other hand, an understanding of the MIM and its techniques allows a clinician to flexibly choose the best couple of techniques that might be most useful for the unique patient at hand and with which the clinician, personally, feels most comfortable. It has been my experience, and the experience of those clinicians who have shared their tips in our MIM workshops, that only one or two techniques can have surprisingly powerful impacts on a patient's medication interest. Familiarity with the MIM allows the clinician to optimize the number of these impacts through the wise utilization of a small number of techniques drawn from his or her knowledge of a large number of potentially effective options.

Just as a surgeon has spent immense amounts of time to perfect a variety of surgical techniques from which to choose only a handful for solving a specific surgical challenge in the most effective fashion in any given operation, with a working knowledge of the MIM the reader can choose the best interviewing techniques to enhance medication interest with any specific patient in any given appointment. In subsequent sessions different MIM techniques may be best used with the same patient. At any point in ongoing care, as with the surgeon, the selection of an effective interviewing technique may greatly relieve a patient's suffering – or perhaps even save the patient's life – for lack of follow-through with needed medications remains the leading cause of preventable treatment failure in most serious diseases.

As we close this section on building a medication alliance with family members, it can be said that, without a doubt, it is useful to all involved – clinicians, patients, and family members – for clinicians to cultivate the most powerful alliance possible with family members through the selective use of the techniques described in this chapter. Once the patient has left the office, it is the opinions of the family members that will continue to be voiced to the patient.

Curiously, and of great significance, their opinions will not be the only voices of importance in determining the patient's medication interest and follow-through.

Friends, Peers, and Interested Bystanders: The Bleachers Are Crowded with Voices

The process of anticipating the opinions of friends or, in subsequent visits, directly uncovering their opinions if they are accompanying the patient may be as important a clinical task as uncovering the views of a spouse or intimate other. On the good side of the continuum, imagine the powerful boost to medication interest if a friend comments, "Oh my gosh, that's the same drug I used for my asthma. It's great. I'm not kidding you; it saved my life." At the other end of the continuum, contrast this with the damage done when a patient hears a best friend say, "Oh my God! Don't you dare take that horrible thing. I tried it once and it was horrendous. I'm not kidding you; it almost killed me!" In the latter instance, we might as well have asked our patient to just drop off that prescription in the trash can as he or she walked out our office door. As time permits, you may find the following question to be valuable:

> **TIP 99 Anticipating Friendly Fire**
>
> "Do you have any friends or colleagues who have taken this medication, and, if so, what did they think of it?"

Friends among teenagers, in middle and high school, represent an entirely new set of influences. Direct peer pressure, which is a major lobbying force in this age group, is not the only issue. Groups and cliques are so powerful, and verbal/physical abuse so common in schools, that the mere association of the prescribed medication with a fellow student seen as being an outcast or undesirable friend can be deadly to medication interest.

In addition, student views on the use of medications have undergone a shift with many, not all, students. In the past, as was the case with adults, students tended to keep the use of medications to themselves for fear of embarrassment or stigmatization. Although still true with some students, others have begun to announce their use.

This open sharing of the use of medications is particularly striking with certain psychiatric medications so that one may hear a student announcing, "I'm on this or I'm on that," or "I'm on Ritalin. I'm selling Ritalin. Locker 287, best prices in the school district! Come one, come all!"

As one might expect, social media has only added to the surprising lack of privacy regarding the use of psychiatric medications. Without understanding the potential import of their actions, some student patients will post their personal use of a medication on Facebook or tweet about it. Yet another disturbing caveat can unfold. If they dislike a patient, another student might tweet about our patient's "need for" a psychiatric medication if they think the "outing" will be a source of embarrassment and harassment. The bottom line is: Teenagers will often know of other teenagers who are on the medications we are prescribing. In addition, in some instances, our patients might be openly ridiculed by their peers once having returned to school.

With the Anticipating Friendly Fire question above, clinicians can uncover the type of direct peer pressure to stop a medication, that is often launched from other students and friends. As mentioned above, peer pressures among teens is so intense that it also becomes important to uncover any personal associations the student may have with taking a medication being prescribed for the first time. Back in Chapter 9 (TIP 57, page 192) we already were introduced to an excellent tip that is tailor-made for this task. If you will recall, the Teenager Bad Drug Inquiry went like this, "Do you have any friends or know anyone at school who takes this medication?"

In this technique, the clinician is not asking directly about what has been said to the patient from other students (they haven't begun the medication). Instead, we are merely searching for potentially damaging associations the student may have with a medication that we are prescribing for the first time. It is important to uncover these associations, which can range from, "Oh yeah, I gotta friend who is on that drug, she thinks it's sweet," to "Oh God, I know a kid on that and he's the biggest dork I've ever met."

Let us just say that it seems unwise to suggest a medication to a teenager who fears it will transform him into a dork. As we've seen before in such situations, if one can find a different medication from the same family with a similar efficacy, it may be wise to change one's recommendation on the spot before wasting paper on a written prescription or time on a useless e-script to the pharmacy.

Adding to today's concerns related to peer input – for both teenagers and adults – one cannot overestimate the power of the web for "good and evil." It seems that any person on a medication may expect a barrage of texts, tweets, and Facebook postings about the pros and cons of using the medication in question. When it comes to the web, everyone seems to be an interested bystander with a medical opinion voiced as firmly as if he or she had graduated from medical or nursing school. Actually, this phenomenon is not limited to the web. It has been around for centuries in the guise of community peer pressure, which sometimes can border on near hysteria.

Community Voices: Powerful, Often Useful, Sometimes Damaging, Always Loud

Uncovering Community Biases Both For and Against Medications: The Real World

Let me begin by describing a community of which I am very familiar – community mental health centers (CMHCs) – for the principles and interpersonal currents alive in these centers present a nice model for the complex rustlings of any community in which the reader may find himself or herself practicing. In addition, some readers will go on to become psychiatrists and many other readers will become integrated into the care of patients coping with severe mental illnesses such as persistent posttraumatic stress disorder, bipolar disorder, and schizophrenia.

CMHCs are unique cultural milieus, with the cultures being greatly shaped by the beliefs of, and the sharing of those beliefs by, the patients themselves. Patients share what they feel about their medications with each other, and they share their views robustly. As informed consumers, it makes sense to do so.

If there is a scuttlebutt at a specific CMHC about a particular medication being "really bad to be on" (e.g., terrible side effects, "doesn't do shit," etc.), in my opinion the clinician should consider recommending a different medication in the same family and with the same efficacy, if at all possible. Prescribing a medication that fellow patients at the CMHC feel is a bad drug is an invitation to a medication interest disaster. Moreover, if, over time, the scuttlebutt at the CMHC is, "You don't want Dr. Harper, he prescribes terrible drugs," Dr. Harper's ability to forge future alliances with patients is dealt a severe blow.

CMHCs are far from the only medical communities where medication gossip is thriving. There are other medical "cultures within cultures" in which it is essential to quickly uncover the scuttlebutt about a particular medication including specialized hospital units dedicated to people coping with diverse illnesses including pediatric oncology units, neurologic disorder units, general oncology units, and surgical units. Depending on the philosophies and resources of these units, varying degrees of "community" evolve, much of it related to patient peer support.

It is hard to put into words how powerfully beneficial such supportive specialized units can be. The positive impact on patients and family members experiencing the emotional and practical support of these specialized units, as well as the reassurance of truly being a part of a collaborative treatment team with the implementation of shared decision making, cannot be overstated. It is also important to remember that part of the supportive milieu created by fellow patients on these units – and it is an excellent component – is the fact that they will share opinions about both the medications being used on the unit and the clinicians prescribing them.

By way of example, on an oncology unit, and in the subsequent outpatient peer-support groups that often follow discharge, there will be opinions regarding the medications used to bring specific cancers into remission. There will be opinions on other medications that maintain these remissions once they are obtained, and yet further opinions on the medications designed to attenuate the side effects of both of these types of medications. Whatever the indication, whatever the medication, patients talk.

Also keep in mind that there are other types of communities in which distinctive biases both for and against specific medications (or all medications in general) will be enthusiastically shared. Prisons and jails have intricately complex mini-cultures as do colleges and universities, fraternities, sororities, and sports teams. In addition, not all communities have walls. But all communities share opinions.

Thus, be aware that your patient may be hearing strong opinions about medication from fellow bikers, musicians, politicians, hipsters, goths, union members, or other identifiable groups such as fellow physicians and nurses (we talk a lot about our personal biases about good and bad drugs!), members of the LGBTQ community, or racial and ethnic groups. With these groups, whether within walls or outside them, I have found the following technique to be of great value, simple as it may be:

TIP 100 The Scuttlebutt Question

"What do other people think about (give the exact common name of the medication in question) around here?"

If the group is without walls, such as bikers or hipsters, one can simply change to, "What do your other biker friends think about (give the exact common name of the medication in question)?"

Also keep in mind that if you are, or end up practicing, in a small community it will have its own rules and gossip channels. A practitioner's use of medications will quickly make the rounds of the local community members, especially if they believe the medications in question are bad drugs or that Dr. Google views them as such, which brings us to our final topic.

Not all communities are brick and mortar. Many are virtual. And these digital communities are rapidly becoming the most powerful. And the members of these communities love to talk about meds. In addition, our more traditional media still remain powerful opinion shapers such as television, radio, magazines, and newspapers.

The patients of today are much more informed about medication choices than patients from previous generations. The "medication grapevine" is vastly improved. The web, in particular, has transformed the grapevine. The patients of today, at a mere click, have access to a plethora of websites, chat rooms, and blogs, both endorsing and opposing medication use. Adding even more potent fertilizer to the grapevine, the presence of social media has boosted the growth of the grapevine to the point where many patients have friends scattered across the world offering both solicited and unsolicited opinions about the medications that you and I have just prescribed. The clinician of today should expect that a large number of his or her patients will go home to post a Facebook question such as, "Has anyone heard anything about this drug (whatever the name of the prescribed medication)?"

In my opinion, for the most part, this turn of events is a good one, but there are a few downsides as well. The internet and other popular media including television, radio, and print sometimes contribute to the stigmatization of medications by presenting false and unwarranted biases against them that can lower medication interest, sometimes precipitously. The following interviewing principle is an important one: *Seek out what the patient has heard about the prescribed medication from the web, television, and other media sources*. While I was delivering a workshop in Tampa, Florida, Bruce Edson, a primary care physician, offered a nice technique for implementing this principle that I call the Grapevine Question:

TIP 101 Grapevine Question

"Sometimes this medication can help with problems like you're having. Have you heard or seen anything good or bad on the web or from television, radio, magazines, or newspapers about this medication?"

By specifically mentioning various channels of cultural bias ("on the web or from television, radio, or magazines"), I believe the clinician increases the likelihood that the patient will provide the whole scoop from the grapevine.

Another workshop participant, Lucius Ripley, suggests something that we have discussed before – providing patients with a list of suggested websites – but with a twist related to timing. He has found that it is often effective to provide this list immediately after using the Grapevine Question. As noted earlier, the clinician can give patients specific websites that are objective and demonstrate neither a bias for nor against the medication in question (such as might be provided by the National Institutes of Health or the National Institute of Mental Health).

As we bring this chapter to a close, we can see that there exist numerous MIM principles and interviewing techniques that can help clinicians to meaningfully engage the families, significant others, and friends of our patients. Through the techniques of the MIM, we can forge a truly collaborative treatment team in which there is a genuine shared decision making. We have also gained insight into the fact that the development of our patient's medication interest is not solely the realm of our interpersonal relationship with our patient. Many other voices are at work. Many other people lobby the patient from intimate individuals (family and friends) to anonymous voices on the web (chatrooms and social media).

Our goal is to sensitively uncover these voices, learn from them, address their misconceptions, if present, and adjust our own suggestions for treatment planning when their opinions prove to be correct. The only true mistake is to not seek out these voices, for these voices will be there whether we are aware of their opinions or ignorant of them.

Afterword: A Personal Note to the Reader

Take a load off Fanny, take a load for free

Take a load off Fanny, and you put the load right on me.

Robbie Robertson and The Band

LYRIC FROM THE WEIGHT

I've always liked the above lyric from The Band. In a simple phrase or two it pinpoints the essence of our mission, the chance to help another fellow traveler on the often arduous journey we call life. As physicians, nurses, physician assistants, clinical pharmacists, and case managers our day-to-day goals revolve about our attempts to lighten the load of our patients. We tend to do so by using complex theories, sophisticated technologies, and the very best of evidence-based practices. Our goal is to apply these methods as effectively as we can. But in a less scientific sense, I like to view our goal in a simpler fashion. In the final analysis, our goal is to soften the world a bit for our patients.

The world can be a very hard place. Yet we can soften it. Sometimes we triumphantly prevent death, sometimes merely delay it, and at other times simply must let it be for we have no effective interventions. We relieve suffering. We minimize fears. We provide comfort and, sometimes, we provide our tears or a reassuring touch. All of which serve to soften the world.

In the pages of this book, I'd like to think that we have continued this tradition, for one of our most effective tools for softening the world is the use of our medications. But as former Surgeon General Koop stated in his Foreword to the First Edition of this book, "No medication works inside a bottle." This book has offered a myriad of ways for helping patients to feel that the medication bottles beside their beds are worth reaching for. It has been a book about creating justifiable hope.

From the perspective of the MIM, we view the patient as an ever-changing, intersecting matrix of forces: biological, psychological, interpersonal, familial, cultural, and spiritual. As we have seen in the previous pages, the MIM allows us to sensitively address the patient's decision making as it pertains to one of the most difficult of all questions, "Should I put this drug in my body?" To help patients find an answer to this question, the MIM provides clinicians with flexible tools for exploring every wing of a patient's matrix from the biological and psychological to the familial, cultural, and spiritual.

In clinical practice, we begin by helping our patients to decide whether a medication is the best choice for them or not. If not, we help them to find the best alternatives that fit their needs and beliefs. If so, we help them to navigate the complexities of the Choice Triad, to understand the pros and cons of the various medications that are available. Throughout this process, we always try to uncover what the patient wants before we share what we think the patient may need. At its best, both parties in this shared decision making gain, as do all those family members who participate with us.

If we are honest with ourselves, to be a physician, nurse, physician assistant, or clinical pharmacist we will have to make sacrifices. The training is often extremely difficult. Many of the readers of this book are in the midst of this rigorous training. And, once leaving your training, the hours will be equally daunting throughout the rest of your careers. Both yourselves and even your families will, undoubtedly, make ongoing sacrifices. But in the end, I would like to assure you that it is all worth it. It is a privilege to become a healer. It is a good thing to wake up each morning and know that the world will be a better place because you are in it. And I know that the world will be a better place because you are in it.

Hopefully, the MIM will provide you with some of the tools you need to soften the world for your patients. I also hope that it will create in you the curiosity and drive to discover new interviewing techniques for talking with patients about their medications, for it is through the art of clinical interviewing that you will bring your science to your healing. And your healing will, ultimately, lead you to your soul.

As I said, it is all worth it in the end.

I am reminded of a quotation by Richard S. Hollis, MD, that resonates with the goals of this book and mirrors the lyric of our closing epigram above:

> It is the patient who carries the burden of illness, but the compassionate physician shares that burden, lifting it when possible and lightening it when that is all that can be done. This sharing of the burden has always been the hallmark of the medical profession.[12]

So it has always been. So it is today. And may the principles and techniques of the MIM help you to make it the hallmark of the future. The mission is in your hands. I have the greatest confidence that you will accomplish it.

REFERENCES

1. Boyle B. The critical role of family in patient experience. *Patient Experience J* 2015;2(2):4–6.
2. Clay AM, Parsh B. Patient- and family-centered care: it's not just for pediatrics anymore. *AMA J Ethics* 2016;18(1):40–44.
3. Bertakis KD, Azari R. Patient-centered care is associated with decreased health care utilization. *J Am Board Fam Med* 2011;24(3):229–239.
4. Aronson PL, Yau J, Helfaer MA, et al. Impact of family presence during pediatric intensive care unit rounds on the family and medical team. *Pediatrics* 2009;124(40):1119–1125.
5. Joint Commission. *Advancing Effective Communication, Cultural Competence, and Patient- and Family-Centered Care: A Roadmap for Hospitals.* Oakbrook Terrace, IL: Joint Commission; 2010. http://www.jointcommission.org/assets/1/6/ARoadmapforHospitalsfinalversion727.pdf. Accessed June 24, 2017.
6. Small DC, Small RM. Patients first! Engaging the hearts and minds of nurses with a patient-centered practice model. *Online J Issues Nurs* 2011;16(2):2.
7. Ciufo D, Hader R, Holly C. A comprehensive systematic review of visitation models in adult critical care units within the context of patient- and family-centered care. *Int J Evid Based Healthc* 2011;9(4):362–387.
8. Philibert I, Patow C, Cichon J. Incorporating patient- and family-centered care into residency education: approaches, benefits, and challenges. *J Grad Med Educ* 2011;3(2):272–278.

9. American Nurses Credentialing Center. *Magnet Recognition Program: A Program Overview.* Silver Spring, MD: American Nurses Credentialing Center; 2011. http://nursecredentialing.org/Documents/Magnet/MagOverview-92011.pdf. Accessed June 24, 2017.
10. Institute for Patient- and Family-Centered Care. Bethesda, MD: Institute for Patient- and Family-Centered Care. http://www.ipfcc.org. Accessed March 5, 2018.
11. Benjamin JM, Cox ED, Trapskin PJ, et al. Family-initiated dialogue about medications during family-centered rounds. *Pediatrics* 2015;135(1):94–101.
12. Hollis RS. Caring: a privilege and our responsibility. *Obstet Gynecol* 1994;83:1–4.

APPENDICES

To the Reader

Appendix A **(a bonus chapter)** appears both in the subsequent pages of this paperback and in the accompanying ebook. Appendices B and C appear as further **bonus material appearing only in the accompanying ebook** (directions for access to the ebook appear on the inside front cover of the book).

Appendix A: The Next Step: A Concise Guide to Enhancing Medication Follow-Through

Appendix B: The Tip Archive (which contains the names and the exact wording of all 101 of the MIM interviewing tips)

Appendix C: Reprinted Journal Article from *Professional Case Management:*

"The Medication Interest Model: An Integrative Clinical Interviewing Approach for Improving Medication Adherence – Part 2: Implications for Teaching and Research"

Appendix A

The Next Step: A Concise Guide to Enhancing Medication Follow-Through

Introduction

Reason to Be, Goals, and Organization

In the pages of this book, we have studied how clinicians can collaboratively work with patients to maximize a patient's personal interest in choosing and staying on a medication. We have seen how the Medication Interest Model (MIM) provides a sound framework for understanding patient choice (the Choice Triad) and a variety of interviewing techniques (over 100) for effectively implementing shared decision making while enhancing motivation and addressing patient concerns.

Although patient choice and motivation stand as prerequisite foundation stones for effective use, patient choice is only the first step in the process of successful ongoing medication use. The next step requires that efforts must be made by all parties involved – not only the patient but also the physicians, nurses, physician assistants, pharmacists, case managers, and other health care providers as well as family members, pharmacies, community support programs and insurance companies – to reduce the numerous *external obstacles* that can prevent the patient from being able to effectively take his or her medications in an ongoing fashion. In this book, we have referred to this second step as the process of "medication follow-through," a term coined by Kim Mueser[1] from whose wisdom on this topic we will frequently borrow in the following pages.

Even though the MIM does not directly address strategies and approaches for navigating the tricky waters of medication follow-through, this appendix – essentially a bonus chapter - has been added to provide medical, nursing, physician assistant, and clinical pharmacy students (as well as more experienced clinicians and case managers), with a concise introduction to the array of promising methods currently available for enhancing medication follow-through. Indeed, such techniques and innovations can only be effective to the degree with which clinicians and case managers *are aware of their existence and importance.*

Let me begin by stating what this appendix is not: (1) It is not a comprehensive review of the literature and research on strategies for improving medication follow-through; (2) it is not intended to describe which approaches have shown the strongest evidence base empirically; (3) it is not intended to comprehensively, nor authoritatively, describe specific ways to effectively implement the numerous approaches currently available for enhancing medication follow-through.

In contrast, it is intended to do the following: (1) metacommunicate – by its very inclusion in this book – the critical importance of addressing medication follow-through; (2) introduce the student reader, as well as more experienced clinicians, to the array of approaches available at present while addressing a few promising ideas for the future; (3) proffer a few practical tips that I have found useful over the years; and (4) provide a reference or two on each of the approaches for the interested reader, including articles regarding the exciting advances being made with the use of texting, chat rooms, tablet and smart phone apps, and other promising innovations afforded by the web and mobile devices.

Although generally well-demarcated from each other, the first step in enhancing medication use (interviewing techniques regarding choice as addressed in the previous 14 chapters of this book) and the second step (enhancing medication follow-through once choice has been made as addressed in this appendix) sometimes exhibit a degree of overlap. More specifically, we have already seen that interviewing techniques may be of use in uncovering and addressing some of the external obstacles to effective medication follow-through. For instance, MIM Tip 41 (Gently Exploring Cost Issues, see page 171) can help clinicians explore patients' concerns related to medication prices. Tips 43, 44, and 45 (Inquiry into General Inconvenience, Inquiry into Timing Inconvenience, and Inquiry into Transportation Inconvenience, see pages 173–175) can help transform specific external roadblocks related to patient inconvenience.

In this appendix, I have tried to provide a practical framework that will introduce the many approaches for improving medication follow-through in an organized fashion. The goal is to provide a concise and handy reference for clinicians as they enter the hectic world of clinical practice. Topics are organized as follows:

Part 1: Strategies for Improving Illness Self-Management

Part 2: Case Management

Part 3: Integrating Care: The Medical Home, Pharmacist-Based Interventions, and Peer Support

Optimism Served with a Note of Caution

As mentioned above, an extensive amount of research has been undertaken regarding methods for improving medication follow-through (with a substantially lesser amount dedicated to improving medication interest, choice, and motivation). Despite the large number of studies, it should be noted that reviews and meta-reviews have indicated that relatively few randomized controlled trials (RCTs) have been done. Moreover, the results of many of these RCT trials have been disappointing. Some methodologies have certainly shown exciting promise, as can be seen in the articles subsequently cited in this appendix, but the evidence base for effective approaches to enhancing medication follow-through – consisting of well-designed and soundly implemented RCTs – is surprisingly small.

I should let the reviewers speak for themselves. Nieuwlaat and colleagues concluded:

> "Across the body of evidence, effects were inconsistent from study to study, and only a minority of lowest risk of bias RCTs improved both adherence and clinical outcomes. Current methods of improving medication adherence for chronic health problems are mostly complex and not very effective, so that the full benefits of treatment cannot be realized."[2]

Costa and colleagues similarly conclude:

> ". . . we identified inconsistent methodology and findings across the studies, different approaches for the same tool. Finally, most of the tools were complex, labor intensive, and not predictably effective. Most of the studies are mainly focused on short-term adherence, and no consistent results were presented for long-term evidence, and the current methods of improving medication adherence for chronic illness are mostly complex and not very effective."[3]

Where does this leave us as clinicians as we search for the best evidence base to help guide our efforts toward improving medication follow-through? At first glance, it might appear a bit disheartening, but I don't think it need be. In essence, the evidence base points out that, despite large amounts of research, the empirical study of methods for increasing medication follow-through (as well as efforts for medication interest and choice) is in its infancy.

Lack of validating empirical research does not mean that effective methods do not exist. It often takes many years, and even decades, to demonstrate both the efficacy and effectiveness of interventions that ultimately prove to be quite useful. Research doesn't create new interventions; it validates them. Digitalis was used for centuries to help relieve the symptoms of congestive heart failure long before any research supported its use.

At times, whether related to the complexity of variables, the statistical demands for an impossible to achieve subject pool size, or compelling ethical concerns, some extremely valuable innovations are never validated by empirical research. To my knowledge, no double-blind studies have substantiated that it is better to jump out of plane at 30,000 feet with a big billowy thing above one's head versus jumping out in one's birthday suit. Despite the lack of a validating empirical evidence base, I believe that qualitative single-case observations have provided a generally agreed upon answer.

Indeed, without substantial empirical support, evidence-based methodology suggests that clinicians should use the best logical interventions currently supported by lower levels of evidence base (such as expert face validity and construct validity as well as personal observation and qualitative support). In short, without a robust empirical evidence base, clinicians need not shrug their shoulders as if nothing can be done. Quite to the contrary, evidence-based methodology suggests that each patient now becomes their own experiment in the sense that clinicians try to determine what works best for *that unique patient* from the best evidence available and the result of direct observation of efficacy.

The following pages are designed to provide readers with a working knowledge of "what might work best." It is hoped that with this knowledge readers can – with any given individual – collaboratively arrive at the best possible approach for solidifying medication follow-through within the limitations of the clinician's resources and those of the patient.

The beauty of this approach is simple: The results are directly observable. Our identified patient either shows improved medication follow-through or not. The challenge may be daunting, but the possible solutions are both numerous and exciting.

Core Medication Follow-Through Principles

Before proceeding with our survey of the potential strategies available for improving medication follow-through, I would like to share a few guiding principles. Over the years, the following principles have proven to be of use for both myself and my colleagues regarding the successful implementation of any of the approaches delineated below. I believe that future research may show that many of the disappointing results mentioned in the review articles above may be caused by a lack of application of the principles below. Such a lack, could, in my opinion, undercut the efficacy and effectiveness of any medication follow-through approach no matter how potentially useful it might be.

First, and, in my opinion, foremost, no matter what plan is developed for implementing medication follow-through, it is critical to remember that patients' levels of motivation frequently lessen over time. Ironically, the single most important principle to remember when securing sound medication follow-through is: *the principles and interviewing techniques of whatever model or combination of models chosen by the clinician for addressing choice and motivation (such as the MIM, motivational interviewing, and cognitive behavioral therapy) these techniques must be assiduously implemented in an ongoing basis while attending to medication follow-through.* Without robust patient motivation, many well-designed medication follow-through plans will falter. One of the easiest mistakes for a treatment team to make is to think, "we've secured buy-in with the patient, now let's focus primarily on approaches to transform obstacles to medication follow-through." To the contrary, patient interest and motivation should never slide into the category of secondary aspects of care.

In addition, if one should choose to peruse the various review articles referenced in this appendix, one will find an aggregate agreement that no single approach to improving medication follow-through has currently proven to be particularly effective. Nor, in my opinion, is it likely that a single panacea will suddenly materialize that will solve the problem of poor follow-through in a generic sense.

In contrast, it appears that clinicians will most likely find the most success by collaboratively working with patients to find the *best combination of approaches for the unique needs, concerns, and preferences of each patient.* In this regard, some patients will find monthly follow-up calls from case managers to be very useful, whereas others may find them to be intrusive; some patients will find weekly pill boxes to be invaluable, whereas others may find them to be prohibitively annoying to set-up; some patients will find smart phone apps to be fun and practical, whereas others will deem them to be confusing and unappealing.

The reality of the situation is that considerable time must be spent in helping a patient develop a sound plan for optimizing medication follow-through. With each patient, a treatment team is faced with the task of developing two separate plans of action via shared decision making. First, the team must collaboratively devise a potentially effective treatment plan. Second, the team must collaboratively develop a sound implementation plan for securing maximum, effective follow-through with the aforementioned treatment plan.

Regarding the use of medications, the two plans consist of (1) helping the patient choose the desired medication (if, indeed, the patient wants to use a medication) and (2) helping the patient decide on the most appealing plan for maximizing medication follow-through. In those patients presenting with particularly difficult clinical challenges, who have been selected for discussion at treatment plan meetings, I have found it to be useful to routinely address both plans, *to weigh them as equally important,* and to concretize the plan regarding medication follow-through once the team has finished brainstorming.

After collaboratively finalizing the plan with the patient, it is important to remember that with *each subsequent meeting with the patient*, it can be invaluable to discuss whether or not the plan is working, collaboratively adjust the plan if it is not working, and continue to do such shared decision making in subsequent appointments until the medication follow-through plan has been optimized to its best achievable degree.

In addition, over time, clinicians can monitor the effectiveness of the plan, for patient situations, resources, and obstacles to medication follow-up often change. A medication follow-through plan that was effective 2 years ago with a patient with diabetes and hypertension may not be currently effective for the patient. The patient may have developed renal failure and poor eyesight secondary to her diabetes with resulting changes in prescribed medications, the ability to read directions effectively, and a host of problems related to increased losses in mobility and transportation needs.

Finally, time concerns must be addressed. The above principles take time to implement, but as with the MIM itself, the time spent can have enormous long-range time savings for clinicians in addition to marked improvements in patient outcomes. In my opinion, it is difficult for any single prescribing clinician to design and implement the best possible medication follow-through plan from the enticing, yet large, selection of interventions described later, but a team can do so. I was on such a team and, as described in Chapter 2, the results in patient satisfaction, medication follow-through, and clinical outcome (as reflected by decreased hospital days) were impressive.

The role for the reader is to bring an active awareness to treatment plan meetings (if one's practice allows enough time to hold such meetings which is not always the case) and/or shared decision-making conversations with patients as to what possible medication follow-through interventions exist. This appendix attempts to foster such awareness.

Such integrative brainstorming (with resulting tasks distributed to varying team members as time and expertise allow) can help teams create follow-through implementation plans that are feasible in the unique health care system, family environment, and clinical milieu of the patient. All systems have limitations. The goal is not to implement all of the interventions that are described below. Nor is it the goal to create an idealized "perfect" plan. The goal is to create – and re-create as necessary over time – the best possible plan that *can actually be done* within the severe time and resource constraints facing all involved. A limited plan done well is much more effective than a "state-of-the-art plan" done poorly.

It is also important to acknowledge that a large number of prescribing clinicians do not have the luxury of a "team." Many prescribing clinicians working in rural areas, poverty-stricken areas in developing countries, or inner cities are "the team." Even in these situations, the knowledge of potential approaches for enhancing medication follow-through provided in this appendix may help a solo clinician to optimize follow-through with a particular patient. Before proceeding, let us review our principles that, if implemented wisely, may increase the likelihood that the following tools will achieve their goals:

1. Always, in a continuous fashion, address the patient's ongoing medication interest and motivation, for his or her motivation will often decrease over time. Without robust motivation, even the best-designed plans for enhancing medication follow-through are often doomed to failure.
2. No single method for enhancing medication follow-through is likely to be adequate by itself. Multiple methods are often a key to success.
3. Use shared decision making to create a plan that is designed specifically to the unique needs, concerns, and preferences of each patient.
4. During team treatment plan meetings develop the habit of designing not only a treatment plan but a medication follow-through implementation plan as well which will be further developed collaboratively with the patient. If no such team meetings exist, try to develop a habit of collaboratively discussing and concretely agreeing on a medication follow-through plan with each patient.

5. Once a plan has been agreed on via shared decision making with the patient, the success of the plan can be monitored at each successive appointment. If necessary, alterations can be collaboratively made until medication follow-through has been maximized (the goal is to maximize implementation realizing that 100% fidelity may not be possible).
6. Once the best possible system is implemented, its effectiveness should be intermittently monitored in an ongoing fashion over time.
7. If available, utilize a team for both brainstorming and division of labor regarding implementation, always keeping in mind that the patient and his or her loved ones are critical extended components of the treatment team.

Part 1: Strategies for Improving Illness Self-Management

Illness self-management is the technical term for helping patients to better understand, manage, and psychologically cope more effectively with both their disease and their illness. Far from suggesting that the patient is "on his or her own" in coping with the illness, the term means quite the opposite.

Effective self-management represents a collaborative undertaking of the patient's health care providers, family members and friends, and community resources with the patient so that the patient is better able to manage symptoms, utilize treatments (including effective medication follow-through), and make useful lifestyle changes, as well as successfully navigate any cultural and spiritual complications associated with their illness.[4] With regard to improving medication follow-through a wealth of tools for use come under its umbrella including: pillboxes and packaging, other methods for tracking medication use such as "shelf-sliding," traditional prompts for taking medications on time such as behavioral tailoring, technological prompts such as apps for mobile devices, and dosage simplification.

Organizing and Tracking Medication Use Via Pillboxes, Packaging, and "Shelf-Sliding"

Pillboxes and Packaging

As Mueser reminds us, other than lack of medication interest, the most common reason people don't take their meds is that they forget to do so. One way to address this problem is to provide devices that help patients organize their pills. Especially when patients are taking multiple pills, the use of pillboxes – as simple and low-tech as these devices may be – in my opinion, should be near the top of the list of interventions for enhancing medication follow-through. They are low cost in money to patients and low cost in time commitment to clinicians and case managers.

A wide variety of pillboxes are available that allow patients to store pills prospectively in specific compartments that are based on both the day of the week and the time of the day. Not only do pillboxes show patients exactly what medications to take and when (a major advantage when patients are faced with numerous medications with varying schedules), but they also show patients if they have missed a dosing, for the unemptied pill compartment will be a hard-to-miss indicator.

Pill organizers may contain pills for a single day (which can be easily carried around in a purse or pocket), a week, or even a month. After the prescription is initially picked-up, various people may fill the pillbox ranging from the patients themselves, family members, case managers, and in some instances even pharmacy staff. Some pill organizers contain alarms or reminder chimes that can prompt patients as to when a dose is to be taken.[5]

Another option occasionally available in sophisticated and well-staffed pharmacies is the prepackaging of pills in blister packs. This pharmacy service can sometimes be provided as a personalized packaging for the patient's dosing schedule.

Shelf-Sliding

Some patients – especially younger adults and those patients taking only a couple of medications – don't want to be bothered with pillboxes and/or they may feel that pillboxes are "just for old people." But truth be told, no matter what age one might be, it is surprisingly easy to find oneself standing at night – bottle in hand – wondering, "Did I take this thing in the morning or not?"

I have found a technique that works well (I use it for myself) – a ploy I call "shelf-sliding." It is particularly useful when one must take medications twice a day for tracking whether one has taken a medication earlier in the day or evening as prescribed.

In this strategy, patients place all of their pill bottles up front on the right side of the shelf. After removing their morning dose from its bottle, they place the pill bottle on the far left of the shelf creating a large space between their bottles of "still to be taken" medications on the far right. The patient then pops the pill and proceeds to repeat the process with each morning dose, placing each subsequent bottle immediately on the far left. If one has three medications to take in the morning, by following this simple procedure, once taken all three of the bottles will be on the left side of the shelf, indicating that they have been taken.

At night, if indeed, the patient has taken the morning doses, all the bottles should be on the left when the cabinet is opened. The patient then removes the night dose from its bottle, immediately places the corresponding bottle back to the far right side of the shelf, and takes the pill. The process is repeated for each of the corresponding medications. If, on opening the cabinet on the next morning, the pill bottles are not on the right side of the shelf, the patient will know that it is likely that he or she missed a previously required night-time dose.

Prompting Reminders

A different approach to the nearly ubiquitous problem of forgetfulness is to remind patients in real time that it is time to take their medications. Pillboxes alone (unless they come with some type of integrated electronic prompting device) can organize what medication to take and when to take it, but do not have the ability to alert the patient that it is time to take it. With regard to prescriptions, themselves, patients can benefit by being prompted as to when a prescription needs to be filled by calls from the pharmacy or case manager. Tools for prompting the time to take a specific dose lie in two broad categories: (1) approaches using traditional strategies and (2) approaches using the web and mobile devices.

Traditional Strategies

One of the simplest methods to prompt oneself is to post a sign in a conspicuous place within the house that "can't be missed." By way of example, a patient can put a homemade sign stating in bold red letters, "Did you take your meds this morning?" on the inside of their front door or on the door to their garage. Patients may vary on the best placement of such signs with common placements being: Beside their coffee pot or Keurig, on their computer keyboard, on a bathroom mirror, on their purse or briefcase, or on closet doors where the necessities of daily routine are kept (such as dog/cat food or a clothes closet).

Behavioral Tailoring

The use of reminder signs in conspicuous places suggests a prompting method that I have found to be one of the simplest yet most effective plans for increasing medication follow-through – behavioral tailoring. Behavioral tailoring involves collaboratively designing medication prompts by fitting the taking of the medication into the patient's usual routine.[6] Rather than posting a prompting sign (although this can also be done as part of a multitiered reminder system) in behavioral tailoring the medication bottles or pillboxes, themselves, are placed in the conspicuous place.

Before proceeding, it is important to remember that behavioral tailoring must be carefully implemented if there are any individuals – from children to the elderly – living in the household that could mistakenly ingest medications if the bottles are out in the open. If such is the case, the medication bottles must be in a location, such as a locked medicine cabinet or locked pillbox where potentially dangerous ingestions cannot occur. *An assessment as to this potential risk should be done with every patient before designing a behavioral tailoring strategy.*

In any case, the art to effectively implementing behavioral tailoring lies in personalizing the trigger location to the exact, and sometimes idiosyncratic, needs and preferences of the patient. Besides enhancing medication follow-through, I have found behavioral tailoring to be popular with many patients, for it is both an enjoyable and engaging example of shared decision making.

One of the most popular and useful pairings is to have patients place their pill bottles beside their toothbrushes and toothpaste. Thus, "you can't brush your teeth until you take your pills." This location is further facilitated by the fact that many patients already have drinking glasses at their bathroom sinks. If they do not normally have a glass sitting at the location, it is wise to have them add one. *Small details, such as this last point, can be surprisingly important in making a behavioral tailoring strategy effective or ineffective.* Anything that makes it easier to take the pills immediately at the point of the prompt can be useful. Mueser notes that the strategy can be further fool-proofed by having the patient attach his or her pillbox to the toothbrush with a rubber band.[7]

Another commonly chosen site is to have patients place their bottles where they pick up their cell phones every morning. Other patients prefer placing their pill bottles or boxes on their pillows in the morning after making their beds, thus they cannot crawl back into bed until they have taken their evening meds. If this method is chosen by the patient, it is often useful to have the patient keep a glass of water on his or her bed stand to expedite the process.

One other common location remains – sometimes missed by clinicians despite its obvious nature. We are a culture and a people obsessed with vitamins and supplements. With the doggedness of alchemists in pursuit of the secret of longevity, many patients are meticulous about taking the miniature fountains of youth that they believe lie within their vitamin capsules and caplets. In many instances, the vitamins, indeed, may enhance health. In all instances, their use can provide a genuine aid for improving medication follow-through. Clinicians typically uncover a patient's vitamin use when taking the initial medication history. If the patient's use of vitamins appears to have become a powerful habit, the clinician can ask the patient to add his or her pill bottles to the shelf of vitamin bottles.

In a similar vein, if we return for a moment to the use of pillboxes, I have had patients that keep a large weekly pillbox filled with their daily schedule of vitamins, a treasure chest that also accompanies them on their vacations and business trips. In such cases, the prescribed medications can simply be added to the appropriate compartments.

No matter what behavioral tailoring strategy is designed, as mentioned in our core principles for enhancing medication follow-through, to maximize a successful outcome it is wise to examine the effectiveness of the behavioral tailoring in subsequent appointments. In this ongoing shared decision making, adjustments can be made if necessary or the strategy abandoned it if it proves to be a failed technique. New techniques can be subsequently brainstormed. *Note that if one is not scheduled to see the patient in the next several weeks following the creation of a plan, it can be invaluable, if staffing allows it, to have a team member call the patient within several days to see how the system is working and to adjust the system if necessary.*

I believe the reader may find that behavioral tailoring becomes one of his or her favorite strategies for securing medication follow-through. It is simple, costs the patient nothing, and requires a minimal cost in staffing time. Moreover, it appears to have a promising evidence base that stretches back several decades. This evidence base is exemplified, qualitatively, by its having been employed for decades by experienced clinicians and case managers and, empirically, by its effectiveness displayed in controlled research with patients, even those patients suffering from severe mental illnesses whose cognitive impairments make remembering medications particularly difficult.[8–11]

Strategies Using the Internet, Mobile Devices, and Other Electronic Medium

Low-Tech Approaches

As we will see in our sections on case management and pharmacy interventions, frequent, personalized contact with a valued clinician can prove to be a pivotal reagent in the complex processes at play in improving medication follow-through. The phone remains a useful tool in this regard, both landlines and smart phones. Enhanced by the development of more high-tech interactive visual formats such as Skyping, these telephone encounters can become more intimate, hopefully enhancing their potency as medication reminders and motivators.

As time and staffing permits, clinicians can select a small number of patients to receive scheduled, brief phone contacts. Patients who are viewed as being particularly high risks for not following up with their meds and whose lack of follow-up poses potential serious morbidity or death are naturals for such a list. Even if a solo practitioner, or a small team, only has available the resources to implement such a strategy with one or a handful of such patients, it is well worth doing if it may save a life.

Smart phones are certainly high-tech in nature and will be, in the next section, the rock-bed of our exploration of high-tech methods for prompting patients to take their medications. But in this section, we will address a low-tech feature of smart phones that may prove to be as effective as the smart phone's more advanced features. In short, smart phones are wonderful alarm clocks as are smart watches.

Patients frequently find the use of the alarm system on their phones to be an excellent way to remind them that it is time to take their medications. Some patients prefer using an alarm tone, others prefer vibration (commonly chosen to avoid drawing attention in workplaces or leisure time public settings), and some prefer both.

Also remember that patients may vary markedly in their sophistication and comfortableness in using various functions of their smart phones. Never assume that a patient knows how to set the alarm system on their cell phone. I have found it useful to gently ask as with, "People vary on what apps they like to use on their phones; by any chance, have you ever used the alarm system on your phone?"

It is important to collaboratively discuss such issues. Patient proclivities can vary significantly with regard to technological advances, not infrequently by generational preferences, and are sometimes surprising. It can be ill-advised to assume what approach a patient would prefer. Even a patient who loves using his or her smart phone – and can do so in a sophisticated fashion – may not want to use the alarm system at home. The patient in question, if they have maintained a home landline, may prefer turning his or her smart phone off once at home where the patient can, at last, get relief from an unwanted string of text messages some of which are arriving late at night.

High-Tech Approaches

The web, especially when coupled with mobile devices, represents another particularly promising frontier. Numerous devices can be used as vehicles for electronic prompting ranging from stationary devices (landline phones and home computers) to mobile devices (laptops, tablets, smart phones, and smart watches). Intelligent home management systems with smart speakers may become a preferred method for medication prompting for some patients. Future mobile devices may include eye-glasses fitted with micro-screens and even implantable communication devices. Returning to the present, a variety of electronic avenues – from low-tech to high-tech – have been studied including reminder phone calls, pagers, text messaging, interactive voice response systems, videotelephone calls, and programmed electronic audiovisual reminder devices (such as pill bottles with miniaturized computer components that create a bottle cap capable of providing a chirping sound and/or light at the time of dosing).

As exciting as these innovations appear to be and I believe will, ultimately, prove to be, it is important to remember that the research is still in its infancy. Moreover, the early indications warrant some caution for the results have been, not infrequently, disappointing. Some of the approaches remain overly complex, costly, and user unfriendly (depending on the user).[12] In many healthcare settings, these high-tech approaches are simply unavailable. Because of these limitations, many current and future readers may not be able to use the high-tech approaches described above.

But this need not be a major concern, for we have seen earlier that many cheap and easy-to-implement strategies, such as behavioral tailoring and smart phone alarms, can be used to create effective plans for enhancing medication follow-through. Indeed, with any specific patient, high-tech interventions may not show any superiority from low-tech interventions when the low-tech interventions are implemented using the core medication follow-through principles outlined earlier in this appendix.

Many of the following high-tech tools may best fulfill their ultimate promise – once they are cost efficient and readily available – not so much as solo interventions but as useful adjuncts and backup systems for already effective traditional and low-tech strategies. In contrast, for other patients, they may become the preferred prompting tool, in which case the more traditional tools can be used for backup and reenforcement. As mentioned in our core principles, future clinicians will have the option to use shared decision making to arrive at the collection of approaches most appealing to the unique patient at hand.

In this regard, another promising aspect of high-tech prompting pertains to its ease of use for patients (future generations of patients will have been using smartphones since toddlerhood), instantaneous conveyance of message, and rather extraordinary geographical reach. Especially in rural and underdeveloped locales, where the availability of clinicians and case managers can be very low (preventing the type of personalized and face-to-face interactions that can enhance more traditional approaches), short, high-tech text messages may prove to be helpful prompts. Of course, such approaches can only work if the patients have the financial means and cell-tower reach to use smart phones.

The most readily available web-based, high-tech approaches to prompting generally involve short message services (SMS) more popularly known as text messaging. These SMS-based approaches can be grouped into two categories: (1) simple text messaging and (2) complex text messaging involving sophisticated apps. We will begin with the simplest and most easily used.

Prompting Via Simple Texting: Texting has become second nature to many, if not most, people and is often viewed as an indispensable aid to daily functioning in our wired world. For those patients for which this is true, text prompts concerning medication use may represent a natural and comfortable fit.[13–16]

In its most basic format, patients may receive a texting prompt at the time of prescribed use such as "John, take Plavix 75 mg at 9:00 AM. Respond with 1." In simple texting, short messages can also be used to influence medication use as well as reenforcing other aspects of follow-up such as, "Remember to see your cardiologist and/or primary care physician 1 to 2 weeks after your hospitalization."[17] More personalized messaging that supports collaboratively agreed-on strategies can also be used as with, "Try to remember to place your medication bottles on your pillow when you make your bed this morning" (reenforcing a behavioral tailoring strategy) or "Good morning Tyra, be sure to reset your alarm prompts today, for we've added a noontime dose" (reenforcing a cell phone prompting strategy).

If such a texting reminder system is available for your use, keep in mind that not all patients will like or use texting. For such patients, it can be disengaging if the clinician assumes that they will enjoy the system. For this reason, during shared decision making it is useful to ask questions such as, "Do you like to text?" "How often in a day do you use texting?" and "Do you think it would be useful if we could arrange to have texts sent to you to prompt you when it's time to take your medication?"

Prompting Via Complex Texting: In complex texting, more sophisticated apps are used to augment medication prompting.[18–25] A patient's medication practices regarding use can be monitored, tracked, and information shared with prescribing clinicians, case managers, and other allied health care providers (all of which will depend on patient agreements regarding confidentiality of care). Short messages, as well as more comprehensive learning modules (sometimes interactive in nature to enhance initial learning and ongoing consolidation) can be added regarding illness awareness and the importance of medication follow-through in relieving symptoms, disability, and risk of death.

Such educational programs can use laptops, tablets, smart phones, and other mobile devices. As is the case with medication use, the patient's time spent using the educational programs can be tracked and adjustments tailored to the patient's interest and learning styles. Personalized coaching and even efforts to address patient motivation – borrowing techniques from approaches such as the MIM, motivational interviewing, and cognitive behavioral therapy – can be employed.

Some of the unfolding promises for integrating high-tech interventions with traditional models for enhancing medication follow-through are dazzling in their potential promise, sometimes seemingly more appropriate in science fiction than clinical practice. What was once science fiction has already begun to morph into science fact. For instance, let us take a look at improving medication follow-through with one of our most deadly killers – diabetes.

Cahn, Akirov, and Raz have created an excellent review of some of the technological advances that are currently available for the management of diabetes as well as insights into potential future innovations.[26] They note that over 150,000 apps at the time of their article were available regarding health care interventions. These apps offered services as diverse as providing educational instruction, recording and displaying data, providing reminders or alerts, and enabling rapid and interactive communication among providers and patients.

With diabetes, wearable sensors now allow for continuous or flash (intermittent) monitoring of glucose levels in real time. Integrated with wearable insulin pumps – in addition to an automated ongoing release of insulin when needed (thus ensuring medication follow-through) – patients can be alerted to shifts in blood glucose levels perhaps related to an unexpected, or unintended, increase in carbohydrate intake. Having been alerted, patients can then supplement insulin dose as needed. Future advances may include progressively more subtle communications between patients and their software regarding potentially programmable alterations in dosing, related to perceived future physical activity level and/or anticipated unusual carbohydrate ingestion.

The medicine of the not-so-distant future may employ such approaches with other disease states where medication follow-through may be of immediate importance in preventing death. Continuous monitoring of physiology with rapid, automatic release of appropriate medications, when potentially life-threatening pathophysiology arises as with dangerous arrhythmias or poorly controlled malignant hypertension, may someday become feasible and even commonplace. Once again, medication follow-through will have essentially become guaranteed.

Returning to the present, as the kinks of high-tech systems have been addressed, the research results regarding both low- and high-tech texting and apps seems to be showing increasingly positive results. I, personally feel that these approaches will eventually prove to be valuable tools for integration into medication follow-through plans. Most likely, such plans will be composed of multiple tools with a seamless integration of direct human-to-human interaction and technological assistance.

But, as mentioned earlier, I believe that the most critical foundation stone will always remain the clinician-patient alliance. Using tools, such as the MIM, to address patient choice and motivation will remain the first, and prerequisite, step in helping medications to move from the bottle to our patient's mouths. Aided with both traditional and high-tech prompting interventions, medication follow-through will hopefully be enhanced. In the meantime, we haven't even exhausted other traditional methods for enhancing patient illness self-management.

Dosage Simplification

Thus far, we have been focusing on methods for increasing a patient's ability to follow-through with the complex medication regimens that appear to be necessitated by the patient's disease processes. Truth be told, our recommended protocols are sometimes unnecessarily complex. Time may be better spent simplifying the regimens themselves. Research has demonstrated that the more complicated the regimen, the greater the difficulty in following it.[27–29]

The complexity of the medication regimen depends on three variables: (1) the number of different medications prescribed, (2) the number of pills of each medication at each dosing, and (3) the number of times per day that each medication must be taken. Every effort should be made to use the least number of doses required to be effective with each medication and with each patient (all of whom have their own rate of metabolism). Pill size is also important to consider.

Patients vary markedly on how comfortable or uncomfortable they may be in swallowing pills. As described in Chapter 9 (see page 181), gagging is a surprisingly common phenomena, especially when patients must take a large number of pills, but – and this is an important "but" – some patients may gag on a small number of pills. It can be valuable to ask patients questions such as, "What has it been like for you to take all of your pills in the morning?" and/or "Martellus, do you ever find yourself gagging when you take your pills?"

When simplifying a dosing schedule, these factors regarding the patient's gag reflex are important to consider. And simplification may not always consist of decreasing the number of pills. Some patients only gag on larger pills (I have found this to be a common phenomenon). If the tablet cannot be divided, such a patient may prefer taking two tablets of a medication in a smaller size as opposed to the same dose in a larger tablet or capsule.

Unfortunately, this solution is not always feasible because some pills do not increase markedly in price in larger milligrams, and hence the price of the medication can increase when two pills are taken instead of one! Once again, the best answer for the patient at hand arises from a shared decision making with the patient regarding all variables involved. A wealthier patient might care very little about the increase in cost, whereas a poorer patient may find the increase prohibitive.

If it is possible to *safely* shift the frequency of dosing (e.g., pills taken all at night rather than two or three times per day), a patient's medication follow-through might improve significantly. Of course, the confounding variable here is the resulting potential for uneven blood levels and subsequent loss of beneficial impact, as well as the potential for an increase in side-effects during peak levels.

Another variable can go unrecognized by clinicians and case managers regarding problems engendered by the number of pills being taken. Curiously, this time the problem is not related to the number of pills being prescribed by the clinician. The problem is caused by the fact that the patient is simultaneously swallowing a large number of vitamins and supplements many of which are quite large in size.

As hinted at earlier, it is not uncommon to find patients swallowing 10 to 20 vitamins in the morning or evening along with their prescribed medications. If the patient is finding it hard to get all of these pills down, once again, shared decision making regarding the priorities of what needs to be taken will generally achieve better results as opposed to authoritarian dictums such as, "Well, you simply have to cut back on your vitamins because you need to take these medications."

Finally, one more option can help with simplification. In patients who have been stabilized on a medication regimen for many months – and whom one anticipates that the patient's doses will not require frequent adjustments in the near future – one can consider combination pills. Such pills take two different medications and combine them into one pill, as is sometimes seen with cardiovascular medications.[30] This alternative can be greatly appreciated by a patient, but obviously it is not viable if either of the medications will frequently need to be adjusted while the other component is best left as is.

Part 2: Case Management

Arguably, the single greatest advancement in enhancing medication follow-through has been the conceptualization and development of case management. Many of the readers of this book are well aware of this point, for they are either students studying case management or are already veteran providers of case management.

For all other readers and prescribers, the number one takeaway from this section is the importance of utilizing the case managers on the treatment team to the utmost effectiveness. In many instances, patients have more contacts with their case managers than with their physicians, advanced practice nurses, or other prescribers. Case managers are often the nexus of the therapeutic alliance as it relates to overall care. In essence, they are frequently the gatekeepers to the patient's views on their medications and are, at times, the voice whose opinion is most valued by the patient regarding medication use.

Depending on the diseases in question, the financial support of the treatment teams involved, the proclivities of administration, and geographic location, various disciplines with varying levels of education provide case management. Nurses and social workers, with both bachelor- or master-level degrees, are often the primary workforce in case management. In other instances, bachelor-level graduates with degrees unrelated to nursing or social work provide case management services. I have also seen nondegreed individuals, working with patients coping with severe mental health problems such as schizophrenia and bipolar disorder, provide excellent services (although potentially limited in scope) if trained and supervised effectively.

The interested reader will find a variety of excellent books devoted to case management.[31–34]

It is also difficult to differentiate the objectives of case management from the objectives of increased illness self-management described in Part 1, for case managers are major players in fostering improved illness self-management. They are agents of change. They are frequently the conduits through which communication occurs throughout the team including the patient, the patient's family, the prescriber, other allied health professionals, and the community at large. As we shall soon see, it is from this communication that patients often achieve an increase in illness self-management. The vectors in which case managers achieve increases in medication follow-through can be conceptualized as follows:

1. Providing logistical support
2. Providing psychological support
3. Helping patients to navigate the health care system
4. Social skills training and enhancing patient skills at communicating their needs and concerns regarding medications
5. Nurturing a user-friendly environment for enhancing medication follow-through

Providing Logistical Support

Depending on resources and staffing, case management can range from infrequent telephone contact to frequent telephone, face-to-face, and, in the best of situations, home visits. Regarding medication follow-through, case managers can help patients who are coping with cognitive deficits (such as dementias, intellectual disabilities) or physical disabilities (such as severe rheumatoid arthritis or the sequelae of strokes) to correctly load their pillboxes. They can help to arrange for transportation or pickup from pharmacies and, in some systems where home visits occur, they sometimes can provide transportation.

Case managers can greatly increase the likelihood of interventions (such as prompting signs and behavioral tailoring) to work effectively. For instance, they can help with the design, creation, and deployment of prompting signs. During a home visit, a case manager can facilitate shared decision making regarding the most effective behavioral tailoring system. In addition, when doing a home visit a case manager can model shelf-sliding and subsequently directly observe a patient using the technique. Even if home visits are not feasible (which is often the case), during face-to-face office visits, approaches such as shelf-sliding can be modelled and the patient asked to demonstrate the process.

It cannot be overemphasized how powerful such focused attention and follow-up on medication follow-through plans can be. A patient leaving a prescriber's office with merely the suggestion of doing behavioral tailoring or shelf-sliding with no follow-up until the next monthly appointment is often a patient doomed to a month of erratic medication follow-through. It is not the selection of the plan that failed. It is the team's implementation of the plan that failed. Sound case management can transform such a supposedly "failed" plan into a resounding success story.

Finally, a case manager might be the best person to judge a patient's ability to perform the activities of daily living that are required to effectively follow-through with a given medication. For instance, if the patient's medication regimen requires that a tablet be cut in half, a case manager can ask the patient to demonstrate doing so directly using the Show-Me Method described in Chapter 10 (see pages 209–211). In such instances, the case manager can assess an aged patient's (perhaps coping with impaired eyesight) or an intellectually impaired patient's (perhaps having problems understanding how to complete the task) ability to complete the task correctly.

Providing Psychological Support

Many of our patients are dealing with severe and chronic, sometimes debilitating diseases. Some of these patients are also socially isolated with few, if any, family or friends for support. Depression is common. As described in Chapter 1 (see page 8) studies have shown that patients suffering with depression are considerably less likely to take their medications, not only for psychiatric diseases, but for their *nonpsychiatric* diseases. Well-trained case managers can help spot such depressions and, subsequently, arrange for appropriate treatment. Such interventions not only address the patient's depression – and perhaps even prevent suicide – but also can directly result in increased medication follow-through with the patient's *nonpsychiatric* medications.

In a less striking fashion, case managers by phone, office appointments, or home visits can provide much needed positive reenforcement for patients who are trying to implement various strategies for improving their medication follow-through. It certainly can be useful to receive a computer-generated e-mail congratulating one on sound follow-through, but it is probably a good deal more motivating to see a warm smile and to hear a hearty congratulations from a trusted case manager commenting, "You know, Anne, you have designed one of the best plans for prompting yourself with the behavioral tailoring I have ever seen. It's really great. If you don't mind, I'm going to share it with some other patients."

Let us recall the gist of our first core principle, mentioned in our chapter's introduction: *During the implementation of follow-through plans, the therapeutic alliance remains the primary tool.* The robust nature of the case manager's therapeutic alliance, as generated by his or her use of the principles and techniques of the MIM, can reap benefits with regard to both unearthing the truth regarding the patient's actual medication practices as well as enhancing motivation. A patient may be more likely to share the number of doses he or she has purposefully, or unintentionally, missed, as well as relaying any increased doubts about using the medication with his or her case manager when compared with other members of the treatment team who are seen less frequently.

Helping Patients to Navigate the Health Care System

Psychological support from a case manager is of further utility in yet another arena – navigating the health care system itself. This navigation is particularly daunting in the United States (my opinion), for it is a health care system composed of a patchwork of multiple, sometimes poorly communicating, subsystems. Patients must run a gauntlet of confusing challenges related to Medicare, Medicaid, the Affordable Care Act, insurance companies, state and federal government regulations, the billing procedures and errors originating from hospital and clinic billing services, and their own sometimes precarious financial status. In my opinion, it is next to impossible for a patient to truly know if he or she is receiving the best possible care at the best price available without the help of a coordinating ombudsman. Case managers are the ombudsmen.

The costs of medications, coupled with the demoralization arising from attempting to navigate the above gauntlet, can markedly decrease patients' motivation to effectively follow-through with their medication regimen. For many patients, the help provided by their case manager is a godsend. Many a patient who would not have been able to "jump through the hoops" to get Medicaid or disability benefits – so as to afford their prescribed medications – do so because of aggressive case management.

Moreover, case managers, as they gain experience with the systems surrounding them often gain an expertise in how to acquire medications for a patient at the lowest cost. Sometimes, the hectic pace and overload of clinical work makes it difficult for prescribing clinicians to be aware of potential cost saving via pharmacy discounts, pharmaceutical discounts, or the availability of samples, for such programs are constantly in flux. Case managers, despite working under their own extreme time demands, often discover creative ideas regarding cost-saving resources.

Social Skills Training

Some patients will lack the prerequisite social and communication skills to communicate their needs and concerns about medication follow-through (as well as their doubts or concerns about their medications and/or their side effects). Various patients cycling through a primary care or specialty clinic will lack effective skills in this area. Obviously, patients coping with dementias, severe mental illnesses such as schizophrenia and bipolar disorder (that often have subtle cognitive disorders), as well as patients with intellectual disabilities or autism often need help with social and communication skills. Frankly, many other patients, such as those patients coming from poorer educational backgrounds, those coping with simple social anxiety, or those lacking in appropriate self-assertiveness will also have trouble conveying their needs.

Case managers can provide simple social skills training that can help patients communicate better with them as well as with prescribers and other treatment team members. Sometimes this training is as simple as helping the patient to write down a list of questions regarding their medications to take to their next follow-up appointment. I strongly recommend this practice for use by all patients, for it can be unsettling once one is in the room with the prescriber and the time constraints intensify.

Occasionally, case managers accompany patients to their visits with their prescribing clinicians, an optimum situation if feasible. This approach is more typically done by case managers working with patients with severe mental illnesses such as schizophrenia, bipolar disorder, or severe intellectual limitations. More complex social skills training (such as self-assertiveness training) and more sophisticated educational approaches (such as role-playing) may be provided as time permits and the skill-set of the case manager allows.

Nurturing a User-Friendly Environment for Enhancing Medication Follow-Through

Creating a Home Environment More Conducive to Effective Medication Follow-Through

If time allocation and job description allow it, during a home visit a case manager has a unique opportunity to directly observe the physical layout and orderliness of a patient's home. Sometimes such direct observations can potentiate the effectiveness of medication follow-through plans that simply could not be done without being in the patient's home. For instance, the case manager may spot potential obstacles to implementing a behavioral tailoring plan.

As Mueser describes, if a patient wants to take his medications when he prepares his morning cup of coffee, problems can arise if the kitchen counter is so cluttered that the pill bottles visually disappear in a mass of dirty plates, food containers, coffee supplies, and a bunch of unread mail. If the patient agrees, the case manager can help the patient organize the counter and coffee supplies and then help the patient decide where to put the pill bottles. During follow-up visits, the case manager can assess whether the behavioral tailoring plan has been maintained.[35]

In a similar fashion, shelf-sliding only works when the area between which the morning and evening bottles slide is kept completely clear. Once again, a single glance by the case manager can determine whether this condition has been met.

Creating an Interpersonal Environment More Conducive to Effective Medication Follow-Through

Many patients live with significant others whether they be partners, spouses, parents, adult children, or housemates sharing the rent. If the patient is comfortable with such intimates being part of the treatment team (with children a parent will always be involved), then case managers can enlist such allies in shared decision making regarding plans for enhancing medication follow-through. One advantage of this process can be an increased support by family members for the use of the medications, an enthusiasm that ensues from their inclusion.

On a practical level, family allies often contribute creative ideas for prompting and behavioral tailoring. They may also point out habitual behavioral patterns of the patient, not spontaneously shared by the patient (such as the fact that the patient does not get out of bed until 11:00 AM). Such behavioral insights may impact on effective dosing schedules or other variables that may impact on medication follow-through planning (such as the patient does not brush his or her teeth daily thus eliminating that prompt for behavioral tailoring).

Family members can also provide powerful positive feedback to the patient regarding the patient's effective implementation of any collaboratively designed plans. In this regard, following the spirit of the MIM, it is *critical* that the patient perceives the positive feedback – not as a form of "parentified monitoring" – but as an effective collaborative excitement about patient healing.

The importance of including family members in the loop regarding medication follow-through has another hidden, but extremely, valuable benefit. As discussed earlier, the time pressures on case managers are often exquisite for their case-loads can be intimidating. If the family member, such as a spouse or perhaps the adult child of a patient in the early stages of dementia, becomes invested in helping with the development and ongoing implementation of the medication follow-through plan, then the case manager has essentially created a new case manager by proxy. Even if no home visits are possible, the creation of this family case manager by proxy can result in outstanding ongoing support for the patient's medication follow-through. If home visits are possible, but must be carefully distributed, one or two home visits resulting in the production of a sound proxy may obviate any need for further home visits.

On a final note, a few well-timed "home" visits to other institutions, such as nursing homes or inpatient units, can help facilitate important clinical communications. Moreover, the unannounced visits of a case manager in a setting, such as a nursing home, may have ramifications in the quality of care being given to that patient within that setting, sometimes rather dramatically.

Part 3: Integrating Care: The Medical Home, Pharmacy-Based Interventions, and Peer Support

Patient-Centered Medical Home

Although not created primarily to help with improving medication follow-through per se, the emphasis on integrating care in the past several decades holds promise in doing so. The concept of integrating care is exemplified by the widely adapted model of the patient-centered medical home (PCMH).[36] In contrast to the MIM (described in the body of this book) and the methods for enhancing medication follow-through (described in this appendix), the concept of the medical home is a more generalized, systems-based approach to improving and coordinating overall clinical services in primary care settings. When implemented with fidelity, it is also designed to effectively address the many problems described earlier regarding our patient's abilities to navigate the daunting challenges of contemporary care.

The patient-centered home model was created to maximize patient/family access and communication with the treating prescribers and other health care providers while integrating care via other community resources, all of which may have a beneficial impact on medication follow-through. Attention is to be given to working with the "whole person" with an emphasis on ongoing patient feedback, quality assurance, and patient satisfaction within the health care system itself.

Ideally, the model utilizes technological advances, such as those described earlier, as well as advances in the electronic medical record and IT. Enhanced communication channels among health care providers, patients, and families are viewed as cornerstones of a sound medical home potentially resulting in an enhancement of medication follow-through. The core principles of the model were outlined succinctly in 2007 being released as the *Joint Principles of the Patient-Centered Medical Home* created by the combined efforts of four professional organizations (American Academy of Family Physicians [AAFP], American Academy of Pediatrics [AAP], American College of Physicians [ACP], and American Osteopathic Association [AOA]).[37]

As with many good ideas on paper, the empirical support for the cost effectiveness and feasibility of the medical home model has shown mixed results when implemented in real-world environments.[38–43] Hopefully, with time, the effective elements of the model will be isolated and operationalized. It would seem to hold promise, via its integrative and ongoing attention to improved clinician/patient communication, for enhancing medication follow-through.

From the reader's perspective, the lesson to be gained is that the practicing clinician, on entering a new job position, should learn about the elements of the medical home that are available in that particular practice, organization, or facility. Depending on where one practices, one may find effective elements of the available medical home that can be used in helping to enhance a patient's medication follow-through.

Pharmacy-Based Interventions

Retail pharmacists can play a significant role in enhancing medication follow-through.[44,45] If integrated as part of an ongoing community-based health care system, retail pharmacists may directly contact prescribers and other health care providers such as case managers (*depending on written consent from the patient to do so*) to expedite and ensure communication regarding patient concerns or problems with medication choice or follow-through. The pharmacist may have state-of-the-art information on side effects, drug-drug interactions, or new formulations of the medication that might minimize the dosage needed or simplify the dosing schedule that can be relayed to treating clinicians. On a more direct level, the pharmacy can alert the patient that a refill date is coming or contact the patient if they are late in procuring a refill, if the patient voices an interest in being so contacted. Earlier in the chapter, we had also discussed the use of individualized, blister packaging of medications for the patient.

In addition, patients with chronic diseases, who are frequent customers at the pharmacy, may become familiar with a specific pharmacist, developing a more robust pharmacist/patient alliance. Such circumstances further increase the likelihood that the patient may relay concerns about his or her medication preferentially to the pharmacist, who can then facilitate the patient raising his or her concerns with the prescribing clinician or case manager.

If the pharmacist notices that a patient is being asked to swallow an inordinately large number of pills or pills of an unusually large size, he or she can inquire whether the patient is having any problems with swallowing or gagging. In addition, pharmacists, as time permits, may indirectly enhance medication follow-through by enhancing the patient's ongoing motivation using principles and techniques from the MIM or motivational interviewing.

Considering the wide variety of interventions that a retail pharmacy can provide, it can be useful when a clinician (or the director of a case management team) has moved into a new location to personally contact the directors of various pharmacies to begin forging a relationship, to discover their available services (or limitations), and to tap their expertise. Pharmacy directors appreciate clinicians/case managers who show a personal interest and respect for their work. The resulting personal relationship between the prescribing clinician and the pharmacy director (and, as a consequence, the director's staff) can pay off nicely with an increased interest by the pharmacy staff in helping a particular team's patients despite the intense time pressures under which the typical retail pharmacist works.

Clinical pharmacists, imbedded in a primary care clinic or joining rounds on an inpatient unit, are invaluable if one's team is lucky enough to have one available. Many of the readers of this book are well aware of this point, for they are either graduate students in a clinical pharmacy program or are already in clinical practice. Besides being able to sometimes prescribe (what medications and under what type of supervision is determined by a variety of governmental and professional organizations), clinical pharmacists can provide a multitude of interventions.[46,47]

Often thoroughly up to date on the most recent advancements and problems with medications, clinical pharmacists can suggest immediate recommendations for more effective pharmacologic interventions. They can be exquisitely aware of potential drug-drug interactions or complex changes in metabolism following liver and kidney dysfunction or other metabolic determinants of serum levels all of which can impact on clinical care. Such metabolizing problems can also impact on a patient's medication follow-through if damaging side effects arise or the patient develops cognitive impairment or a frank delirium at home.

Clinical pharmacists can also be used to provide ongoing monitoring of the medication practices of patients, often forging powerful therapeutic alliances. In such situations, they may be highly effective at uncovering patient concerns or side effects that were missed in the hectic atmosphere of rounding or during a time-limited clinic appointment. Even more so than a retail pharmacist, because they may have more time to be with the patient, they can be leveraged to indirectly enhance medication follow-through by fostering the patient's ongoing medication interest using the principles and techniques of the MIM or motivational interviewing. They can also provide educational sessions with teams to update prescribers and other team members on pharmacologic advances with regard to specific diseases, as well as helping a team to sort through the marketing messages of pharmaceutical sales personnel.

Clinical pharmacists, in collaboration with retail pharmacists, can implement ongoing systems known as Medication Therapy Management (MTM) in which pharmacists engage in a structured, ongoing assessment, planning, and careful monitoring of a patient's use and progress on his or her medications. MTM emphasizes the importance of the ongoing pharmacist/patient alliance with a clear emphasis on enhancing medication follow-through (as well as motivation).[48]

Peer-Support Interventions

One group whose expertise and participation can be easily missed by busy treatment teams are patient peers. The integration of peer support can be a powerful aspect of the ongoing enhancement of medication follow-through.[49,50] As much as we clinicians can provide valued consultation and recommendations to our patients, there is something different about hearing encouraging information from fellow patients taking the same or similar drugs. The trust, credibility, and comradery developed among peers can be a potent force in both enhancing motivation and medication follow-through.

Peer support can be provided in groups, individual contacts, and via a variety of conduits. Face-to-face contact by peers is sometimes supplemented or replaced by telephone support, chat rooms, text messaging, and social media. Especially in web-based groups patients must be careful about the possibility of misinformation being promulgated.

In patients who have an interest, another related potential resource is the use of face-to-face medication support groups (as well as face-to-face groups designed for support regarding a specific disease). In such groups, a trained health professional can provide both education and answer generic questions regarding the medication in question and/or its use in a specific disease. Focused time can be spent on various methods patients have discovered, or are available, for easing medication follow-through. Appropriate fears and concerns can be discussed and processed. Inappropriate fears – based on misinformation – can also be effectively addressed.

Depending on the style of the support group, patients may also share experiences and provide emotional support for each other. Empathy and encouragement is sometimes communicated regarding the appearance of side effects or a slowness in the appearance of beneficial effects. Patients may share prompting techniques, such as unique styles of behavioral tailoring, that they have found useful.

Sometimes, if members of a group have bonded over time, they may offer concrete, logistical support such as, "Don't worry Mohammed, I can give you a ride to the pharmacy next Saturday" or "For heaven's sake, Sally, don't go to that pharmacy, that medication is much cheaper at Drake's Pharmacy [fictitious name]."

CONCLUSION

As can be seen from this appendix, a multitude of strategies for enhancing medication follow-through are available. Generally, a combination of strategies is useful. Almost always, a collaboratively designed approach – fitted specifically to the unique needs and desires of the patient – is most effective. Surprisingly simple approaches are often effective (such as behavioral tailoring coupled with the use of reminder prompting via a smart phone), many of which require minimal time from the treatment team or financial resources from the patient. Perhaps the single greatest key to success, after shared decision making with regard to developing a strategy, is to follow up as quickly as feasible after initiating a medication follow-through plan to adapt it until success is consolidated. The results are often satisfying, and, in some instances, lifesaving.

TRANSITIONAL DIRECTIONS TO APPENDICES B AND C

Interested readers may proceed to the ebook for access to Appendices B and C, which appear as bonus material in the ebook (directions for access to the ebook appear on the inside of the front cover of the book).

Appendix B: The Tip Archive

The Tip Archive was created to provide quick access, **via laptops, cell phones, and other mobile devices**, to the MIM interviewing techniques for students during their clinical rotations and future careers. With the specially designed digital Tip Archives, readers can conveniently access all 101 of the MIM interviewing techniques **in their exact wording** as they appeared in the text of the book.

Appendix C: Reprinted Journal Article from Professional Case Management

Shea SC. The medication interest model: an integrative clinical interviewing approach for improving medication adherence – part 2: implications for teaching and research. *Professional Case Management* 2009;14(1):1–19.

REFERENCES

1. Mueser K. Improving medication adherence in schizophrenia through innovations in medication follow-through and antipsychotic design. The third installment of a 3-part series entitled "Enhancing medication interest and medication follow-through in the treatment of schizophrenia." *Counseling Points* 2008;1(3):1–19.
2. Nieuwlaat R, Wilczynski N, Navarro T, et.al. Interventions for enhancing medication adherence [review]. *Cochrane Database Syst Rev* 2014;(11):1–22. doi:10.1002/14651858.CD000011.pub4.
3. Costa E, Giardini A, Savin M, et. al. Interventional tools to improve medication adherence: review of literature. *Patient Prefer Adherence* 2015;9:1303–1314. doi:10.2147/PPA.S87551.
4. Wilkinson A, Whitehead L. Evolution of the concept of self-care and implications for nurse: a literature review. *Intl J Nurs Stud* 2009;46:1143–1147.
5. Mueser K. Improving medication adherence in schizophrenia through innovations in medication follow-through and antipsychotic design. The third installment of a 3-part series entitled "Enhancing medication interest and medication follow-through in the treatment of schizophrenia." *Counseling Points* 2008;1(3):5.
6. Mueser K. Improving medication adherence in schizophrenia through innovations in medication follow-through and antipsychotic design. The third installment of a 3-part series entitled "Enhancing medication interest and medication follow-through in the treatment of schizophrenia." *Counseling Points* 2008;1(3):5.

7. Mueser K. Improving medication adherence in schizophrenia through innovations in medication follow-through and antipsychotic design. The third installment of a 3-part series entitled "Enhancing medication interest and medication follow-through in the treatment of schizophrenia." *Counseling Points* 2008;1(3):5
8. Mueser K. Improving medication adherence in schizophrenia through innovations in medication follow-through and antipsychotic design. The third installment of a 3-part series entitled "Enhancing medication interest and medication follow-through in the treatment of schizophrenia." *Counseling Points* 2008;1(3):5
9. Azrin NH, Teichner G. Evaluation of an instructional program for improving medication compliance for chronically mentally ill outpatients. *Behav Res Ther* 1998;36: 849–861.
10. Cramer JA, Rosenheck. Enhancing medication compliance for people with serious mental illness. *J Nerv Ment Dis* 1999;187:53–55.
11. Kelly GR, Scott JE. Medication compliance and health education among outpatients with chronic mental disorders. *Med Care* 1990;28:1181–1197.
12. Fenerty SD, West C, Davis SA, et al. The effect of reminder systems on patients' adherence to treatment. *Patient Prefer Adherence* 2012;6:127–135. doi:10.2147/PPA.S26314.
13. Miller CW, Himelhoch S. Acceptability of mobile phone technology for medication adherence interventions among HIV-positive patients at an urban clinic. *AIDS Res Treat* 2013;2013:670525. doi:10.1155/2013/670525.
14. Deglise C, Suggs LS, Odermatt P. SMS for disease control in developing countries: a systematic review of mobile health applications. *J Telemed Telecare* 2012;18(5):273–281.
15. Thakkar J, Kurup R, Laba TL, et.al. Mobile telephone text messaging for medication adherence in chronic disease. *JAMA Intern Med* 2016;176(3):340–349. doi:10.1001/jamainternmed.2015.7667.
16. Jones KR, Lekhak N, Kaewluang N. Using mobile phones and short message service to deliver self-management interventions for chronic conditions: a meta-review. *Worldviews Evid Based Nurs* 2014;11(2):81–88. doi:10.1111/wvn.12030.
17. Park LG, Howie-Esquivel J, Chung ML, et al. A text messaging intervention to promote medication adherence for patients with coronary heart disease: a randomized controlled trial. *Patient Educ Couns* February 2014;94(2):261–268. doi:10.1016/j.pcc.2013.10.027.
18. Dayer L, Heldenbrand S, Anderson P, et.al. Smartphone medication adherence apps: potential benefits to patients and providers. *J Am Pharm Assoc* 2013;53(2):172–181. doi:10.1331/JAPhA.2013.12202.
19. Brzan PP, Rotman E, Pajnkihar M, et al. Mobile applications for control and self-management of diabetes: a systematic review. *J Med Syst* 2016;40(9):210. doi:10.1007/s10916-016-0564-8.
20. Pandeyl A, Krumme A, Patel T, et al. The impact of text messaging on medication adherence and exercise among postmyocardial infarction patients: randomized controlled pilot trial. *JMIR Mhealth Uhealth* 2017;5(8):e110. doi:10.2196/mhealth.7144.
21. Hayakawa M, Uchimura Y, Omae K, et al. A smartphone-based medication self-management system with real-time medication monitoring. *Appl Clin Inform* 2013;4:37–52. doi:4338/ACI-2012-10-RA-0045.
22. Patel S, Jacobus-Kantor L, Marshall L, et al. Mobilizing your medications: an automated medication reminder application for mobile phones and hypertension medication adherence in a high-risk urban population. *J Diabetes Sci Technol* 2013;7(3):630–639.

23. Mistry N, Keepanasseril A, Wilczynski NL, et al. Technology-mediated interventions for enhancing medication adherence [review]. *J Am Med Inform Assoc* 2015;22(e1):177–193. doi:10.1093/jamia/ocu047.
24. Badawy S, Thompson AA, Kuhns LM. Medication adherence and technology-based interventions for adolescents with chronic health conditions: a few key considerations. *JMIR Mhealth Uhealth* 2017;5(12):e202. doi:10.2196/mhealth.8310.
25. Shan V, Dileep A, Dickens C, et.al. Patient-centered tablet application for improving medication adherence after a drug-eluting stent. *Front Public Health* 2016;4:272. doi:10.3389/fpubh.2016.00272.
26. Cahn A, Akirov A, Raz I. Digital health technology and diabetes management. *J Diabetes* 2018;10(1):10–17. doi:10.1111/1753-0407.12606.
27. Mueser K. Improving medication adherence in schizophrenia through innovations in medication follow-through and antipsychotic design. The third installment of a 3-part series entitled "Enhancing medication interest and medication follow-through in the treatment of schizophrenia." *Counseling Points* 2008;1(3):5.
28. Claxton AJ, Cramer J, Piere C. A systematic review of the associations between dose regimens and medication compliance. *Clin Ther* 2001;23:1296–1310.
29. Conn VS, Taylor SG, Kelley S. Medication regimen complexity and adherence among older adults. *Image J Nurs Sch* 1991;23:231–235.
30. Nieuwlaat R, Wilczynski N, Navarro T, et.al. Interventions for enhancing medication adherence [review]. *Cochrane Database Syst Rev* 2014;(11):14–15. doi:10.1002/14651858.CD000011.pub4.
31. Summers N. *Fundamentals of Case Management Practice: Skills for the Human Services*, 5th Ed. Pacific Grove, CA: Brooks Cole; 2015.
32. Powell SK, Hussein AT. *Case Management: A Practical Guide for Education and Practice*, 3rd ed. Philadelphia, PA: Lippincott Williams & Wilkins; 2009.
33. Cesta TG, Tahan HM. *The Case Managers Survival Guide: Winning Strategies in the New Healthcare Environment*, 3rd ed. Lancaster, PA: DESTech Publications, Inc.; 2016.
34. Mullahy CM. *The Case Manager's Handbook*, 6th ed. Burlington, MA: Jones & Bartlett Learning; 2016.
35. Mueser K. Improving medication adherence in schizophrenia through innovations in medication follow-through and antipsychotic design. The third installment of a 3-part series entitled "Enhancing medication interest and medication follow-through in the treatment of schizophrenia." *Counseling Points* 2008;1(3):8.
36. National Committee for Quality Assurance (NCQA). *Patient-Centered Medical Home (PCMH) Recognition*. 2018. http://www.ncqa.org/programs/recognition/practices/patient-centered-medical-home-pcmh. Accessed February 02, 2018.
37. American College of Physicians. *Joint Principles of the Patient-Centered Medical Home*. https://www.acponline.org/system/files/documents/running_practice/delivery_and_payment_models/pcmh/demonstrations/jointprinc_05_17.pdf. Accessed February 12, 2018.
38. Patient-Centered Primary Care Collaborative. *The Impact of Primary Care Practice Transformation on Cost, Quality, and Utilization: A Systematic Review of Research Published in 2016*. https://www.pcpcc.org/sites/default/files/resources/pcmh_evidence_es_071417%20FINAL.pdf.
39. Jackson GL, Powers BJ, Chatterjee R, et al. Improving patient care. The patient-centered medical home. *Annals Int Med* 2013;158(3):169–178.
40. van den Berk-Clark C, Doucette E, Rottnek F, et al. Do patient-centered medical homes improve health behaviors, outcomes, and experiences of low-income patients? A systematic review and meta-analysis. *Health Ser Res* July 2017. doi:10.1111/1475-6773.12737/full.

41. Franz BA, Murphy JW. The patient-centered medical home as a community-based strategy. *Perm J* 2017;21. doi:10.7812/TPP/17-002.
42. Rosenthal TC. Are we learning more about patient-centered medical homes (PCMHs), or learning more about primary care? *J Am Board Fam Med* 2016;29(1):4–7. doi:10.3122/jabfm.2016.01.150352.
43. Oh A, Martsolf GR, Freidberg MW. Association between sponsorship and findings of medical home evaluations. *JAMA Intern Med* 2017;177(9):1375–1376. doi:10.1001/jamainternmed.2017.3188.
44. Pringle J, Coley K. Improving medication adherence: a framework for community pharmacy-based interventions. *Integr Pharm Res Pract* 2015;4:175–183. doi:10.2147/IPRP.S93036.
45. Shah D, Simms K, Barksdale D, et al. Improving medication adherence of patients with chronic heart failure: challenges and solutions. *Res Rep Clin Cardiol* 2015;6:87–95.
46. Morgado M, Rolo S, Castelo-Branco M. Pharmacist intervention program to enhance hypertension control: a randomized controlled trial. *Int J Clin Pharm* 2011;33(1):132–140.
47. Francis J, Abraham S. Clinical pharmacists: bridging the gap between patients and physicians. *Saudi Pharm J* 2014;22(6):600–602. doi:10.1016/jsps.2014.02.011.
48. American Pharmacists Association and the National Association of Chain Drug Stores Foundation. *Medication Therapy Management in Pharmacy Practice: Core Elements of an MTM Service Model, Version 2.0.* March 2008. https://www.pharmacist.com/sites/default/files/files/core_elements_of_an_mtm_practice.pdf.
49. Simoni JM, Pantalone DW, Plummer MD, et. al. A randomized controlled trial of a peer support intervention targeting antiretroviral adherence and depressive symptomatology among HIV-positive men and women. *Health Psychology* 2007;26(4):488-495. MEDLINE: 17605569.
50. Simoni JM, Huh D, Frick PA, et. al. Peer support and pager messaging to promote antiretroviral modifying therapy in Seattle: a randomized controlled trial. *J Acquir Immune Defic Syndr* 2009;52(4):465-473. MEDLINE: 19911481.

Index

D

R

S